Human Poliovirus

Human Poliovirus

Guest Editors

Mark A. McKinlay
Walter A. Orenstein

MDPI

Basel • Beijing • Wuhan • Barcelona • Belgrade • Novi Sad • Cluj • Manchester

Guest Editors
Mark A. McKinlay
Center for Vaccine Equity
The Task Force for Global Health
Decatur
USA

Walter A. Orenstein
Department of Medicine
Emory University School of Medicine
Atlanta
USA

Editorial Office
MDPI AG
Grosspeteranlage 5
4052 Basel, Switzerland

This is a reprint of the Special Issue, published open access by the journal *Pathogens* (ISSN 2076-0817), freely accessible at: https://www.mdpi.com/journal/pathogens/special_issues/human_poliovirus.

For citation purposes, cite each article independently as indicated on the article page online and as indicated below:

Lastname, A.A.; Lastname, B.B. Article Title. *Journal Name* **Year**, *Volume Number*, Page Range.

ISBN 978-3-7258-5527-8 (Hbk)
ISBN 978-3-7258-5528-5 (PDF)
https://doi.org/10.3390/books978-3-7258-5528-5

Contents

Preface

In 1988 when the polio eradication effort began, there were an estimated 350,000 cases of paralytic polio and 123 countries were considered endemic. Polioviruses cause paralysis by destroying the anterior horn cells of the spine, resulting in denervation of muscles and flaccid paralysis. When the muscles involved in respiration are paralyzed, breathing is compromised and can lead to death. The worldwide polio eradication effort has successfully led to the eradication of two of the three wild poliovirus serotypes (Types 2 and 3) and a >99% reduction in cases caused by wild poliovirus type 1. However, the program faces significant challenges and failure to achieve the goal could lead to a major global resurgence. This reprint describes the reasons for the success of the polio eradication effort to date, the challenges to finally achieving eradication, and the means to overcome them. The benefits of a polio free world would be substantial.

Mark A. McKinlay and Walter A. Orenstein
Guest Editors

pathogens

MDPI

Article

Establishment of a Poliovirus Containment Program and Containment Certification Process for Poliovirus-Essential Facilities, United States 2017–2022

Christy Ottendorfer [1], Bryan Shelby [1], Cecelia A. Sanders [1], Anna Llewellyn [2], Christy Myrick [3], Christye Brown [4], Suganthi Suppiah [1], Kortney Gustin [1] and Lia Haynes Smith [1,*]

1 Centers for Disease Control and Prevention, Office of Readiness and Response, U.S. National Authority for Containment of Poliovirus, Atlanta, GA 30329, USA; uyk0@cdc.gov (C.O.); zfg0@cdc.gov (C.A.S.)
2 Centers for Disease Control and Prevention, National Center for Emerging and Zoonotic Infectious Diseases, Atlanta, GA 30329, USA; gif7@cdc.gov
3 Centers for Disease Control and Prevention, Office of Laboratory Science and Safety, Atlanta, GA 30329, USA
4 Morehouse School of Medicine, Atlanta, GA 30310, USA; cybrown@msm.edu
* Correspondence: loh5@cdc.gov; Tel.: +1-404-718-4639

Abstract: Upon declaration of poliovirus (PV) type 2 eradication in 2015, the World Health Organization (WHO) published PV containment requirements in the Global Action Plan III (GAPIII) for mitigating the risk of a facility-associated release post eradication. In 2018, the 71st World Health Assembly resolution urged member states retaining PV to appoint a National Authority for Containment (NAC), reduce the number of PV facilities, and submit applications for containment certification. The United States (US) NAC was established in 2018 for containment oversight, and two paths to WHO GAPIII containment certification were developed. Facilities retaining PV were identified through national poliovirus containment surveys. The US NAC conducted 27 site visits at 18 facilities (20 laboratories: A/BSL-2 (65%), A/BSL-3 (20%), and storage-only (15%)) to verify the implementation of US NAC's preliminary containment measures. The NAC identified areas for improvement in seven categories: primary containment, decontamination, hand hygiene, security, emergency response, training, and immunization practices. Sixteen facility applications were endorsed to pursue poliovirus-essential facility (PEF) certification, whereas four facilities opted to withdraw during the containment certification process. The US made noteworthy progress in PV containment to enhance biosafety and biosecurity practices at US PV facilities to safeguard the polio eradication effort.

Keywords: polio; GAPIII; poliovirus containment; NAC; poliovirus-essential facility; PEF

1. Introduction

Two of the three wild poliovirus (WPV) serotypes, type 2 and type 3, were declared eradicated in 2015 and 2019, respectively [1]. Wild poliovirus type 1 remains endemic in only two countries (Afghanistan and Pakistan) [1]. In the United States (US), the last wild poliovirus outbreak occurred in 1979 [2]. Wild polioviruses were eliminated in the US due to successful childhood immunization programs with the live-attenuated oral poliovirus vaccine (OPV) that was later replaced with an inactivated injectable intramuscular formulation in 2000 [2,3]. Since the Global Polio Eradication Initiative (GPEI) was founded in 1988, the global incidence of wild poliovirus has declined from 350,000 cases a year in 176 countries to 22 cases in 2 countries in 2022, with an additional 8 cases in Mozambique linked to importation of virus circulating in Pakistan [1]. Globally, continued use of OPV contributed to outbreaks of neurovirulent circulating vaccine-derived poliovirus (cVDPV) in areas with low population immunity [1]. Since most cVDPV outbreaks were caused by OPV/Sabin strain type 2 (OPV2) [4], World Health Organization (WHO) member states synchronized a global switch in April 2016 from trivalent OPV (tOPV, contains Sabin strain types 1, 2, 3) to bivalent OPV (bOPV, contains Sabin strain types 1 and 3) for routine and supplementary immunization programs [5]. The global cessation of routine OPV2 use triggered stringent containment requirements for all poliovirus type 2 (PV2) materials to minimize the risk of reintroduction of PV2 from facilities back into communities [6–9].

The *WHO Global Action Plan to minimize poliovirus-facility-associated risk after type-specific eradication of wild polioviruses and sequential cessation of oral polio vaccine use*, 3rd ed. (GAPIII), outlines facility containment requirements to mitigate the risks of a facility-associated release of poliovirus [10], and in 2022, WHO released the *Global Action Plan for Poliovirus Containment*, 4th ed. (GAPIV) [11], to address public comments received on GAPIII with full implementation anticipated by 2026. The World Health Assembly (WHA) resolution 71.16 in May 2018 urged countries retaining polioviruses to (1) reduce the number of facilities, (2) appoint a National Authority for Containment (NAC) for oversight of containment activities, and (3) have facilities selected to retain polioviruses to submit applications for participation in the containment certification program no later than December 2019 [12]. Countries are working to implement GAPIII/GAPIV containment guidelines including appointing NACs and conducting national surveys to identify facilities retaining poliovirus infectious materials (e.g., seed stocks and virus isolates) and potentially infectious materials (PIMs [13], e.g., stool or upper respiratory specimens not known to contain poliovirus that were collected in a time and place when poliovirus was circulating or OPV was used) [6]. Further, countries must identify and approve a limited number of facilities as designated poliovirus-essential facilities (PEFs) permitted to retain polioviruses in accordance with GAPIII/GAPIV [10,11] and applicable national laws, regulations, or standards. These facilities must be certified against GAPIII/GAPIV requirements via an auditing process described in the WHO GAPIII Containment Certification Scheme (CCS) [14]. The WHO and GPEI's Global Commission for the Certification of Poliomyelitis Eradication (GCC) provides oversight and uses an independent committee, the GCC Containment Working Group (GCC-CWG), to make recommendations to the GCC for endorsement of PEF containment certificates. A GCC-endorsed and NAC-countersigned application provides assurance to the global community that the facility's implementation of GAPIII/GAPIV is appropriate and consistent worldwide [14].

While US poliovirus survey activities began in 2002 with the first national survey [15], in January 2017, the Poliovirus Containment Activity was established within the U.S. Centers for Disease Control and Prevention (CDC) to perform the global poliovirus containment functions in the United States. In January 2018, the US Department of Health and Human Services Acting Assistant Secretary of Health approved the designation of the Poliovirus Containment Activity as the US NAC. The US NAC operates with eight full-time government employees responsible for the national poliovirus inventory (surveys) and oversight of GAPIII containment certification. The US NAC's director also has oversight responsibilities as the US National Poliovirus Containment Coordinator, who oversees the national survey and inventory. We report the establishment of a national poliovirus containment program, describe a voluntary containment certification process for poliovirus-essential facilities, and share preliminary results of poliovirus laboratory containment implementation in the United States.

2. Materials and Methods

2.1. US Poliovirus Containment Program

A national program was established within the CDC Office of Readiness and Response to provide oversight of poliovirus containment in the United States. US NAC created a website, guidance, and a containment certification process for facilities retaining eradicated poliovirus materials. PV2 infectious materials (i.e., wild, vaccine-derived poliovirus (VDPV), OPV/Sabin viruses) and, since 2019, wild and vaccine-derived poliovirus type 3 materials (WPV3/VDPV3) are subject to WHO's GAPIII containment requirements and should be held only in PEFs [16]. Poliovirus-essential facility containment certification is overseen by the US NAC audit team. The audit team is composed of four auditors with expertise in microbiology and biosafety, and prior experience performing regulatory inspections of US select agent laboratories. Auditors also completed the WHO GAPIII auditor training course and maintain ISO45001:2018 [17] and ISO19011:2018 [18] certifications. Auditors disclose any potential conflicts of interest to the NAC Director consistent with the certification scheme [14].

2.2. Facility Identification and Outreach

US facilities retaining PV materials were identified through three national surveys conducted by CDC between 2002 and 2022, which were used to determine the national inventory of PV materials [15,19,20]. US NAC used survey results to identify and contact facilities reporting PV materials and perform outreach with webinars and site visits to provide training on WHO GAPIII containment certification. Facilities not entering the WHO Containment Certification Scheme submitted documentation to the US NAC attesting to the destruction, inactivation, or transfer of PV materials. Facilities reporting materials that were not yet subject to containment (e.g., OPV/Sabin 1) could retain their inventory without registering as a PEF. Facilities reporting storage of potentially infectious materials subject to GAPIII/IV (e.g., WPV2/VDPV2 PIM) were not designated as PEFs by US NAC and have been excluded from this report. These facilities were requested to contact US NAC for additional guidance prior to starting work with these specimens.

2.3. Certification Process

As the first step in the certification process, GCC requested that facilities complete a Certificate of Participation (CP) application, provide a description of preliminary containment conditions/risk mitigation strategies used to safeguard PV materials, and provide a time-bound action plan describing progress in the implementation of GAPIII containment or a commitment to conclude work prior to the established global CP expiry date [14]. Once a facility's CP application information was endorsed by US NAC, the application was submitted to WHO for additional processing and release to the GCC-CWG for review and GCC endorsement. Facilities that perform critical national or international activities with PV materials and plan to retain PV for an extended period were enrolled to be audited against GAPIII/GAPIV to become fully certified PEFs. Two paths for CP in the GAPIII/GAPIV PEF auditing scheme are available for a phased transition to WHO GAPIII/GAPIV containment in the United States (Figure 1).

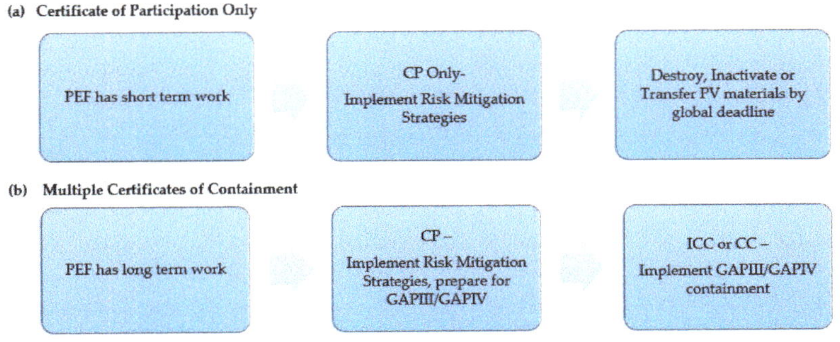

Figure 1. Two certification paths for the phased transition to WHO GAPIII/GAPIV containment in the United States: (**a**) certification path for PEFs planning to conclude work prior to the global CP expiry date; (**b**) certification path for PEFs planning to continue work and implement GAPIII/GAPIV containment. CP—Certificate of Participation; ICC—Interim Certificate of Containment; CC—Certificate of Containment.

2.4. Site Visits

Site visits were conducted for verification of facility CP application information and for periodic monitoring once the CP was awarded. Site visits consisted of laboratory tours, personnel interviews, completion of a facility questionnaire, and document review by US NAC auditors and CDC technical subject matter experts to assess preliminary containment conditions/risk mitigation strategies, laboratory design/features based on *Biosafety in Microbiological and Biomedical Laboratories* (BMBL) 5th edition guidance [21] and GAPIII [10], and inventory of PV materials during 2018–2022. In lieu of an onsite visit, two virtual site visits were conducted in October and November 2020 with adapted assessment criteria due to the COVID-19 pandemic. Findings were communicated to the facility in writing following each site visit, and, when applicable, the facility submitted information on corrective actions taken to resolve identified findings.

2.5. Information Collection and Analysis

CDC determined that the national survey, facility questionnaire, and CP application information collection activities conducted under the project are exempt from the requirements of the Paperwork Reduction Act (PRA) as they fall under the activities authorized under the National Childhood Vaccine Injury Act (NCVIA) in Section 2102(a)(6)-(a)(7) of the Public Health Service Act (42 USC 300aa-2(a)(6)-(a)(7). This activity was reviewed by CDC and was conducted consistent with applicable federal law and CDC policy. §See, e.g., 45 C.F.R. part 46, 21 C.F.R. part 56; 42 U.S.C. §241(d); 5 U.S.C. §552a; 44 U.S.C. §3501 et seq. Descriptive statistical analyses (median, frequency) on PEF data sets were performed in Microsoft 365 Excel v2102; maps were created in Microsoft Power BI v2.95.804.0.

3. Results

3.1. Facility Identification and Outreach

A total of 30 potential PEFs (retaining WPV2/VDPV2, OPV2, and/or WPV3/VDPV3 infectious materials) located in 15 states were identified via national poliovirus containment surveys and correspondence to CDC between 2017 and 2022. Following US NAC initial outreach, facility leadership at ten facilities (10/30, 33%) opted to destroy, inactivate, or transfer PV infectious materials rather than seek certification as a PEF. As of 31 December 2022, a total of 10 PEFs in seven states remained active in the containment certification process (Figure 2). The annual number of potential PEFs in the United States fluctuated between 2017 and 2022, with the largest decrease (20 to 12, 40% reduction) occurring in 2018 following initial US NAC outreach (Figure 3).

3.2. Certificate of Participation Application

US NAC developed a fillable CP application adapted from the WHO CP form [14]. The US NAC CP application collected facility information on essential work, virus type (wild, vaccine-derived, OPV, and novel oral polio vaccine (nOPV)), viral propagation volume, the number of essential personnel, laboratory locations, a time-bound action plan to either complete work under a CP or implement GAPIII/GAPIV, and final certification goal (i.e., plans to complete PV work or to be audited against GAPIII/GAPIV standards for certification as a PEF). The US NAC CP application required approval and signatures from the facility's principal investigator, institutional biosafety officer, and a senior institutional representative (e.g., Director, University President) to affirm full commitment by facility partners to engage in the containment certification process.

A total of 20 potential PEFs submitted CP applications to US NAC as of 31 December 2022, where two of the facilities operated PV laboratories at different physical addresses. Two of twenty CP applications were withdrawn at the facilities' request prior to US NAC verification of risk mitigation strategies and excluded from this analysis. Eighteen potential PEFs comprised academic, commercial, and government facility types. No PV vaccine manufacturers operate in the United States. Most US facilities (12/18, 67%) will complete critical work with PV prior to the CP global expiry date, while six facilities will seek additional GAPIII certification as PEFs.

(**a**)

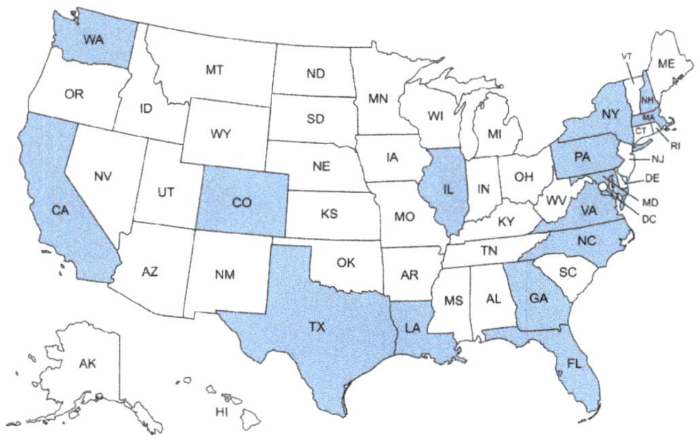

(**b**)

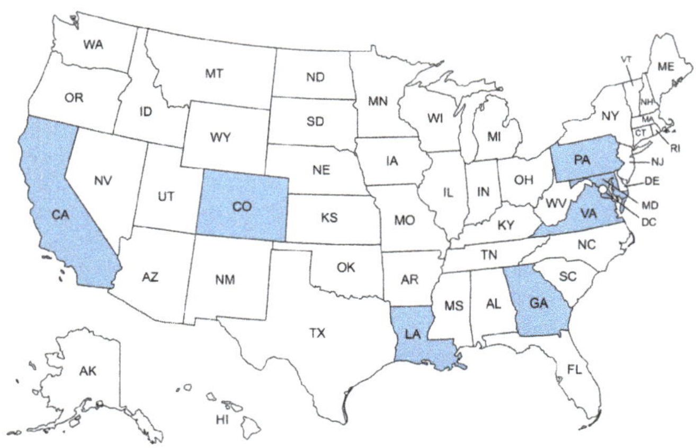

Figure 2. US states hosting poliovirus-essential facilities between 2017 and 2022: (**a**) US states hosting potential PEFs between 2017 and 2022 as reported by respondents to national poliovirus containment surveys or direct communication of facilities with CDC, and (**b**) US states hosting PEFs (WPV2/VDPV2, OPV2, and WPV3/VDPV3 materials) endorsed by US NAC and GCC as of 31 December 2022.

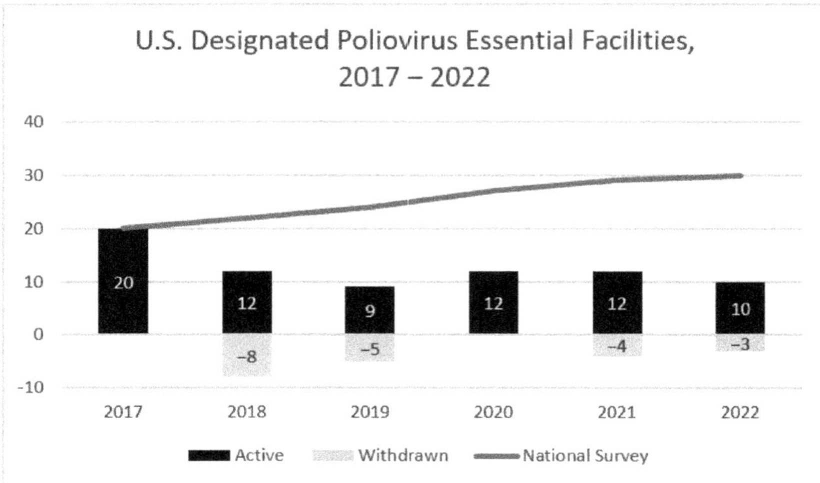

Figure 3. Trends in poliovirus-essential facilities designated in the United States, 2017–2022. Number of active and withdrawn PEFs by year compared to cumulative count of potential PEFs (N = 30) identified in national survey.

3.3. Preliminary Containment Conditions—Risk Mitigation Strategies

An external US working group was established under a CDC federal advisory committee with subject matter expertise in biosafety, containment laboratories, public health, emergency response, and infectious diseases. Seven experts provided input to US NAC on best practices to safeguard polioviruses in domestic laboratories. In 2018, US NAC developed 35 laboratory risk mitigation strategies adapted from GAPIII elements and BMBL 5th edition guidance 21], and, in 2020, the list of risk mitigation strategies was updated with 15 additional containment strategies (Table 1). These strategies were developed in consultation with the external working group and feedback from PEFs. Risk mitigation strategies were selected based on gaps identified during US NAC facility outreach, focused on enhanced biosafety practices considered most likely to mitigate the risk of potential PV occupational exposure or release, and, in the 2020 revision, to address potential biosecurity and emergency management risks and expand containment to WPV3/VDPV3 infectious materials. US NAC provided training on risk mitigation strategies to facilities and requested progress on their implementation during the CP application process, at a minimum of two months later. The risk mitigation strategies were the recommended minimum safeguards for PV infectious materials in US laboratories effective until the global CP expiry date. An overview of the implementation timeline and US approach to enroll facilities in containment certification is shown in Figure S1.

Table 1. US National Authority for Containment's risk mitigation strategies for poliovirus materials, 2018–2022.

No.	Hazard Control [a]	Category	Risk Mitigation Strategy for Poliovirus Materials [b]	Containment Strategies Observed by US NAC	
				Frequency/No. Visits	Percent(%)
1	Elimination	Biosafety	Destroy unneeded poliovirus materials	20/27	74
2	Elimination	Biosafety	Inactivation, fixation or extraction of poliovirus materials	8/27	30

Table 1. *Cont.*

No.	Hazard Control [a]	Category	Risk Mitigation Strategy for Poliovirus Materials [b]	Containment Strategies Observed by US NAC	
				Frequency/No. Visits	Percent(%)
3	Engineering	Biosafety	Dedicated room (e.g., an isolation room within a larger laboratory) used for poliovirus	8/27	30
4	Engineering	Biosafety	Two doors are present between public areas and the laboratory room	25/27	93
5	Engineering	Biosafety	Certified BSC used for poliovirus work	18/27	67
6	Engineering	Biosafety	Centrifuge safety cups/sealed rotors that are loaded and unloaded in a BSC for poliovirus work	11/27	41
7	Engineering	Biosafety	Containment caging system with HEPA filtered exhaust used for housing PV-infected animals	2/13	15
8	Administrative	Biosafety	Risk assessments for poliovirus containment	9/13	69
9	Administrative	Biosafety	Risk assessments for animal work	2/13	15
10	Administrative	Biosafety	PV work reviewed/approved by institutional committees (i.e., institutional biosafety committee (IBC), institutional animal care and use committee (IACUC))	4/13	31
11	Administrative	Biosafety	Dedicated BSC and incubator used for poliovirus	10/27	37
12	Administrative	Biosafety	Dedicated caging system used for PV-inoculated animals	1/13	8
13	Administrative	Biosafety	Shared laboratory uses PV spatial and temporal separation with appropriate decontamination procedures	9/27	33
14	Administrative	Biosafety	Personnel trained in poliovirus biosafety and security practices	10/27	37
15	Administrative	Biosafety	Personnel receive annual refresher training	5/13	38
16	Administrative	Biosafety	Personnel provide proof of poliovirus immunization	12/27	44
17	Administrative	Biosafety	Personnel enrolled in occupational health program	12/27	44
18	Administrative	Biosafety	Personnel competent in good microbiological techniques	17/27	63
19	Administrative	Biosafety	Personnel wash hands prior to exit of the laboratory	19/27	70
20	Administrative	Biosafety	Protective clothing and gloves removed prior to exit from the laboratory	16/27	59
21	Administrative	Biosafety	Reusable PPE is decontaminated prior to storage and reuse	12/27	44
22	Administrative	Biosafety	Disposable PPE is treated as biohazardous waste	22/27	81
23	Administrative	Biosafety	Durable leak proof transport container used when poliovirus is removed from primary containment	17/27	63
24	Administrative	Biosafety	Dedicated reagents used for poliovirus	15/27	55
25	Administrative	Biosafety	Segregate poliovirus from all other materials (e.g., in own clearly labeled freezer box)	22/27	81
26	Administrative	Biosafety	Perform work with one poliovirus serotype at a time to minimize potential cross-contamination (when possible)	6/13	46
27	Administrative	Biosafety	Decontamination of work surfaces	18/27	67
28	Administrative	Biosafety	All materials leaving the laboratory are decontaminated using an appropriate method (autoclave, incinerator)	18/27	67
29	Administrative	Biosafety	Periodic validation of autoclave decontamination procedures	21/27	78
30	Administrative	Biosafety	Containers with poliovirus are surface disinfected prior to removal from the BSC	13/27	48
31	Administrative	Biosafety	Procedures for decontamination of equipment are implemented	14/27	52

Table 1. *Cont.*

No.	Hazard Control [a]	Category	Risk Mitigation Strategy for Poliovirus Materials [b]	Containment Strategies Observed by US NAC	
				Frequency/No. Visits	Percent(%)
32	Administrative	Biosafety	Chemical treatment known to inactivate poliovirus implemented	7/27	26
33	Administrative	Security	Locked freezer where poliovirus is stored (when stored outside a dedicated, secured laboratory)	18/27	67
34	Administrative	Security	Locked laboratory	20/27	74
35	Administrative	Security	Limit access to personnel identified as essential by the facility	18/27	67
36	Administrative	Security	Poliovirus inventory records are current, accurate and complete	7/13	54
37	Administrative	Security	Poliovirus animal tracking and infected tissue inventory records	1/13	8
38	Administrative	Security	Security policies implemented for controlled access to poliovirus materials and areas	9/13	69
39	Administrative	Security	Individual entries into poliovirus areas are documented (e.g., electronic record, manual logbooks)	8/13	61
40	Administrative	Security	Visitor policy for entering poliovirus areas	6/13	46
41	Administrative	Emergency Response	Emergency response plans developed, including measures to protect personnel and the environment in the event of a release [c]	23/27	85
42	Administrative	Emergency Response	Personnel report accidents or incidents with PV per institutional policy	20/27	74
43	Administrative	Emergency Response	Notify appropriate state and local agencies of possession of PV materials	8/13	61
44	Administrative	Emergency Response	Develop and coordinate emergency response plans with first responders	7/13	54
45	Administrative	Emergency Response	Develop response procedures for PV-infected escaped animals	1/13	8
46	PPE [d]	Biosafety	Protective laboratory clothing with a solid-front (e.g., disposable wrap-around gown, scrubs, coverall)	21/27	78
47	PPE	Biosafety	Gloves (double gloves are recommended)	27/27	100
48	PPE	Biosafety	Face or surgical mask or respirator	19/27	70
49	PPE	Biosafety	Eye and face protection for anticipated splashes or sprays (e.g., safety glasses, face shield)	21/27	78
50	PPE	Biosafety	Shoe covers or dedicated shoes	20/27	74

[a] Adapted from Hierarchy of Controls = elimination, substitution, engineering controls, administrative controls, and personal protective equipment (PPE) in Hierarchy of Controls Workplace Safety & Health Topics website; CDC/The National Institute for Occupational Safety and Health (NIOSH), 2015. Available at https://www.cdc.gov/niosh/topics/hierarchy/default.html (accessed on 6 December 2023). [b] U.S. NAC risk mitigation strategies (n = 35) were implemented for poliovirus type 2 in 2018; additional risk mitigation strategies (n = 15, numbers 7–10, 12, 15, 26, 36–40, 43–45) were implemented in late 2020 for WPV2/VDPV2, OPV2, and WPV3/VDPV3 materials. [c] In October 2021, the risk mitigation strategy for emergency response plans was updated to align response procedures for potential poliovirus exposures with WHO guidance. [d] PPE—personal protective equipment.

3.4. Certification Process

The results for facilities identified in the national survey and participation in containment certification are shown in Table 2. The first step in the PEF containment certification process has multiple steps including (1) US NAC endorsement, (2) WHO review, (3) GCC-CWG review and recommendation to GCC, (4) GCC endorsement, and (5) US NAC issuance of CP to PEF. Prior to endorsement, US NAC assessed PEFs based on critical national or international work activities, laboratory features, and the implementation of preliminary containment conditions/risk mitigation strategies during site visits. US NAC also communicated with facilities to resolve incomplete CP application information, site visit findings, and requests for clarification resulting from reviews by the WHO and the GCC-CWG during the certification process.

Table 2. US poliovirus-essential facilities' participation in containment certification and application processing times, 2018–2022.

CCS [a] Process	PEF Participation in Certification	Frequency (N = 30)	Percent (%)	Time (Days)	
				Median	Range
Option A	Facility submits CP application	20	67	-	-
USA requirement	i. Implement risk mitigation strategies	18/20	90	83	3–418
Step 1	ii. NAC endorsement	17/20	85	84	3–418
Step 2	iii. WHO review	17/20	85	10	1–128
Step 3	iv. GCC-CWG review	17/20	85	22	1–77
Step 4	v. GCC endorsement [b]	16/20	80	12.5	1–463
Step 5	vi. CP issued [c]	15/20	75	233	91–678
Step 6	vii. Facility withdraws from certification [d]				
-	• Before US NAC endorsement	3/20	15	39	38–373
-	• Before GCC endorsement	1/20	5	608	-
-	• Ends work under valid CP	6/20	30	841.5	151–1471
Option B	No participation, destroy or transfer PV	10	33	-	-

[a] CCS—Containment Certification Scheme [14]. [b] GCC returned 3 applications as 'unsatisfactory'; 2 of 3 facilities reapplied and received GCC endorsement. [c] One GCC-endorsed PEF plans to destroy WPV2 and WPV3 and retain WPV1 only, US NAC issuance of certificate pending (data as of June 2023). [d] Three potential PEFs withdrew from containment certification scheme prior to US NAC endorsement (n = 2 destroyed PV materials, n = 1 opted not to receive PV materials). One PEF opted to transfer PV materials to another PEF instead of reapplication to achieve GCC endorsement. Six PEFs concluded work with containment PV strains under a valid CP and were withdrawn from containment certification as of 31 December 2022.

Characteristics for eighteen PEFs (n = 20 PV laboratory sites), laboratory designs, and 27 laboratory features are shown in Table 3. US PEFs that enrolled in the CP process used and/or stored PV in A/BSL-2 (65%), A/BSL-3 (20%), and storage (15%) areas. Some PV laboratories had enhanced features, including GAPIII facility requirements such as a ventilation system maintaining inward directional airflow (55%), a double-door personnel airlock/anteroom (35%), a personal walk-through exit shower (10%), and an effluent decontamination system (5%) (Table 3).

Table 3. Characteristics, laboratory design, and laboratory features of US poliovirus-essential facilities (PEFs).

PEF Characteristics [a]			27 Laboratory Features [b]		
N = 18 PEFs	Frequency (N = 18)	Percent (%)	PV Laboratory Sites (Operated in 18 PEFs)	Frequency (n = 20)	Percent (%)
Facility primary work objective			*Containment boundary*		
Biomedical research	9	50	Containment perimeter sealable for gaseous decontamination	5	25
Clinical diagnostic laboratory	1	6	Facility is equipped with a double-door personnel airlock/anteroom	7	35
Public health laboratory	4	22	Double doors are interlocked (physical or procedural)	5	25
Industrial/production laboratory	2	11	Backflow prevention on all services/utilities passing across the boundary	2	10
Other	2	11	*Sinks and Showers*		
Virus type [c]			Hands-free/automated hand washing sink	8	40
WPV2/VDPV2	9	50	Personal exit shower	4	20
WPV3/VDPV3	6	33	Personal walk-through exit shower	2	10
OPV/Sabin 2	12	67	Emergency shower	16	80
nOPV2	6	33	*Ventilation System*		

Table 3. *Cont.*

PEF Characteristics [a]			27 Laboratory Features [b]		
N = 18 PEFs	**Frequency (N = 18)**	**Percent (%)**	**PV Laboratory Sites (Operated in 18 PEFs)**	**Frequency (n = 20)**	**Percent (%)**
Work type(s) [d]			Controlled air system maintains inward directional airflow	11	55
Research	12	67	Exhaust air is HEPA filtered	7	35
Vaccine production	0	0	Dedicated ventilation system to PV area (exhaust and supply)	2	10
Clinical trials	3	17	Backflow protection on supply air	4	20
Animal model	4	22	Ductwork sealable for gaseous decontamination	4	20
Diagnostics	3	17	Monitors/alarms to ensure directional airflow can be readily validated	5	25
QC testing [e]	3	17	*Decontamination Systems*		
Storage only	3	17	Single door autoclave	7	35
Certification goal [f]			Pass-through autoclave	5	25
Certificate of Participation (CP)	12	67	Material airlock/decontamination chamber sealable for gaseous decontamination	1	5
Interim Certificate of Containment (ICC)	1	5	Dunk tank containing sufficient active compound to inactivate poliovirus	1	5
Certificate of Containment (CC)	5	28	Effluent decontamination system	1	5
			Security		
			Entry door(s) equipped with lock/lock cylinder rated as burglary resistant	17	85
Laboratory Design	Frequency (n = 20)	Percent (%)	Lock(s) fail secure and allow egress only	11	55
Design [g]			Locked door with two-factor access control measure	6	30
A/BSL-3	4	20	Video surveillance	13	65
A/BSL-2	13	65	Two-person system for PV work	7	35
Storage only	3	15	Intrusion detection system	8	40
			Facility perimeter is subject to constant monitoring	13	65
			Facility is located on a secure site with perimeter control	9	45

[a] PEFs (N = 18, operated in 20 PV laboratory sites) with CP applications and preliminary containment conditions verified by US NAC. [b] Physical laboratory features, when available, were reported with a list of preliminary containment conditions to GCC. These 27 laboratory features were not required by US NAC for endorsement of a CP. [c] WPV—wild poliovirus; VDPV—vaccine derived poliovirus; OPV—oral polio vaccine; nOPV—novel oral polio vaccine. Ten PEFs retain a combination of virus types. [d] Work type(s)—11 PEFs with one work type, 7 PEFs with more than one work type. [e] QC—quality control. [f] Certification goal—three facilities changed between CC- and CP-only goals, one facility changed from ICC- to CP-only goal compared to initial CP applications received. [g] A/BSL = animal/biosafety level. Data as of 31 December 2022.

3.5. Site Visits

During 2018–2022, US NAC conducted a total of 27 site visits at 20 PV laboratories in 18 PEFs to verify preliminary containment conditions/risk mitigation strategies. From June 2018 to June 2020, US NAC assessed 35 risk mitigation strategies and found US PEFs adopted preliminary containment conditions (median = 22.5; max = 30; min = 3) during 14 site visits. US NAC also found a similar trend (median = 29; max = 43; min = 15) when the number of risk mitigation strategies was increased to 50 (n = 13 visits), with an increase from a minimum of 3 to 15 strategies observed during these visits. The results for the risk mitigation strategies assessed and the PEF containment practices verified during site visits are shown in Table 1.

US NAC found PEFs separated the PV laboratory room from public areas with two doors (25/27, 93%), reduced the quantities of polioviruses stored (20/27, 74%), segregated PV from all other materials (22/27, 81%), and dedicated reagents used for PV work (15/27, 56%). In the United States, a limited number of PEFs perform animal studies with PV serotypes subject to containment, and, thus, animal containment criteria were not applicable to most facilities. US NAC observed animal-specific risk assessments and HEPA-filtered exhaust on containment caging systems at two PEFs performing animal work, but one of the two PEFs did not fully implement the recommended animal PV containment practices (i.e., a dedicated caging system, animal recordkeeping through final disposition, and emergency response plans for an escaped animal) (Table 1).

Areas for improvement included the use of certified primary containment devices for manipulation of PV materials, appropriate decontamination of solid and liquid biohazardous waste, hand hygiene practices, training, and proof of PV immunization records for essential personnel granted access to PV laboratories and materials (Figure 4). Some PV laboratory sites (8/20, 40%) fully implemented the recommended personal protective equipment (PPE) for laboratory staff. For PPE, a nose and mouth covering had the lowest implementation observed by US NAC during site visits (8/27, 30%) (Figure 4). Similarly, facility security controls and emergency response protocols needed modifications to address poliovirus containment (Figure 4). For example, US NAC observed that PV laboratories did not restrict access only to essential personnel for PV laboratory and storage areas (9/27, 33%). Facilities implemented corrective actions to resolve US NAC findings prior to issuance of CPs. US NAC also conducted periodic monitoring after the CP was awarded for several PEFs (7/18, 39%) to ensure containment practices were maintained.

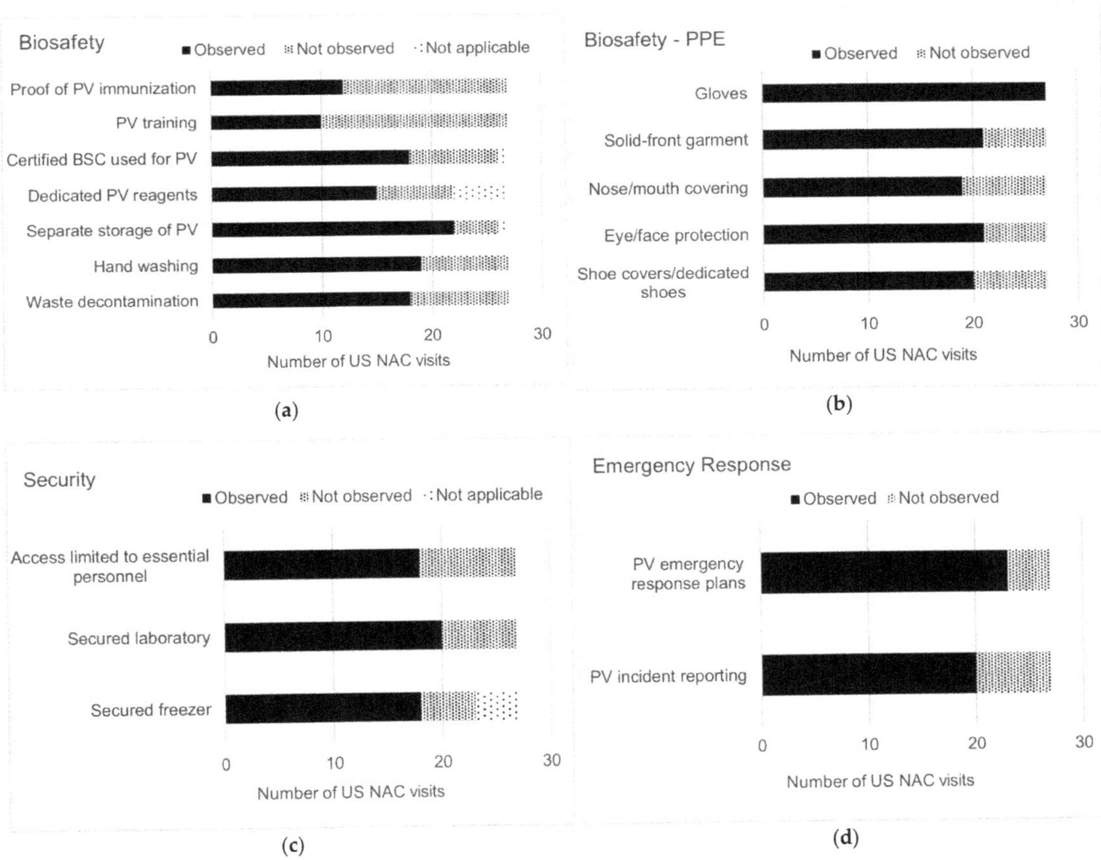

Figure 4. Risk mitigation strategies implemented by U.S. PEFs at time of site visit (n = 27), by category: (**a**) Biosafety category—seven key biosafety containment strategies. For storage-only PEFs or PEFs that did not store PV, certain containment strategies were not applicable. (**b**) Biosafety category—five personal protective equipment (PPE) containment strategies. (**c**) Security category—three containment strategies. For freezers located in a PV-dedicated secured laboratory, a secured freezer is not applicable. (**d**) Emergency response category—two containment strategies.

3.6. US NAC and GCC Endorsement

National and global endorsement and associated processing times for facility CP applications are shown in Table 2. US NAC received completed CP application information (i.e., CP application, preliminary containment conditions/risk mitigation strategies, time-bound action plan, material inventory, resolution of site visit findings) for 17 of 18 PEFs. GCC-CWG requested clarification on eight applications and returned three CP applications as 'unsatisfactory', requiring PEF reapplication. A total of sixteen PEFs were endorsed by GCC in the United States as of June 2023. Extended processing times (median days = 233; min = 91; max = 678) were observed for US PEFs to achieve NAC- and GCC-endorsed CP applications (Table 2).

3.7. Withdrawal of PEFs

Following GCC endorsement, six PEFs completed essential work with WPV2, WPV3, and OPV/Sabin 2, and/or received a temporary waiver from WHO to exclude research activities with nOPV2 from the Containment Certification Scheme resulting in ten active PEFs as of 31 December 2022 (Figure 3). To withdraw from containment certification, PEFs submitted a written statement signed by the principal investigator or institutional representative requesting to withdraw from containment certification, documentation with two witness signatures of the transfer, inactivation or destruction of WPV2/WPV3 and OPV2 materials, and a description of validated decontamination methods used to decommission laboratory areas. US NAC reviewed the documentation and notified WHO of the withdrawal. Overall, a substantial reduction (20/30, 67%) in the number of potential US PEFs has occurred since the appointment of US NAC.

4. Discussion

Poliovirus containment is a key goal of the poliovirus eradication strategy and a prerequisite for future certification of a poliovirus-free world [22]. As of November 2023, WHO reported a total of 22 countries with plans to retain PV materials in 69 PEFs, with 42 designated PEFs awarded GCC-endorsed CPs to become audited against GAPIII [6,23]. While some countries experienced delays in appointing an NAC [6,23], US NAC was established in January 2018 following a process initiated by CDC. The rapid implementation of containment activities in the US was likely due to existing partnerships between CDC and WHO, monthly coordination meetings between US NAC and WHO, the establishment of an external working group, and allocation of CDC resources and full-time staffing to US NAC. These activities supported the engagement of PV laboratories in the certification process and safeguarded PV infectious materials with enhanced safety and security practices. Notably, all US PV laboratories reporting WPV2/VDPV2, OPV2, and WPV3/VDPV3 infectious materials in the national survey participated in the containment certification process or opted to destroy, inactivate, or transfer these materials to comply with GAPIII/GAPIV. We report on progress made towards a successful transition to more stringent GAPIII/GAPIV containment in the United States.

Poliovirus does not currently meet the criteria for classification as a select agent in the United States, and, as a result, the United States does not have a legal framework to require containment of polioviruses as of November 2023 [24]. Further, poliovirus has previously been classified as a risk group 2 agent with recommended biosafety level 2 (BSL-2) laboratories and containment practices as described in BMBL guidelines [21], whereas poliovirus containment is closely aligned with enhanced BSL-3 laboratories and practices [10,11]. These issues presented a challenge to the immediate implementation of GAPIII containment by US facilities performing essential work with polioviruses. Most US PEFs planned to complete work under a CP and not seek additional certification. Thus, the United States developed a phased approach to manage a voluntary program of facilities retaining WPV2/VDPV2, OPV2, and WPV3/VDPV3 to work with and store these viruses safely and securely while progressing toward stringent containment measures outlined in GAPIII/GAPIV.

The total number of PEFs in the United States fluctuated between 2017 and 2022, with the largest decrease occurring in 2018. The PEFs reported GAPIII containment requirements as a deterrent for the retention of PV materials. However, since 2019, a modest reduction in PEFs was balanced with newly identified facilities. Globally, the United States continues to have the largest number of facilities retaining polioviruses that entered WHO's Containment Certification Scheme as of November 2023 [23]. Several US PEFs did not modify operations to comply with GAPIII containment, consistent with the 2018 WHA resolution [12], until contacted by US NAC. As a result, US NAC developed recommendations for preliminary containment conditions/risk mitigation strategies in consultation with an independent US working group and PEF partners that were realistic for facilities to achieve in a short time. The US NAC risk mitigation strategies were standardized for transparency and consistency in the certification process due to the large number of US PEFs. US NAC found that site visits and discussions with facility personnel were critical to raise awareness of containment requirements and to verify the implementation of practices prior to endorsement of CP applications.

US NAC also observed gaps in PEF biocontainment practices during site visits, including some fundamental GAPIII principles. For example, many PEFs had not verified PV immunizations for essential personnel, ensured stringent adherence to hand hygiene practices, or required use of certified primary containment devices for all manipulations of PV infectious materials. These site visit findings, along with a reported 21 incidents of PV release at research laboratories and vaccine production facilities that have occurred globally since 2000, resulting in 16 poliovirus infections [25], suggest current containment practices in PV laboratories should be reviewed and strengthened. US NAC site visits were instrumental in observing PV biocontainment practices, and although gaps were identified, facilities resolved findings and improved poliovirus containment practices in designated US PEFs. These results show that a transition from decades of poliovirus research using BSL-2 laboratories and practices to higher biocontainment standards required time, engagement, and collaboration by all partners, particularly for enhanced laboratory containment of attenuated OPV2 vaccine viruses [7].

US NAC found that its PEF certification process resulted in consistent implementation of enhanced safety and security practices beyond BSL-2 standards for PV infectious materials. US NAC acknowledges that the risk mitigation strategies (preliminary containment conditions) reported here were not a substitute for WHO's GAPIII/GAPIV containment requirements. In addition, the approach taken was risk-based and may not be applicable to all PEF-hosting countries globally. For example, poliovirus vaccines are not manufactured in the United States; this is a higher risk activity with multiple reported containment breaches [9,25–27]. The United States also complies with GAPIII/GAPIV requirements for national high population immunization coverage (93% inactivated poliovirus vaccine, third dose, as of 2022 [28,29]) as well as sanitation system safeguards to mitigate the transmission of diseases such as those due to wild polioviruses.

US NAC continues to improve its guidance for PEFs and the risk mitigation strategies were updated with more descriptive information in 2020–2021, including containment of WPV3/VDPV3 and additional emergency response and security strategies aligned to the GAPIII/GAPIV standard. US NAC identified similar gaps in PEF readiness for these enhancements. As a result, PEF readiness for site visits and the implementation of recommended enhanced containment conditions were factors that contributed to delays in the certification process. While our recommended preliminary containment conditions were adapted from GAPIII, PEF conformance to a more complex and system-based GAPIII/GAPIV standard suggests that additional time may be necessary for PEFs to achieve full conformance to GAPIII/GAPIV than currently outlined in the WHO Containment Certification Scheme [14]. Most PEF-hosting-country NACs have been established; however, no designated PEFs have been fully certified to GAPIII/GAPIV containment worldwide [6,23].

Poliovirus-essential facility CP applications required nearly 8 months (median days = 233; range 91–678) for endorsement by both US NAC and GCC from the date of submission to US NAC. Currently, the WHO Containment Certification Scheme recommends that NACs review CP applications to determine if the PEF can potentially meet GAPIII criteria, but does not specify site visit assessments for this first step [14]. US NAC incorporated site visits prior to its endorsement of PEFs, a significant contributing factor in longer processing times. While PEFs averaged less than three months to implement enhanced containment practices, one PEF required 418 days to implement the recommended risk mitigation strategies due to limited availability of BSL-3 space during the COVID-19 pandemic. Despite a longer processing time, US NAC deemed these visits necessary before giving its endorsement of a designated PEF and instrumental in responding to WHO and/or GCC requests for clarification during their review processes. US NAC also found longer processing times were needed when GCC returned a few CP applications as unsatisfactory and requiring reapplication. These CP applications required additional correspondence with WHO and GCC for resolution of reviewer feedback and resulted in an extended approval process. The CP processing times improved to less than six months for four US PEFs enrolled during 2020–2022, suggesting that, despite challenges and the COVID-19 pandemic, US NAC's processes are effective for the identification and certification of PEFs.

Overall, the United States successfully appointed an NAC, reduced the number of potential PEFs by 67%, and ensured all facilities retaining WPV2/VDPV2, OPV2, and WPV3/VDPV3 infectious materials in the national survey submitted CP applications. Notably, the United States is complying with the May 2018 World Health Assembly resolution 71.16 [12] without a national legal framework requiring containment of polioviruses. As of June 2023, one US PEF achieved an Interim Certificate of Containment against GAPIII to advance beyond the initial CP process ([30] unpublished data, manuscript in preparation). The United States is one of only three countries achieving this accomplishment. The results reported suggest that US NAC's outreach and phased approach for the implementation of stringent GAPIII/GAPIV containment measures, engagement of laboratory partners in preliminary containment recommendations, and to raise facility awareness of the risks posed by retaining eradicated polioviruses has led to the adoption of enhanced laboratory safeguards. US NAC will continue to monitor its national survey, PEFs, and report on the transition to GAPIII/GAPIV containment audits aligned with the anticipated global CP expiry date.

Limitations

The findings in this report are subject to at least three limitations. First, we were unable to account for possible under-reporting of facilities retaining poliovirus materials in national surveys used for the identification of PEFs. Second, and related to the first limitation, the United States does not maintain a registry of laboratories, and thus the unknown total number of laboratories limited the ability to perform an independent verification of laboratories retaining poliovirus materials. Third, the GAPIII and BMBL guidelines were sampled to develop risk mitigation strategies focused on biosafety practices, and thus do not represent other mitigation measures that PEFs may use to reduce risks in the retention of polioviruses.

5. Conclusions

The United States made noteworthy progress on the implementation of the WHO GAPIII/GAPIV Containment Certification Scheme. Globally, the United States was the second country to receive an endorsement of poliovirus-essential facility CP applications by the GCC and has the highest number of PV facilities endorsed as designated poliovirus-essential facilities as of June 2023. US PEFs established a community of practice committed to the implementation of containment certification and adopted enhanced biosafety and biosecurity containment practices for PV materials exceeding routine BSL-2 practices during the transition to WHO GAPIII/GAPIV containment, and US NAC engaged institutional leadership, biosafety professionals, and investigators in global poliovirus containment goals.

Supplementary Materials: The following supporting information can be downloaded at https://www.mdpi.com/article/10.3390/pathogens13020116/s1: Figure S1: Poliovirus containment timeline and steps for enrollment of facilities in containment certification, United States.

Author Contributions: The findings and conclusions in this report are those of the authors and do not necessarily represent the official position of the U.S. Centers for Disease Control and Prevention (CDC). C.O., B.S., C.A.S., A.L., C.M., S.S. and K.G. performed containment site visits and reviewed the manuscript; C.B. led development of NAC website, performed outreach activities, and reviewed the manuscript; C.O., C.A.S. and L.H.S. led the experimental design, collection, and analysis of data; C.O. and C.A.S. prepared the figures and wrote the manuscript; L.H.S. directed the poliovirus containment program. All authors have read and agreed to the published version of the manuscript.

Funding: The authors did not receive external funding to support the work reported in this manuscript.

Institutional Review Board Statement: CDC determined this activity (HSR#18110601) to be public health non-research; thus, Institutional Review Board review was not required.

Informed Consent Statement: Not applicable.

Data Availability Statement: The datasets generated and analyzed during the current study are not publicly available due to privacy concerns for the poliovirus-essential facilities. Aggregated data are available from the corresponding author on reasonable request.

Acknowledgments: We thank the poliovirus-essential facilities for collaboration and participation in poliovirus containment; Daniel Sosin, Alison Mawle, and Olen Kew (CDC) for leadership and US poliovirus containment program development; Mark Pallansch (CDC) for technical expertise and manuscript review; Cassandra Tansey (CDC) for the technical expertise and development of animal containment guidance; and the CDC/ORR Board of Scientific Counselors Poliovirus Containment Working Group for the review, technical expertise, and support of US NAC policy recommendations.

Conflicts of Interest: The authors declare they have no conflicts of interest. The findings and conclusions in this report are those of the authors and do not necessarily represent the views of the US Centers for Disease Control and Prevention.

References

1. Lee, S.E.; Greene, S.A.; Burns, C.C.; Tallis, G.; Wassilak, S.G.; Bolu, O. Progress Toward Poliomyelitis Eradication—Worldwide, January 2021–March 2023. *Morb. Mortal. Wkly. Rep.* **2023**, *72*, 517–522. [CrossRef] [PubMed]
2. Strebel, P.M.; Sutter, R.W.; Cochi, S.L.; Biellik, R.J.; Brink, E.W.; Kew, O.M.; Pallansch, M.A.; Orenstein, W.A.; Hinman, A.R. Epidemiology of poliomyelitis in the United States one decade after the last reported case of indigenous wild virus-associated disease. *Clin. Infect. Dis.* **1992**, *14*, 568–579. [CrossRef] [PubMed]
3. Advisory Committee on Immunization Practices (ACIP). Revised Recommendations for Routine Poliomyelitis Vaccination. *Morb. Mortal. Wkly. Rep.* **1999**, *48*, 590.
4. Jorba, J.; Diop, O.M.; Iber, J.; Sutter, R.W.; Wassilak, S.G.; Burns, C.C. Update on vaccine-derived polioviruses—Worldwide, January 2015–May 2016. *Morb. Mortal. Wkly. Rep.* **2016**, *65*, 763–769. [CrossRef] [PubMed]
5. Hampton, L.M.; Farrell, M.; Ramirez-Gonzalez, A.; Menning, L.; Shendale, S.; Lewis, I.; Rubin, J.; Garon, J.; Harris, J.; Hyde, T.; et al. Cessation of Trivalent Oral Poliovirus Vaccine and Introduction of Inactivated Poliovirus Vaccine—Worldwide, 2016. *Morb. Mortal. Wkly. Rep.* **2016**, *65*, 934–938. [CrossRef] [PubMed]
6. Moffett, D.B.; Llewellyn, A.; Singh, H.; Saxentoff, E.; Partridge, J.; Boualam, L.; Zaffran, M. Progress Toward Poliovirus Containment Implementation—Worldwide, 2019–2020. *Morb. Mortal. Wkly. Rep.* **2020**, *69*, 1330–1333. [CrossRef] [PubMed]
7. Dowdle, W.R.; Gary, H.E.; Sanders, R.; van Loon, A.M. Can post-eradication laboratory containment of wild polioviruses be achieved? *Bull. World Health Organ.* **2002**, *80*, 311–316. [PubMed]
8. Bandyopadhyay, A.S.; Singh, H.; Fournier-Caruana, J.; Modlin, J.F.; Wenger, J.; Partridge, J.; Zaffran, M.J. Facility-Associated Release of Polioviruses into Communities-Risks for the Post eradication Era. *Emerg. Infect. Dis.* **2019**, *25*, 1363–1369. [CrossRef] [PubMed]
9. Duizer, E.; Ruijs, W.L.; Hintaran, A.P.; Hafkamp, M.C.; van der Veer, M.; Te Wierik, M.J. Wild poliovirus type 3 (WPV3)-shedding event following detection in environmental surveillance of poliovirus essential facilities, the Netherlands, November 2022 to January 2023. *Eurosurveillance* **2023**, *28*, 2300049. [CrossRef] [PubMed]

10. World Health Organization. *WHO Global Action Plan to Minimize Poliovirus Facility-Associated Risk after Type-Specific Eradication of Wild Polioviruses and Sequential Cessation of Oral Polio Vaccine Use—GAPIII*, 3rd ed.; World Health Organization: Geneva, Switzerland, 2015.
11. World Health Organization. *WHO Global Action Plan for Poliovirus Containment*, 4th ed.; World Health Organization: Geneva, Switzerland, 2022.
12. Seventy First World Health Assembly. WHA Resolution 71.16: Poliomyelitis—Containment of Polioviruses. 2018. Available online: https://polioeradication.org/wp-content/uploads/2019/05/A71_R16-en.pdf (accessed on 6 December 2023).
13. World Health Organization. *Guidance to Minimize Risks for Facilities Collecting, Handling or Storing Materials Potentially Infectious for Polioviruses (PIM Guidance)*; World Health Organization: Geneva, Switzerland, 2018.
14. World Health Organization. *Containment Certification Scheme to Support the WHO Global Action Plan for Poliovirus Containment (GAPIII-CCS)*; World Health Organization: Geneva, Switzerland, 2017.
15. Centers for Disease Control and Prevention (CDC). National laboratory inventory for global poliovirus containment—United States, November 2003. *Morb. Mortal. Wkly. Rep.* **2004**, *53*, 457–459.
16. Global Polio Eradication Initiative. Poliovirus Type 3 (PV3) Containment after Declaration of Wild Poliovirus Type 3 (WPV3) Eradication. 2019. Available online: https://polioeradication.org/wp-content/uploads/2016/07/PV3-containment-statement-20190930.pdf (accessed on 17 January 2024).
17. *ISO Standard No. 45001:2018*; Occupational Health and Safety Management Systems—Requirements with Guidance for Use. International Organization for Standardization (ISO): Geneva, Switzerland, 2018.
18. *ISO Standard No. 19011:2018*; Guidelines for Auditing Management Systems. International Organization for Standardization (ISO): Geneva, Switzerland, 2018.
19. Centers for Disease Control and Prevention (CDC), United States National Authority for Containment. Past Poliovirus Surveys of U.S. Laboratories. Available online: https://www.cdc.gov/orr/polioviruscontainment/us-containment.htm (accessed on 6 December 2023).
20. Centers for Disease Control and Prevention (CDC). *National Inventory for Poliovirus Containment: Minimizing Risk of Poliovirus Release from Laboratories in the United States*; Federal Register: Washington, DC, USA, 2019; Volume 84.
21. US Department of Health and Human Services (HHS); CDC. *Biosafety in Microbiological and Biomedical Laboratories*, 5th ed.; HHS Publication no. (CDC) 21-1112; CDC: Atlanta, GA, USA, 2009.
22. Global Polio Eradication Initiative. *Polio Endgame Strategy 2022–2026: Delivering on a Promise*; World Health Organization: Geneva, Switzerland, 2021.
23. World Health Organization. Country Progress towards Poliovirus Containment Certification (Website, Data as of 20 November 2023). Available online: https://polioeradication.org/polio-today/preparing-for-a-polio-free-world/containment/ (accessed on 6 December 2023).
24. U.S. Government Publishing Office. Electronic Code of Federal Regulations Title 42 Chapter 1 Subchapter F Part 73. Available online: https://www.ecfr.gov/current/title-42/chapter-I/subchapter-F/part-73 (accessed on 6 December 2023).
25. Irwin, A. Polio is on the brink of eradication. Here's how to keep it from coming back. *Nature* **2023**, *623*, 680–682. [CrossRef] [PubMed]
26. Jeannoël, M.; Antona, D.; Lazarus, C.; Lina, B.; Schuffenecker, I. Risk Assessment and Virological Monitoring Following an Accidental Exposure to Concentrated Sabin Poliovirus Type 3 in France, November 2018. *Vaccines* **2020**, *8*, 331. [CrossRef] [PubMed]
27. Duizer, E.; Ruijs, W.L.; van der Weijden, C.P.; Timen, A. Response to a wild poliovirus type 2 (WPV2)-shedding event following accidental exposure to WPV2, the Netherlands, April 2017. *Eurosurveillance* **2017**, *22*, 30542. [CrossRef] [PubMed]
28. Centers for Disease Control and Prevention (CDC). Polio Vaccination Coverage Among Children 19–35 Months by State, HHS Region, and the United States, National Immunization Survey-Child (NIS-Child), 1995 through 2020. Available online: https://www.cdc.gov/vaccines/imz-managers/coverage/childvaxview/interactive-reports/index (accessed on 6 December 2023).
29. World Health Organization. Immunization Data Portal, Polio 3rd dose Coverage Estimates. Available online: https://immunizationdata.who.int/pages/profiles/usa.html (accessed on 6 December 2023).
30. Ottendorfer, C.; Sanders, C.A.; Suppiah, S.; Gustin, K.; Smith, L.H. Implementation of GAPIII Laboratory Containment in Poliovirus-Essential Facilities—United States, 2017–2023. *Preprints* 2024. *in draft*.

pathogens

MDPI

Review

Population Immunity and Polio Eradication

Paul E. M. Fine

Department of Infectious Disease Epidemiology and International Health, London School of Hygiene and Tropical Medicine, Keppel St., London WC1E 7HT, UK; paul.fine@lshtm.ac.uk

Abstract: The Global Polio Eradication Initiative made immense progress after its establishment in 1988 as a consequence of high coverage with various poliovirus vaccines in all populations of the world. Problems have arisen in recent years, however, related to security issues in some countries, to the circulation of vaccine-derived polioviruses, and to the recognition that individuals with certain immune deficiencies can remain infected and infectious for many months or years. As natural infection and different vaccines have different effects on the immune system, the patterns of humoral and mucosal immunity to polioviruses in the world today are complex but are crucial to the ultimate success of the eradication initiative. This paper describes the background of the current situation and current immunological patterns and discusses their implications for managing population immunity to polioviruses in the years ahead.

Keywords: Polio; eradication; immunity; herd immunity; vaccination

1. Introduction

The global polio eradication initiative was established as a millennium target by the World Health Assembly in 1988. Its justification was based upon a mixture of theory and experience. The theory claimed that, by raising immunity above a defined "herd immunity threshold" level, infection incidence should decline—ultimately to zero, if that high immunity level could be maintained. The experience had been provided by the successful eradication of smallpox, as achieved and certified in the late 1970s. In addition, the Pan American Region of the WHO was making impressive progress toward a regional polio elimination target, set in 1985, after discovering the effectiveness of vaccination campaigns. The argument for the feasibility of eradication was bolstered by the presence of the Expanded Programme on Immunisation (EPI), which was providing routine immunisation services to all populations. The argument was also supported by economic models, which showed that the additional costs of a targeted programme could be more than recovered by future savings if polioviruses ceased to circulate and vaccinations could be discontinued worldwide [1,2].

As documented in the several papers in this issue, there was dramatic progress towards the eradication goal for 12 years after it was set. The incidence of poliomyelitis disease declined globally by approximately 99% by the year 2000. Types 2 and 3 wild virus stopped circulating in 1999 and 2012, respectively, and their eradication has been certified. However, major difficulties have appeared: political problems disrupting vaccination programmes in several countries, the appearance and extensive spread of vaccine-derived polioviruses, now circulating in some 20 countries, and the recognition of the long-term secretion of polioviruses by individuals with certain immune deficiencies. These observations have challenged the theoretical and practical arguments that had been used to support the eradication initiative.

The declines in infection and disease incidence have been brought about entirely by vaccination, on a massive scale, in every population in the world. The nature and extent of the immunity induced by this vaccination initiative are complex but critical for the ultimate success or failure of the entire initiative. This paper summarises the theoretical and practical background to the evolving circumstances, mentions some outstanding gaps in our understanding of population immunity to polioviruses, and considers their implications.

2. Theoretical Background

There is a large library of literature devoted to the theory of infection eradication by means of vaccines [3]. Much of this literature emphasises the concept of "herd immunity", defined as a threshold level of immunity in a population above which infection incidence should decline, ultimately (if levels above that threshold are maintained) to zero.

The basic argument is simple. It starts with a recognition that the level of immunity required in a population to reduce or stop transmission of an infectious agent is related to the transmissibility of that infection: the more transmissible it is, then the higher the level of immunity required. Transmissibility in this context is most appropriately described by the "basic reproduction number", typically symbolised as R_0, and defined as the average number of transmissions by each infected individual in a totally susceptible population. In numerical terms, if each infected individual would transmit the agent on average to R_0 others in a totally susceptible population, then infection incidences would be constant if all but one of the R_0 (i.e., $[R_0 - 1]$ out of the R_0) individuals exposed to each infectious individual were immune and protected against infection. This gives a threshold for the critical proportion immune, often called the herd immunity threshold:

$$(R_0 - 1)/R_0 = 1 - 1/R_0 \quad (1)$$

This relationship is illustrated in Figure 1. The implication of such a threshold is that, as long as the proportion immune is above this threshold, then incidences of infection should decline in the population, ultimately to zero.

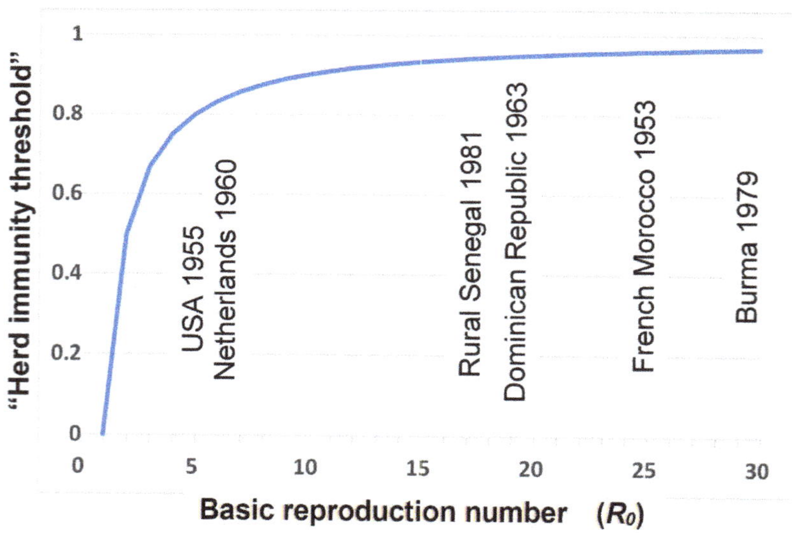

Figure 1. Estimates of the basic reproduction numbers and simple theoretical "herd immunity thresholds" (calculated as: $1 - 1/R_0$) for wild poliovirus, in different populations, from References [4,5].

Because of this relationship, there has been much interest in estimating the R_0 of different infections, including polioviruses. These estimations were based upon the age patterns of infection and immunity in populations in which the infection was at a stable endemic level (as constant incidences imply that the proportion immune in the population is at the herd immunity threshold). Starting with the simplest possible assumption, if everyone became infected (and, thus, naturally immune) at age A and lived for L years, then A/L would give the proportion of everyone's life spent susceptible and $1 - A/L$ would be the proportion immune. Equating this to the herd immunity threshold (expression 1) gives $A/L = 1/R_0$ and thus $R_0 = L/A$. In other words, the basic reproduction number should be equal to the average life expectancy divided by the average age at infection. It was later shown by Dietz that this estimate can be improved by assuming that mortality is constant by age rather than assuming everyone lives for L years; in which case, the basic reproduction number should be $R_0 = L/A + 1$ [3,6].

The application of this theory to poliovirus serological data, from studies carried out before vaccines were introduced, provided estimates of R_0 ranging from approximately 4 for wealthy countries up to 30 for poor populations (see Figure 1). One should not expect precision in such estimates, but this range of values makes intuitive sense, given the faecal–oral mode of transmission of polioviruses, which means that transmission is far more efficient (R_0 is far higher) in poor populations with inadequate standards of hygiene than in wealthy populations with high standards of sewage disposal and hygiene practices [4,5,7].

On the basis of such logic, it was estimated that the herd immunity threshold for poliovirus eradication ranges from approximately 75% in wealthy high-hygiene populations to 97% in poor populations [4–6]. The theoretical challenge of the eradication programme was thus to achieve, and maintain, these levels of immunity with vaccines.

Such simple logic appears in many textbooks. It may be appealing, but reflection reveals a variety of problems in terms of its applicability to actual circumstances. It implies several crucial assumptions.

1. There is an assumption that immunity is 100% effective in preventing infection and infectiousness. However, immunity versus poliovirus infection is complicated, depending upon whether it is attributable to natural infection, inactivated vaccines or oral vaccines, or to combinations of these over time [5,8]. It is well known that immunity induced by oral poliovirus vaccine (OPV) is qualitatively very different from that induced by inactivated poliovirus vaccine (IPV) and that OPV induces far stronger intestinal mucosal IgA-mediated protection than IPV [9]. Thus, while both types of vaccines may be highly effective in preventing disease, OPV is far more effective in preventing infection and infectiousness, which are essential for stopping their transmission and, hence, eradication. This is a major reason why most countries relied upon OPV in their eradication programmes, the only exceptions being a few countries (e.g., the Netherlands) with very high standards of hygiene and hence very low R_o for polioviruses. The distinction was illustrated dramatically by circumstances in Israel, which shifted from OPV to IPV in 2005, and where a wild virus circulated for several months in the absence of the clinical disease in 2013, necessitating the national programme to revert to the use of OPV vaccines [10].

Though OPV-derived intestinal mucosal immunity is far stronger than that generated by IPV, challenge studies have shown that it is not complete or 100% protective, i.e., OPV-vaccinated individuals still become infected when challenged and still excrete small numbers of polioviruses. Interestingly, it may be that enhanced-potency IPV vaccines are more effective in providing pharyngeal rather than intestinal mucosal immunity [11]. There is also heterogeneity in vaccine responses between populations. Unfortunately, the responses to OPV are weaker in low-income tropical populations than in high-income temperate zone areas, perhaps because of interference from other enteric infections. This means they perform least well in those areas with the highest poliovirus transmissibility [5].

A further complexity arises with reference to poliovirus immunity in that there is some level of cross-protection between types. This is a complex issue that has proved difficult to study but might have to be considered in a thorough assessment of population immunity.

2. There is an assumption in discussions of herd immunity and eradication that immunity persists and does not wane. The duration of protection induced by IPV vaccines is still under discussion, but several high-income countries recommend boosters for adults [8]. Studies in India have revealed that mucosal immunity declines appreciably with time after OPV [12]. The recognition of the long-term excretion of polioviruses by individuals

with particular immune deficiencies means that the duration of protection is a crucially important issue for the eradication initiative [13].

3. There is also an assumption in basic herd immunity calculations that populations are homogeneous and that they mix at random. This is, of course, far from true in real populations. People and communities are heterogeneous, and they do not mix at random. There are subsets in all populations made up of individuals who mix more intensely than others in terms of the sorts of contact required for the transmission of polioviruses. These characteristics are typically associated with socioeconomic conditions and mean that certain subsets of any large population can continue to transmit and maintain an infection to which many others in the larger population are effectively no longer at risk. This circumstance is exacerbated in many populations by the fact that vaccination coverage levels differ between different groups, and it is often the fact that relatively poor and underserved segments of populations have relatively low levels of vaccination coverage, as well as relatively low levels of sanitation and hygiene. The growth of vaccine hesitancy sentiment in many populations adds a further complexity to this issue—illustrated, for example, by the recently documented circulation of vaccine-derived viruses—and a clinical case in a population in New York with low level of vaccine uptake [14]. The fact that the large majority of wild polio virus activity in Pakistan has been concentrated in the Pashto ethnic group, who constitute only some 15% of the national population, is a particularly important example of this heterogeneity today [15].

For all these reasons, simplistic estimations of herd immunity thresholds are misleading and typically underestimate the actual levels of immunity required to continually reduce the incidence of infection in populations. It is possible to make "improved" theoretical estimates based upon the incorporation of a range of assumptions relating to the quality of immune response and non-random distribution of risk and of vaccines into the equation, but the variety of potential and actual circumstances is large and difficult to define with any confidence. Given the complexity of the different vaccines and schedules in the past and current use and the variety of immunological measures, it is very difficult to define the level of immunity in any population. No single measure would suffice.

Many studies have provided measures of IgG seroprevalence in different populations [16,17]. While useful as indicators of previous exposure to natural infection and to vaccines, these seroprevalence levels are difficult to interpret for two reasons. First, they do not measure mucosal immunity, which is crucial for protection against infection transmission. Secondly, these levels typically differ by age and social group, but the roles of these different groups in maintaining infection transmission relate to their hygiene and other risk behaviour and are unclear.

Notwithstanding such criticisms, the basic principle of herd immunity has proved valid in the context of the polio eradication programme, as demonstrated by the dramatic declines in poliovirus circulation achieved in many populations around the world and the fact that several high-income countries have been free of poliovirus circulation for many years. But the simple herd immunity theory is no longer helpful with the challenge facing the polio eradication initiative today. The real focus of the eradication programme needs to be on achieving and maintaining high routine immunisation coverage against polio in all populations and high coverage during supplemental immunisation activities (SIAs) and assuring high-quality surveillance to detect the virus when it is circulating so that rapid action can be taken to terminate transmission.

3. Practical Realities—Current

The current vaccination policies do not aim to achieve some specified prevalence level of some particular measure of population immunity. There has been little discussion of numerical herd immunity thresholds in recent years. It is now more appropriate to discuss different aims and challenges of polio vaccination dependent upon national or regional circumstances. This may be considered in terms of three broad sets of circumstances, analogous to the "goals" as described in the current WHO Strategic Plan 2022–2026 [18].

3.1. Populations with Continued Transmission of the Wild Virus (i.e., Afghanistan and Pakistan Today)

The manifest difficulty in stopping the last chains of wild poliovirus type 1 (WPV1) transmission in these countries reflects a particularly complex interaction of social diversity (for example, the concentration of wild virus transmission in the Pashto population), epidemiological risk factors associated with contact and hygiene (and thus high R_0), political insecurity, and an extreme resistance to vaccination in certain population groups. The national programmes have worked hard to carry out both acute flaccid paralysis (AFP) and environmental surveillance in their populations and to raise coverage as high as possible using the bivalent 1–3 OPV vaccine—in particular, in those communities where wild virus is found. This vaccine is used because it is available, though the type 3 component is no longer needed in this context. Though the challenge of stopping WPV1 circulation has stymied these national programmes for several years, there is now some hope of success in that case numbers are lower in 2023 than ever before, and we may hope that the control efforts will at last succeed. Once the WPV1 virus is no longer found, there will be a need to maintain a high level of OPV-derived immunity for at least three years of intensive surveillance until WPV1 eradication is certified. There are arguments to shift to type 1 novel oral poliovirus vaccine (nOPV1) (and perhaps, also, nOPV3 vaccines), when available, to minimise the risk of generating type 1 or 3 vaccine-derived polio viruses (VDPVs).

3.2. Populations with Circulating VDPVs

This applies now (late 2023) to some 23 countries, 4 with circulating cVDPV1 and 20 with cVDPV2. The incidence of cVDPV2 increased dramatically, especially in Africa, after the removal of Sabin type 2 from trivalent OPV in 2016. The response to these events was initially to carry out monovalent OPV2 campaigns, but the availability of nOPV2 vaccines has provided a better alternative, with appreciably less risk of generating further VDPVs [19]. More than 800 million doses of nOPV2 have been used in 16 countries by late 2023, reducing the number of (reported) cVDPV2 cases from 689 in 2022 to 364 in 2023. Whether nOPV2 use will be sufficient to stop all cVDPV2 circulation is not yet known, as there is some evidence that nOPV2 can itself produce new vaccine-derived strains [20]. There has been a recent substantial increase in cVDPV1, which increases the need for regulatory approval of the nOPV1 vaccine with a low tendency to revert towards wild-type virulence.

3.3. Populations with No Circulating Polioviruses

The majority of countries are now in this category. All continue routine poliovirus vaccination, with a variety of vaccines and schedules [5]. Most low- and middle-income countries (LMICs) have a schedule involving three doses of bivalent 1–3 OPV, starting at a minimum of 6 weeks, supplemented with a dose of trivalent IPV administered from a minimum of 14 weeks of age (with DTP3 or Penta3). High-income counties use only trivalent IPV, typically combined with other antigens (e.g., as a hexavalent product with diphtheria, tetanus, pertussis, *Haemophilus*, and hepatitis B antigens). Several of these countries have found evidence of the circulation of VDPV in recent years by means of environmental surveillance and have responded in a variety of ways. In addition to the New York example mentioned above, type 2 VDPV was identified in sewage in North London in 2022, which led to a response whereby 370,000 children ages 1–9 received an additional dose of either hexavalent or trivalent (with diphtheria and tetanus) IPV vaccine [21].

The overall implication of these activities and history is an immensely complex pattern of immunity to polioviruses in today's world. Immunity levels are high, but the precise prevalence of particular immunoglobulins and intestinal immunity to particular virus types varies considerably within and between populations.

4. Practical Implications—Future

Given the high level of international travel in today's world, as long as any wild or vaccine-derived poliovirus continues to circulate anywhere, the entire global population will remain at risk of poliovirus infection and polio disease, and it is likely that all countries will consider it necessary to continue vaccination of their populations to maintain a high level of protective "immunity". The vaccines used will differ between different regions of the world.

It is likely that high-income countries (HICs) will continue to use only IPV, as they are highly effective against disease and have been shown to provide sufficient mucosal immunity to stop poliovirus transmission where standards of hygiene are high. In addition, they avoid the risk of vaccine-associated paralytic polio (VAPP) or of generating VDPVs. These vaccines are relatively expensive, but HICs are relatively risk-averse and able to afford them. The recent experiences of Israel, the USA, and the UK with the circulation of polioviruses (WPV1 in Israel, cVDPV2 in the USA, and the UK) in populations with IPV-only policies are important indicators here. They demonstrate that IPV can mask continued poliovirus transmission by selective prevention of the disease. IPV can only stop poliovirus transmission if at high coverage in populations with very high standards of hygiene, but even in these circumstances, there may be subpopulations with low coverage and/or particular socioeconomic-related risk factors in which circulation can persist.

In contrast to the HICs, most LMICs are likely to continue with live oral vaccines for the foreseeable future. Perhaps the most important outstanding question is whether the newly developed nOPV vaccines will be able to stop the circulation of the current cVDPV viruses without introducing new circulating VDPVs themselves.

This presents a dilemma, as the continued use of OPV vaccines of any sort in LMICs means that live transmissible viruses continue to be introduced with the attendant risk of generating new cVDPVs. Opinions differ as to the long-term implications of this situation. Chumakov et al. recently argued that one should plan for the continued use of new OPV vaccines with a minimal tendency to create cVDPVs and that the overall goal of the programme should shift from the eradication of infection to the prevention of disease. They note that there is some evidence that oral polio vaccines can have beneficial nonspecific effects and that this should be taken into consideration in setting policies [22,23].

A major determinant of future policies, and of the global epidemiological circumstances, will be determined by the properties and availability of different sorts of vaccines [5,8]. The development and introduction of nOPV2 in recent years has helped to reduce the transmission of type 2 VDPVs. Analogous nOPV1 and nOPV3 vaccines are in development and will hopefully be available in the near future. In addition, there are efforts to develop other sorts of vaccines, including based upon mRNA or vaccine-like particle (VLP) technology. We may hope that one or another of these vaccines proves able to provide mucosal protection but avoid any risk of generating further VDPVs.

Whatever vaccines are available, several complex issues must be taken into consideration in determining poliovirus vaccination policies.

1. The properties of the available poliovirus vaccines. This includes their production properties and cost, as well as type specificity, effectiveness, and safety profile, and the willingness of international agencies such as the Global Alliance for Vaccines and Immunisation (GAVI) to provide them to LMICs.
2. The capabilities of different countries to provide vaccines to their populations with high routine coverage.
3. The need for campaigns or "national immunisation days" (NIDs). These have been a regular feature of polio control for the past 20 years at considerable cost and disruption. Costs for these activities should not fall only on LMICs, where poliomyelitis is not among the highest-priority health concerns.
4. Concerns over the reintroduction of polioviruses in the future. This raises issues of (a) containment of polioviruses in laboratories and vaccine production facilities through-

out the world, (b) the presence of long-term and immune deficient virus excretors, and (c) the risk of the de novo synthesis of new polioviruses and bioterrorism
5. The extent and effectiveness of global poliovirus surveillance, both AFP and environmental surveillance. This is a major global undertaking and is expensive.
6. The acceptability of polio vaccines in a world with increasing vaccine hesitancy, recognising that polio vaccines have been the targets of particular distrust in some populations.
7. The nature and credibility of strategies for a stepwise focus upon one or another poliovirus type, e.g., withdrawal of type 3 antigens from OPVs and IPVs. These strategies have major implications for vaccine production and supply.
8. The credibility of evidence that OPV vaccines can have beneficial nonspecific effects on child mortality.
9. The propensity of nOPV vaccines to produce cVDPVs, albeit at a markedly reduced rate.
10. Competing public health issues (COVID-19 has provided a dramatic example).
11. The contribution of polio programme resources to other public health problems. This has long been recognised as necessary for the acceptability of polio eradication activities—in particular, in low-income settings.
12. The need to intensify surveillance, including water and sewage surveillance, to detect any polioviruses, which can lead to appropriate responses to stop transmission before it becomes widespread.
13. The future of special funding for polio at the global level.

Consideration of all these issues together is immensely challenging and made even more difficult by the fact that the debate is held in a world in which many other important health and political issues compete for resources. Polio eradication has held a special place among global health priorities for more than three decades, but this cannot continue forever.

5. Discussion

The goal of global polio eradication was set 35 years ago. We may remain committed to having it succeed, but that outcome is by no means certain.

Regardless of the long-term outcome of the initiative, it is important to acknowledge the success in reducing a major cause of disability from some 350,000 cases per year by at least 99% [5]. For that, the world may and should be grateful. But it is also important to learn many lessons from the experience of the initiative: that eradication is far more difficult and complicated to achieve than is expressed in simple herd immunity thresholds.

In this context, it is appropriate to harken back to the smallpox eradication example [24]. It was achieved in just eleven years after the WHO set a ten-year target in 1966 and was thus relatively simple compared to the polio experience, But it is notable that the leaders of that initiative all commented on how lucky they were, given a variety of unforeseen political and financial challenges [25,26].

Though global success with smallpox eradication provided an example for establishing the global polio eradication initiative, the viruses and associated challenges were very different for the two diseases. In particular, the low case-to-infection ratio of polioviruses contrasts with the fact that virtually all variola infections are/were clinically manifest and relatively easy to diagnose. Surveillance was thus vastly simpler for variola than for polioviruses. In addition, a single dose of variola vaccine was sufficient. Further, smallpox virus transmission was predictable. Field workers could identify cases and their contacts with relative ease. They could then focus their immunisation efforts on those contacts. However, the transmissibility of polioviruses is appreciably greater than that of variola in poor populations, and the location of transmission is not predictable, given that the vast majority of transmitters have no symptoms at all. For these reasons, many countries were confident about discontinuing smallpox vaccination some years prior to global eradication. This has not been the case for polio. Few, if any, countries will be willing to stop poliovirus vaccination until after a certification of global eradication, and some may recommend vaccination in their populations for some years thereafter.

There remains a question of the levels of population immunity against polioviruses that will or would be called for in different populations if eradication is not achieved and wild or vaccine-derived viruses continue to circulate. There will be an argument for all countries to maintain very high routine coverage with vaccines similar to those used today (e.g., IPV in HICs and OPV supplemented by IPV in LMICs). In the absence of eradication, there will continue to be outbreaks in high-risk population subsets with low vaccination coverage, requiring responses. These outbreaks may become large, affecting many countries, if high vaccine coverage levels, good surveillance, and a strong response capacity are not maintained. The nature of the responses will be dependent upon the virus involved, the size and nature of the affected group, and the vaccination policy preferred by the population and is likely to mean targeted campaigns with IPV or a type-specific nOPV (or some new sort of vaccine). The coverage requirement will depend on the environmental and social circumstances and vaccination history. Optimising the management of these outbreaks will call upon the accumulated wisdom from experience of poliovirus control in many settings over recent decades.

Should polio eradication not occur in the near future, we may hope for a future world in which socioeconomic conditions and public health infrastructures are improved everywhere and sufficient mucosal immunity is achievable, so that the final eradication of polioviruses can be achieved as readily as in the high- and middle-income countries of today.

Funding: This research received no external funding.

Data Availability Statement: Not applicable.

Acknowledgments: The author wishes to thank the Academic Editors and Kathleen O'Reilly for their helpful comments on this paper.

Conflicts of Interest: The author declares no conflicts of interest.

References

1. Musgrove, P. Is polio eradication in the Americas economically justified? *Bull. Pan Am. Health Organ.* **1988**, *22*, 1–16. [PubMed]
2. Bart, K.; Foulds, J.; Patriarca, P. Global eradication of poliomyelitis: Benefit-cost analysis. *Bull. World Health Organ.* **1996**, *74*, 35–45. [PubMed]
3. Fine, P.E.M.; Mulholland, K.; Scott, J.A.; Edmunds, W.J. Community Protection. In *Vaccines*, 8th ed.; Orenstein, W.A., Offit, P.A., Edwards, K.M., Plotkin, S.A., Eds.; Elsevier Inc.: Philadelphia PA, USA, 2024; Chapter 78, pp. 1063–1624.
4. Patriarca, P.A.; Sutter, R.W.; Oostvogel, P.M. Outbreaks of paralytic poliomyelitis, 1976–1995. *J. Infect. Dis.* **1997**, *175* (Suppl. 1), S165–S172. [CrossRef] [PubMed]
5. Estivariz, C.F.; Burns, C.C.; Macklin, G.R. Poliovirus vaccine–Live. In *Plotkin's Vaccines*, 8th ed.; Orenstein, W.A., Offit, P.A., Edwards, K.M., Plotkin, S.A., Eds.; Elsevier Publishers: Philadelphia, PA, USA, 2024; Chapter 50.
6. Dietz, K. Transmission and control of arbovirus diseases. In *Epidemiology*; Ludwig, D., Cooke, K.L., Eds.; Society for Industrial and Applied Mathematics: Philadelphia, PA, USA, 1975; pp. 104–121.
7. Fine, P.E.M.; Carneiro, I.A.M. Transmissibility and persistence of oral polio vaccine viruses: Implications for the global poliomyelitis eradication initiative. *Am. J. Epidemiol.* **1999**, *150*, 1001–1021. [CrossRef]
8. Vidor, E.J.; Modlin, J.F. Poliovirus vaccine–inactivated. In *Vaccines*, 8th ed.; Orenstein, W.A., Offit, P.A., Edwards, K.M., Plotkin, S.A., Eds.; Elsevier Inc.: Philadelphia, PA, USA, 2024; Chapter 49, pp. 890–913.
9. Parker, E.P.K.; Molodecky, N.A.; Pons-Salort, M.; O'Reilly, K.M.; Grassly, N.C. Impact of inactivated poliovirus vaccine on mucosal immunity: Implications for the polio eradication endgame. *Expert Rev. Vaccines* **2015**, *14*, 1113–1123. [CrossRef]
10. Yaari, R.; Kaliner, E.; Grotto, I.; Katriel, G.; Moran-Gilad, J.; Sofer, D.; Mendelson, E.; Miller, E.; Huppert, A.; POG Group; et al. Modeling the spread of polio in an IPV-vaccinated population: Lessons learned from the 2013 silent outbreak in southern Israel. *BMC Med.* **2016**, *14*, 95. [CrossRef]
11. Onerato, I.M.; Modlin, J.F.; McBean, A.M.; Thoms, M.L.; Losonsky, G.A.; Bernier, R.H. Mucosal immunity induced by enhanced-potency inactivated and oral polio vaccines. *J. Infect. Dis.* **1991**, *163*, 1–6. [CrossRef] [PubMed]
12. Grassly, N.C.; Jafari, H.; Bahl, S.; Sethi, R.; Deshpande, J.M.; Wolff, C.; Sutter, R.W.; Aylward, R.B. Waning intestinal immunity after vaccination with oral poliovirus vaccines in India. *J. Infect. Dis.* **2012**, *205*, 1554–1561. [CrossRef] [PubMed]
13. Macklin, G.; Liao, Y.; Takane, M.; Dooling, K.; Gilmour, S.; Mach, O.; Kew, O.M.; Sutter, R.W.; The iVDPV Working Group. Prolonged Excretion of Poliovirus among Individuals with Primary Immunodeficiency Disorder: An Analysis of the World Health Organization Registry. *Front Immunol.* **2017**, *8*, 1103. [CrossRef] [PubMed]

14. Tanne, J.H. Polio emergency declared in New York State over virus found in wastewater. *BMJ* **2022**, *378*, o2211. [CrossRef] [PubMed]
15. Ataullahjan, A.; Ahsan, H.; Soofi, S.; Habib, M.A.; Bhutta, Z.A. Eradicating polio in Pakistan: A systematic review of programs and policies. *Expert Rev. Vaccines* **2021**, *20*, 661–678. [CrossRef] [PubMed]
16. Alfonso, V.H.; Voorman, A.; Hoff, N.A.; Weldon, W.C.; Gerber, S.; Gadoth, A.; Halbrook, M.; Goldsmith, A.; Mukadi, P.; Doshi, R.H.; et al. Poliovirus immunity among adults in the Democratic Republic of the Congo: A cross sectional serosurvey. *BMC Infect. Dis.* **2022**, *22*, 30. [CrossRef] [PubMed]
17. Hussain, I.; Mach, O.; Hamid, N.A.; Bhatti, Z.S.; Moore, D.D.; Oberste, M.S.; Khan, S.; Khan, H.; Weldon, W.C.; Sutter, R.W.; et al. Seroprevalence of anti-polio antibodies in children from polio high risk area of Afghanistan: A cross sectional survey 2017. *Vaccine* **2018**, *36*, 1921–1924. [CrossRef] [PubMed]
18. WHO. Polio Eradication Strategy 2022–2026: Delivering on a Promise. Available online: https://polioeradication.org/wp-content/uploads/2022/06/Polio-Eradication-Strategy-2022-2026-Delivering-on-a-Promise.pdf (accessed on 1 November 2023).
19. Davlantes, E.; Jorba, J.; Henderson, E.; Bullard, K.; Deka, M.A.; Kfutwah, A.; Martin, J.; Bessaud, M.; Shulman, L.M.; Hawes, K.; et al. Notes from the Field: Circulating Vaccine-Derived Poliovirus Type 2 Emergences Linked to Novel Oral Poliovirus Vaccine Type 2 Use—Six African Countries, 2021–2023. *MMWR Morb. Mortal. Wkly. Rep.* **2023**, *72*, 1041–1042. [CrossRef] [PubMed]
20. Fortner, R. Polio vaccines: Hope, hype, and history repeating? *BMJ* **2023**, *382*, 1763. [CrossRef] [PubMed]
21. Klapsa, D.; Wilton, T.; Zealand, A.; Bujaki, E.; Saxentoff, E.; Troman, C.; Shaw, A.G.; Tedcastle, A.; Majumdar, M.; Mate, R.; et al. Sustained detection of type 2 poliovirus in London sewage between February and July, 2022, by enhanced environmental surveillance. *Lancet* **2022**, *400*, 1531–1538. [CrossRef] [PubMed]
22. Choumakov, K.; Ehrenfeld, E.; Agol, V.I.; Wimmer, E. Polio eradication at the crossroads. *Lancet Glob. Health* **2021**, *9*, e1172–e1175. [CrossRef] [PubMed]
23. Lund, N.; Andersen, A.; Hansen, A.S.K.; Jepsen, F.S.; Barbosa, A.; Biering-Sørensen, S.; Rodrigues, A.; Ravn, H.; Aaby, P.; Benn, C.S. The effect of oral polio vaccine at birth on infant mortality: A randomized trial. *Clin. Infect. Dis.* **2015**, *61*, 1504–1511. [CrossRef] [PubMed]
24. Fenner, F.; Henderson, D.A.; Arita, I.; Jezek, Z.; Ladnyi, I.D. *Smallpox and its Eradication*; WHO: Geneva, Switzerland, 1988.
25. Henderson, D.A.; Klepac, P. Lessons from the eradication of smallpox: An interview with D. A. Henderson. *Philos. Trans. R. Soc. B Biol. Sci.* **2013**, *368*, 20130113. [CrossRef] [PubMed]
26. Arita, I.; Nakane, M.; Fenner, F. Is polio eradication realistic. *Science* **2006**, *312*, 852–854. [CrossRef] [PubMed]

pathogens

MDPI

Article

A Low-Cost, Integrated Immunization, Health, and Nutrition Intervention in Conflict Settings in Pakistan—The Impact on Zero-Dose Children and Polio Coverage

Amira M. Khan [1], Imran Ahmed [2], Muhammad Jawwad [2], Muhammad Islam [1], Rehman Tahir [3], Saeed Anwar [4], Ahmed Ali Nauman [4] and Zulfiqar A. Bhutta [1,2,*]

1 Centre for Global Child Health, Hospital for Sick Children, Toronto, ON M5G OA4, Canada; amira.khan@sickkids.ca (A.M.K.); muhammad.islam@sickkids.ca (M.I.)
2 Centre of Excellence in Women and Child Health, Aga Khan University, Karachi 74800, Pakistan; imran.ahmed@aku.edu (I.A.); muhammad.jawwad@aku.edu (M.J.)
3 Trust for Vaccines and Immunization, Al Sehat Centre, Rafiqui Shaheed Road, Karachi 74350, Pakistan; rehman@tvi.org.pk
4 Prime Foundation, Peshawar Medical College, Warsak Road, Peshawar 25160, Pakistan; sanwar@piph.prime.edu.pk (S.A.); program@piph.prime.edu.pk (A.A.N.)
* Correspondence: zulfiqar.bhutta@sickkids.ca

Abstract: Pakistan is one of two countries globally still endemic for poliovirus. While increasing immunization coverage is a concern, providing equitable access to care is also a priority, especially for conflict-affected populations. Recognizing these challenges, *Naunehal*, an integrated model of maternal, newborn, and child health (MNCH), immunization, and nutrition services delivered through community mobilization, mobile outreach, and private-sector engagement was implemented in conflict-affected union councils (UCs) with high poliovirus transmission, including Kharotabad 1(Quetta, Balochistan) and Bakhmal Ahmedzai (Lakki Marwat, Khyber Pakhtunkhwa). A quasi-experimental pre–post-design was used to assess the impact of the interventions implemented between April 2021 and April 2022, with a baseline and an endline survey. For each of the intervention UCs, a separate, matched-control UC was identified. At endline, the proportion of fully immunized children increased significantly from 27.5% to 51.0% in intervention UCs with a difference-in-difference (DiD) estimate of 13.6%. The proportion of zero-dose children and non-recipients of routine immunization (NR-RI) children decreased from 31.6% to 0.9% and from 31.9% to 3.4%, respectively, with a significant decrease in the latter group. Scaling up and assessing the adoption and feasibility of integrated interventions to improve immunization coverage can inform policymakers of the viability of such services in such contexts.

Keywords: polio eradication; zero dose; immunization; integrated interventions; conflict-affected; health systems

1. Introduction

Pakistan remains one of only two countries globally with a continued endemic transmission of wild poliovirus [1]. While the national-level coverage of fully immunized children is around 76%, it remains much lower in certain regions with the data showing coverage at 37.6% and 42.8% in the provinces of Balochistan and Southern Khyber Pakhtunkhwa (KP), respectively, where being fully immunized refers to children (12–23 months old) who have completed routine immunization till Measles dose 1 (except the Rotavirus vaccine) as per the Expanded Program on Immunization (EPI) schedule [2]. Additionally, despite the slow progress in improving maternal, neonatal, and child health (MNCH) and nutrition indicators, Pakistan has the highest neonatal mortality rate globally at 39 deaths per 1000 live births and an under-five-years-old mortality rate of 63 deaths per 1000 live births [3]. Alarmingly, more than one-third of children under five years old in the country are stunted [4]. During 2020–2022, COVID-19 and its related mitigation strategies further challenged population health and health systems, with a sustained impact on both [5]. Although ensuring the provision of quality healthcare services is a concern, providing equitable access to care poses a challenge, especially for conflict-affected and marginalized populations. The shortage of healthcare staff and deliberate attacks on healthcare workers, especially those administering polio vaccinations, has hindered the distribution of MNCH services. Importantly, an escalation in violence and safety concerns have had a significant impact on community care-seeking behaviors, especially in KP and Balochistan [6]. Climate-related emergencies and food insecurity further exacerbate the situation.

Given the multitude of issues and challenges in the context of polio and beyond, it is critical to implement innovative, low-cost strategies that can increase vaccination coverage, and improve accessibility to health services in insecure and conflict-affected contexts. The polio vaccination program in Pakistan, like most other health delivery strategies, is vertical and largely focuses on urban areas or refugee camps, with limited community buy-ins, and missed remote and internally scattered, displaced populations [7]. Additionally, the strategies for community mobilization and service delivery in such contexts are largely divided between implementing agencies, potentially increasing transaction costs while making the interventions quite complicated.

Nearly all polio cases reported in Pakistan continue to be from seven polio-endemic districts in southern KP, where 1.1 million vaccine-eligible, under-five-years-old children are located [8]. Close to 50,000 of these children are missed in the government's annual supplementary immunization activities (SIAs) as a result of refusals based on vaccine misconceptions, mistrust in health workers, and an emerging "polio fatigue" [1,9,10]. Researchers have linked community "polio fatigue" with weariness and cynicism regarding repeated polio immunization activities when the same community's access to basic health and nutrition services remains limited [11]. Thus, it is not only critical to engage, educate, and mobilize communities, particularly community elders and religious leaders, but also to provide these populations with much-needed health and nutrition services.

The disruption caused by COVID-19 halted vaccination drives and polio supplementary immunization activities in 2020, causing a further setback to polio vaccine coverage as well as routine vaccination rates, particularly in fragile, conflict-affected areas [12–14]. In such circumstances, implementing low-cost integrated strategies for providing health and immunization services where most required was critical. Recognizing these challenges and opportunities, *Naunehal*, an 18-month pilot project, was implemented in three high-risk union councils (UCs) of Pakistan, in 2021–2022. Previous work indicates that we have been working on community-based models for integrating polio, other immunizations, and MNCH interventions, and have been steadily working to simplify the approach and associated costs [15,16]. Thus, the *Naunehal* project adopted a low-cost, integrated model of MNCH, immunization, and nutrition services delivered through community mobilization, mobile outreach, and private-sector engagement strategies. The objective of this paper is to examine the coverage and utilization of the intervention and its impact on immunization coverage (including routine immunizations and oral polio vaccines (OPVs) administered during SIAs) in children under five years old, care-seeking practices, and nutrition behaviors, while exploring the impact on zero-dose children.

2. Materials and Methods

2.1. Study Setting

Naunehal was implemented in three UCs of Pakistan. Kharotabad 1 (Quetta District, Balochistan Province) and Bhana Mari (Peshawar District, (KP) Province) were classified as super-high-risk UCs (SHRUCs) by the Pakistan Polio Eradication Programme, while UC Bakhmal Ahmedzai in district Lakki Marwat, KP, is an area that has experienced polio outbreaks in recent years. In addition to their high poliovirus transmission rates, the UCs also struggled with sub-optimal immunization coverage, maternal and children-under-five-years-old health, and nutrition indicators (Figure 1). Kharotabad-1, a peri-urban UC, and Bakhmal Ahmedzai, a rural UC, are also impacted by sectarian violence and regional insecurity, while Bhana Mari is in an area historically housing refugees. The three UCs were, thus, selected, given their complex contexts and high poliovirus transmission rates.

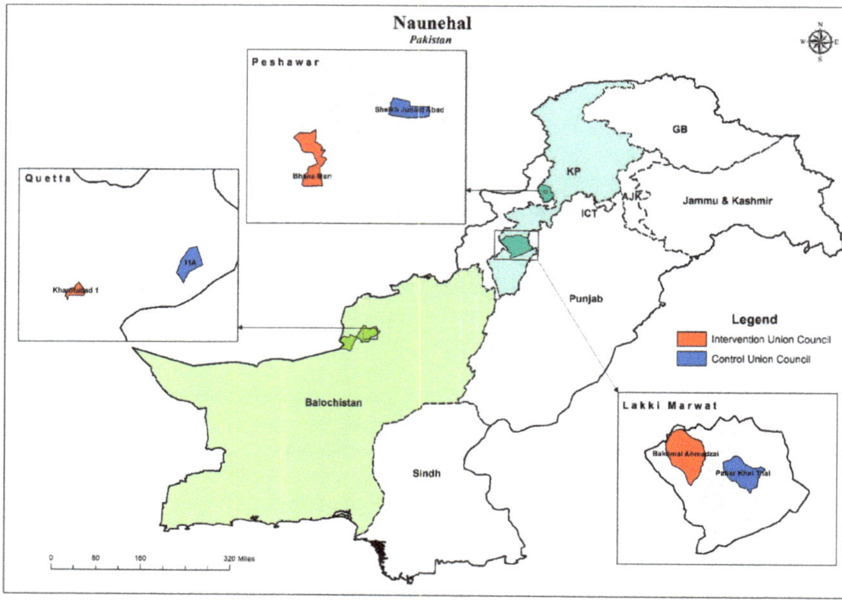

Figure 1. Map showing the control and intervention union councils.

2.2. Study Design

The project adopted a quasi-experimental pre–post design to assess the impacts of the interventions implemented between April 2021 and April 2022. The baseline survey was conducted in Feb–March 2021, while the endline survey was conducted in May 2022. The study protocol has been previously published by Ataullahjan et al. [17].

The three UCs were the intervention sites, and for each of these target UCs, a separate, matched-control UC of a comparable size, population, and location, and coverage indicators were identified, with propensity score matching and in consultation with local partners. The control UCs were Ward-11-A (Quetta District), Pahar Khel Thal (Lakki Marwat District), and Sheikh Junaidabad (Peshawar District), which, though always in the same district, never bordered the target UC.

The project implemented three main strategies in the intervention UCs, including community mobilization, mobile health services, and the engagement of private healthcare providers (HCPs). Community engagement and mobilization included raising awareness via health information sessions that focused on routine childhood immunization; optimal infant and young child feeding (IYCF) practices; water, sanitation, and hygiene; optimal diarrhea management; and appropriate care seeking for both pregnant women and young children. A key component of the community mobilization was ongoing engagement with local leaders and religious scholars to gain their support and buy-ins for the project activities and health messages.

The mobile health services included one team per UC, comprised of a female health worker, a vaccinator, and a facilitator, who visited pre-determined areas of the UC six days a week. The team provided basic health services, routine government-recommended immunization and health services, and IYCF counseling, targeted toward children under five years old and women of reproductive age (WRA). Additionally, the project also identified private HCPs in the intervention UCs to provide age-appropriate routine vaccinations to all under-five-years-old children visiting their clinics. The HCPs were trained in collaboration with the government's District Health Office and EPI. The project also liaised with the EPI to supply the HCPs with vaccines free of cost on a regular, as-needed basis. During the 12-month intervention period, the government's SIAs continued as scheduled both in the intervention and control UCs.

Baseline, midline, and endline surveys were conducted using the 30 × 7 technique in the intervention and control UCs. Thirty clusters demarcated by the government's polio program from each UC were randomly selected and 15 households with children under five years old were selected from each cluster. For each round of the survey, an updated listing of all households was generated for each cluster. The selection of households was performed through systematic random sampling. To achieve an optimal sample size, the target was to survey 450 households from each of the intervention and control UCs. The baseline that was to serve as the basis for targeting and tracking progress focused on household characteristics, immunization practices, health, nutrition, and care-seeking behaviors. As well, the survey examined the community's awareness of and attitude toward COVID-19. The endline survey focused on the same indicators, but also assessed the household's uptake and attitude toward the intervention. Immunization status was determined using the vaccination card. However, if the card was not available, parental recall was used to obtain the information.

The survey inclusion criteria for a household were consent from the family, at least one child under 5 years of age in the household, and that the family had lived in that high-risk UC for at least 6 months (including the child in the household) before the day of the interview. However, the household was also eligible if the only child in the household was born in the last six months. Any household where a parent or caregiver was not available to answer questions related to the child's health and immunization was excluded. The data collected were processed and analyzed at the Aga Khan University, Karachi. A consent form outlining the objectives of the study, how privacy concerns would be handled, and how the data would be used was shared with the participants.

2.3. Statistical Analysis

Data related to demographics, clinical knowledge, attitude and practices, and MNCH-related indicators were compiled and analyzed using STATA version 18.0. To assess the independent effect of interventions, propensity score matching was employed to identify similar UCs based on the geographical location of the UC, population density, size of the children-under-five-years-old population, number of health facilities and health workers, and immunization coverage. Through this process, three matched UCs were also surveyed. Among the predictors, exact matching was enforced to achieve a balance for all the predictors between the intervention and non-intervention groups. Descriptive and inferential statistics were used to characterize the study sample and test hypotheses. Frequency and percentage were calculated for categorical variables and the mean (SD) was calculated for continuous variables.

The mean and percentage point difference in the coverage between the baseline and endline was estimated using a generalized linear model with an identity link and binomial distribution.

We compared the change in prevalence of immunization, antenatal care, postnatal care, and newborn care indicators from the baseline to endline in the two arms using difference-in-difference (DiD) estimates. The DiD estimates were obtained from mixed linear regression models with an interaction term between the variables for arms (intervention vs. control) and time (endline vs. baseline).

The predictors of "zero-dose" and "non-recipient of routine immunization" (NR-RI) children were determined by the multivariable logistic regression after an initial univariable analysis. Variables significant at $p < 0.2$ in the univariable analysis were included in the fully adjusted model. The final model was constructed using a backward elimination, with variables being retained if $p < 0.05$. A p-value less than 0.05 was taken as significant. It is important to mention here that, for our analysis, "NR-RI" was defined as children who did not receive any routine vaccinations (BCG, OPV0, OPV1, Pentavalent (Penta) 1, Pneumococcal Conjugate Vaccine (PCV) 1, OPV2, Penta2, PCV2, OPV3, Inactivated Poliovirus Vaccine (IPV) 1, Penta3, PCV3, and Measles 1), while "zero dose" referred to children who did not receive any routine vaccinations and did not receive OPVs during SIAs. Thus, the NR-RI group was a sub-group of "zero-dose children". On the other hand, "fully immunized" was defined as children who received age-appropriate doses for routine vaccines till Measles 1.

The clustered nature of the data was accounted for by including each cluster as a random effect. Estimates were adjusted for the survey design and sampling weights by treating each UC as strata and clusters as primary sampling units.

2.4. Outcomes

The primary outcomes of this study were the coverage of OPVs and routine EPI vaccines, changes in the proportion of zero-dose children, changes in IYCF practices, and changes in care-seeking behaviors.

3. Results

At baseline, 1286 and 1277 households were visited in the intervention and control UCs, respectively, and the data for 4387 under-five-years-old children were collected. The baseline demographic characteristics of children under five years old at both sites were predominantly similar (Table 1). The male-to-female ratio for under-five-years-old children was almost equal, with a slight male preponderance. A significant majority of mothers (85.1%) in households surveyed at all intervention sites at baseline had no formal schooling—nearly 96% in UC Bakhmal Ahmedzai. Overall, for the intervention UC, 16.8% and 15.2% of the respondents belonged to the poorest and richest quintiles, respectively. However, this varied between UCs with the predominant population in Bhana Mari (intervention UC in Peshawar) belonging to the "rich" (44.1%) quintile, in Kharotabad-1 (intervention UC in Quetta) belonging to the "middle" quintile (46.8%), while in Bakhmal Ahmedzai (intervention UC in Lakki Marwat), most of the population belonged to the "poorest" quintile (64.8%) (Table 1).

While nearly all intervention areas and control households in Lakki Marwat and Peshawar had an improved source of drinking water, the proportions were much lower in the intervention (32.1%) and control (46.1%) areas in Quetta. The improved source of sanitation in households was higher in the intervention and control UCs of Peshawar (99.8%, 99.8%), as compared to Quetta (87.5%, 96.9%) and Lakki Marwat (78.9%, 87.4%) (Table 1). As is apparent, the household characteristics and socioeconomic and education status were markedly better for Peshawar compared to the other districts.

The main study outcomes also included IYCF practices and other health-related care-seeking behaviors related to women and children. Given their distinct determinants and relevance, the findings related to these outcomes and practices will be submitted and discussed in a separate manuscript. In this manuscript, we focused on vaccination-related practices and behaviors.

As shown in Table 2, the mobile health services data from the three sites show that there is a total of 30,768 beneficiaries for the 829 mobile health camp days, with the most camp days (319) in Kharotabad-1. An estimated 13,931 under-five-years-old children were provided services at the mobile health camps, with more than 18,000 immunization doses administered at all intervention sites. There were 73 vaccine refusals, of which 70 were for the oral polio vaccine, and the majority (n = 56) were in Kharotabad-1.

Table 1. Baseline sociodemographic characteristics of households surveyed and under-five-years-old children.

	Overall		Peshawar		Quetta		Lakki Marwat	
	Control	Intervention	Control	Intervention	Control	Intervention	Control	Intervention
Household Characteristics	N = 1277	N = 1286	N = 411	N = 401	N = 433	N = 446	N = 433	N = 439
Finished floor	773 (69.4)	696 (59.3)	404 (97.6)	390 (96.2)	344 (79.0)	253 (56.2)	25 (5.9)	53 (12.0)
Finished roof	1139 (87.9)	998 (76.2)	411 (100.0)	403 (99.2)	373 (84.5)	298 (63.0)	355 (82.3)	297 (65.7)
Finished walls	831 (69.0)	730 (59.7)	409 (98.9)	389 (96.1)	325 (71.8)	244 (52.1)	97 (23.2)	97 (20.9)
Solid fuel	443 (20.6)	464 (26.2)	5 (1.9)	14 (2.6)	6 (1.6)	11 (2.6)	432 (99.7)	439 (100.0)
Single room for sleeping	231 (12.3)	221 (13.9)	47 (14.6)	44 (10.0)	9 (2.3)	22 (5.3)	175 (38.8)	155 (33.9)
Improved source of drinking water	1053 (69.6)	972 (71.1)	410 (99.8)	406 (99.8)	210 (46.1)	141 (31.9)	433 (100.0)	425 (96.7)
Improved source of sanitation	1208 (95.7)	1147 (89.7)	410 (99.8)	406 (99.8)	423 (96.9)	392 (87.5)	375 (87.4)	349 (78.9)
Father's Education								
No formal schooling	350 (33.3)	317 (28.8)	106 (26.3)	79 (24.2)	179 (42.1)	145 (35.5)	65 (16.2)	93 (24.0)
Primary	306 (23.5)	310 (24.0)	16 (6.0)	28 (5.9)	107 (24.6)	166 (37.2)	183 (42.2)	116 (27.6)
Secondary	387 (27.5)	389 (27.5)	142 (35.0)	158 (36.2)	99 (22.4)	96 (19.6)	146 (33.0)	135 (28.5)
Intermediate or above	237 (15.8)	278 (19.7)	147 (32.7)	142 (33.6)	51 (10.9)	41 (7.8)	39 (8.6)	95 (19.9)
Mother's Education								
No formal schooling	1091 (86.1)	1109 (85.1)	271 (65.1)	285 (71.0)	396 (91.0)	406 (90.8)	424 (98.3)	418 (95.7)
Primary	35 (3.9)	58 (5.0)	10 (2.8)	17 (4.6)	23 (5.6)	29 (6.6)	2 (0.4)	12 (2.7)
Secondary	71 (5.2)	69 (5.5)	55 (14.5)	56 (13.0)	14 (2.9)	9 (1.9)	2 (0.3)	4 (0.8)
Intermediate or above	83 (4.8)	58 (4.4)	75 (17.6)	49 (11.4)	3 (0.6)	4 (0.7)	5 (1.0)	5 (0.8)
Wealth Index (Quintiles)								
Poorest	223 (10.1)	292 (16.8)	0 (0.0)	6 (1.1)	1 (0.2)	7 (1.6)	222 (51.9)	279 (64.8)
Poor	253 (16.3)	262 (19.5)	6 (2.1)	14 (2.6)	58 (13.3)	121 (28.8)	189 (43.0)	127 (27.8)
Middle	218 (27.1)	297 (26.1)	17 (5.4)	52 (14.5)	181 (44.1)	212 (46.8)	20 (4.7)	33 (7.4)
Rich	260 (25.2)	255 (22.4)	120 (32.7)	174 (44.1)	139 (30.5)	81 (17.4)	1 (0.2)	0 (0.0)
Richest	326 (21.2)	188 (15.2)	268 (59.8)	161 (37.6)	57 (11.8)	27 (5.4)	1 (0.2)	0 (0.0)
Children Under Five Years Old	N = 2175	N = 2212	N = 542	N = 574	N = 992	N = 946	N = 641	N = 692
Gender								
Male	1133 (51.5)	1124 (50.9)	288 (52.4)	273 (48.1)	502 (50.9)	498 (52.3)	343 (53.4)	353 (51.0)
Female	1042 (48.5)	1088 (49.1)	254 (47.6)	301 (51.9)	490 (49.1)	448 (47.7)	298 (46.6)	339 (49.0)
Age (Months)								
0–5	178 (7.9)	193 (8.2)	52 (9.3)	52 (8.3)	76 (7.6)	70 (7.2)	50 (7.8)	71 (10.2)
6–11	187 (8.9)	204 (10.0)	61 (12.5)	77 (14.1)	80 (8.4)	85 (9.5)	46 (7.4)	42 (5.8)
12–23	405 (18.7)	380 (17.2)	115 (20.6)	126 (21.0)	181 (18.6)	156 (16.6)	109 (17.0)	98 (13.7)
24–59	1405 (64.4)	1435 (64.7)	314 (57.7)	319 (56.5)	655 (65.3)	635 (66.8)	436 (67.9)	481 (70.3)

Table 2. Mobile health services data.

	Overall	Bhana Mari	Bakhmal Ahmedzai	Kharotabad
Mobile health camp days	829	252	258	319
Total beneficiaries	30,768	7524	7225	16,019
Women of a Reproductive Age (WRA) in camps	10,572 (34.4%)	1851 (24.6%)	3039 (42.1%)	5682 (35.5%)
Pregnant women in camps	4416 (41.8%)	661 (35.7%)	824 (27.1%)	2931 (51.6%)
Children under five years old at camps	13,931 (45.3%)	5550 (73.8%)	4157 (57.5%)	4224 (26.4%)
Children under 5 years old provided with routine immunization	5193 (37.3%)	962 (17.3%)	3082 (74.1%)	1149 (27.2%)
Children under 5 years old provided with an OPV	7684 (55.2%)	4310 (77.7%)	1402 (33.7%)	1972 (46.7%)
Total number of immunization doses administered				
BCG	890 (6.4%)	74 (1.3%)	648 (15.6%)	168 (4.0%)
OPV	3721 (26.7%)	532 (9.6%)	2739 (65.9%)	450 (10.7%)
Penta	3541 (25.4%)	471 (8.5%)	2654 (63.8%)	416 (9.8%)
PCV	3526 (25.3%)	466 (8.4%)	2645 (63.6%)	415 (9.8%)
IPV	1344 (9.6%)	211 (3.8%)	1031 (24.8%)	102 (2.4%)
Rota	2554 (18.3%)	293 (5.3%)	1941 (46.7%)	320 (7.6%)
Measles	2501 (18.0%)	421 (7.6%)	1313 (31.6%)	767 (18.2%)
Vaccine Refusals				
Routine immunization	3 (0.0%)	2 (0.0%)	0 (0.0%)	1 (0.0%)
OPV	70 (0.5%)	7 (0.1%)	7 (0.2%)	56 (1.3%)

The immunization coverage component of the post-intervention endline survey for all three districts showed a proportion of fully immunized children that significantly increased from 27.5% to 51.0%, with a DiD estimate of 13.6% (4.5%, 22.8%), with a significant decrease in NR-RI children from 31.9% to 3.4% with a DiD estimate of −20.4% (−32.4, −8.5) (Table 3). The intervention UCs showed an overall decrease in zero-dose children from 31.6% to 0.9%; however, the decreasewas not significant given a similar decrease in the control areas (41.3% to 5.0%).

In comparison to the rural/peri-urban intervention UCs in the districts of Quetta and Lakki Marwat, Bhana Mari was an urban UC with a population with a higher educational and socioeconomic status (Table 1) and significantly higher immunization coverage at baseline (Supplementary Materials, Table S1). Given these differences, the authors performed an additional, separate analysis for the intervention and control UCs in Quetta and Lakki Marwat considering their similar contexts, conflict-affected environments, and sub-optimal health and immunization indicators (Supplementary Materials, Tables S2 and S3).

For these two districts, the proportion of fully immunized children increased significantly, from baseline to endline, from 20.2% to 43.2%, respectively, in intervention UCs with a DiD estimate % diff of 25.2 (17.1, 33.3) (p-value: <0.0001) (Table 4). The coverage for all routine vaccines from birth till 9 months of age increased significantly at endline. Similar to the all-site analysis, the proportion of zero-dose and NR-RI children in intervention UCs decreased from 46% to 1.1% and from 46.0% to 4.2%, respectively, with a significant decreased in the NR-RI category (Table 4). The UC-specific immunization coverage data are included in the Supplementary Materials.

Table 3. Routine immunization coverage at baseline and endline for children under three years old in intervention and control UCs in all three districts.

	Baseline		**Endline**		**Control—% Diff (95% CI)**	**Intervention—% Diff (95% CI)**	**DID Estimate—% Diff (95% CI)**	**DID Estimate—*p*-Value**
	Control	**Intervention**	**Control**	**Intervention**				
	N = 1122	N = 1160	N = 961	N = 1000				
Immunization Status								
Fully immunized	210 (15.9)	305 (27.5)	282 (25.8)	478 (51.0)	9.9 (3.2, 16.6)	23.6 (17.2, 29.9)	13.6 (4.5, 22.8)	0.0038
Partially immunized	463 (42.5)	430 (40.6)	393 (40.7)	473 (45.6)	−1.8 (−9.2, 5.6)	5.0 (−2.6, 12.6)	6.8 (−3.7, 17.3)	0.2039
Non-recipients of routine immunizations	449 (41.6)	425 (31.9)	286 (33.5)	49 (3.4)	−8.1 (−18.3, 2.1)	−28.6 (−34.9, −22.2)	−20.4 (−32.4, −8.5)	0.0009
Zero dose	447 (41.3)	422 (31.6)	47 (5.0)	13 (0.9)	−36.3 (−43.6, −29.0)	−30.8 (−37.4, −24.1)	5.5 (−4.3, 15.4)	0.2676
Ever had a vaccination card	537 (44.5)	640 (60.6)	616 (57.3)	912 (93.2)	12.8 (2.2, 23.4)	32.6 (25.6, 39.6)	19.8 (7.2, 32.4)	0.0022
At Birth								
	N = 1122	N = 1160	N = 961	N = 1000				
BCG	665 (57.8)	722 (66.9)	664 (65.4)	919 (92.9)	7.6 (−2.8, 18.0)	26.0 (19.4, 32.5)	18.3 (6.1, 30.6)	0.0034
OPV0	631 (53.8)	708 (65.6)	576 (53.5)	873 (89.0)	−0.4 (−11.2, 10.4)	23.4 (16.7, 30.0)	23.8 (11.1, 36.4)	0.0003
At 6 Weeks								
	N = 1093	N = 1134	N = 942	N = 980				
OPV1	335 (26.6)	456 (41.8)	544 (50.9)	799 (81.4)	24.4 (14.5, 34.3)	39.6 (32.4, 46.8)	15.2 (3.1, 27.4)	0.0141
Penta 1	559 (47.2)	557 (51.8)	562 (52.1)	850 (86.4)	4.8 (−5.4, 15.0)	34.6 (26.9, 42.4)	29.8 (17.1, 42.5)	<0.0001
PCV 1	538 (45.2)	545 (50.5)	563 (52.2)	845 (85.9)	7.0 (−3.2, 17.2)	35.4 (27.5, 43.3)	28.4 (15.6, 41.3)	<0.0001
Rota Virus 1	531 (43.9)	566 (52.8)	558 (51.8)	827 (83.7)	7.8 (−2.3, 18.0)	30.9 (23.0, 38.8)	23.0 (10.3, 35.8)	0.0005
At 10 Weeks								
	N = 1056	N = 1111	N = 909	N = 956				
OPV 2	259 (21.6)	403 (38.7)	378 (36.3)	642 (69.2)	14.7 (6.2, 23.2)	30.5 (23.5, 37.6)	15.9 (5.0, 26.8)	0.0046
Penta 2	295 (23.8)	430 (40.8)	491 (47.4)	710 (74.7)	23.6 (14.4, 32.8)	33.9 (26.2, 41.7)	10.3 (−1.6, 22.3)	0.0891
PCV 2	292 (23.6)	425 (40.4)	488 (47.2)	703 (73.9)	23.6 (14.5, 32.8)	33.5 (25.7, 41.3)	9.8 (−2.1, 21.8)	0.1056
Rota Virus 2	288 (23.3)	412 (39.2)	483 (46.6)	700 (73.3)	23.3 (14.2, 32.3)	34.1 (26.5, 41.7)	10.9 (−0.9, 22.6)	0.0695
At 14 Weeks								
	N = 1024	N = 1080	N = 882	N = 921				
OPV 3	229 (19.7)	343 (34.0)	315 (30.3)	563 (63.7)	10.6 (2.6, 18.7)	29.7 (22.8, 36.6)	19.1 (8.5, 29.6)	0.0004
Penta 3	209 (18.1)	338 (33.4)	309 (30.3)	530 (60.6)	12.2 (4.0, 20.4)	27.2 (19.9, 34.6)	15.0 (4.1, 25.9)	0.0071
PCV 3	209 (18.1)	330 (32.5)	298 (29.3)	527 (60.4)	11.2 (3.2, 19.2)	27.9 (20.8, 35.0)	16.7 (6.1, 27.3)	0.0022
IPV 1	432 (36.3)	460 (44.5)	448 (44.4)	654 (71.6)	8.1 (−1.3, 17.5)	27.1 (19.2, 34.9)	19.0 (6.8, 31.2)	0.0024
At 9 Months								
	N = 853	N = 875	N = 763	N = 767				
Measles 1	331 (32.4)	397 (47.7)	420 (47.5)	591 (76.0)	15.1 (5.9, 24.3)	28.4 (20.9, 35.8)	13.3 (1.5, 25.1)	0.0269
At 15 Months								
	N = 639	N = 662	N = 598	N = 565				
Measles 2	164 (19.8)	230 (35.1)	247 (37.7)	307 (54.6)	17.9 (9.1, 26.7)	19.5 (11.3, 27.6)	1.6 (−10.3, 13.4)	0.7963

Table 4. Routine immunization coverage at baseline and endline for children under three years old in intervention and control UCs in the districts of Quetta and Lakki Marwat.

	Baseline		Endline		Control—% Diff (95% CI)	Intervention—% Diff (95% CI)	DID Estimate—% Diff (95% CI)	DID Estimate—*p*-Value
	Control	Intervention	Control	Intervention				
	N = 789	N = 810	N = 597	N = 700				
Immunization Status								
Fully immunized	74 (9.6)	144 (20.2)	60 (7.4)	270 (43.2)	−2.1 (−6.0, 1.8)	23.0 (15.8, 30.2)	25.2 (17.1, 33.3)	<0.0001
Partially immunized	275 (38.7)	250 (33.7)	257 (42.7)	384 (52.6)	4.0 (−5.6, 13.6)	18.9 (10.3, 27.4)	14.8 (2.1, 27.5)	0.0225
Non-recipients of routine immunizations	440 (51.8)	416 (46.0)	280 (49.9)	46 (4.2)	−1.9 (−13.6, 9.8)	−41.9 (−49.8, −34.0)	−40.0 (−54.0, −26.0)	<0.0001
Zero dose	438 (51.4)	416 (46.0)	42 (6.8)	12 (1.1)	−44.6 (−52.6, −36.5)	−45.0 (−53.3, −36.7)	−0.4 (−11.8, 11.0)	0.9432
Ever had a vaccination card	258 (35.7)	335 (47.1)	265 (37.3)	632 (93.2)	1.6 (−9.4, 12.6)	46.1 (37.8, 54.4)	44.5 (30.9, 58.1)	<0.0001
At Birth								
	N = 789	N = 810	N = 597	N = 700				
BCG	342 (47.6)	390 (53.7)	309 (48.9)	622 (90.5)	1.2 (−10.6, 13.1)	36.8 (28.5, 45.2)	35.6 (21.3, 49.9)	<0.0001
OPV0	312 (42.8)	369 (50.6)	231 (32.0)	590 (87.1)	−10.8 (−21.6, 0.0)	36.5 (28.4, 44.5)	47.2 (34.0, 60.5)	<0.0001
At 6 Weeks								
	N = 766	N = 786	N = 589	N = 683				
OPV1	152 (18.3)	253 (34.8)	226 (31.3)	528 (77.8)	13.0 (3.4, 22.7)	43.0 (34.2, 51.7)	29.9 (17.1, 42.8)	<0.0001
Penta 1	258 (35.5)	288 (40.1)	243 (32.9)	580 (85.1)	−2.6 (−13.1, 7.8)	45.0 (35.4, 54.6)	47.6 (33.6, 61.6)	<0.0001
PCV 1	242 (33.2)	281 (39.1)	243 (32.9)	578 (84.7)	−0.3 (−10.6, 10.0)	45.6 (36.0, 55.3)	45.9 (31.9, 59.9)	<0.0001
Rota Virus 1	228 (31.2)	277 (38.6)	243 (32.9)	565 (82.1)	1.7 (−8.5, 11.9)	43.5 (33.5, 53.5)	41.8 (27.7, 55.9)	<0.0001
At 10 Weeks								
	N = 744	N = 768	N = 572	N = 663				
OPV 2	100 (13.8)	218 (32.2)	106 (14.4)	393 (62.2)	0.5 (−5.5, 6.5)	30.0 (21.5, 38.5)	29.5 (19.2, 39.8)	<0.0001
Penta 2	129 (15.8)	233 (33.8)	210 (29.9)	456 (69.6)	14.1 (4.7, 23.5)	35.8 (26.3, 45.3)	21.7 (8.4, 35.0)	0.0015
PCV 2	126 (15.5)	229 (33.4)	208 (29.7)	453 (69.0)	14.2 (4.8, 23.6)	35.6 (26.0, 45.1)	21.4 (8.1, 34.6)	0.0017
Rota Virus 2	125 (15.5)	225 (32.8)	209 (29.8)	449 (68.0)	14.3 (4.9, 23.8)	35.2 (25.6, 44.7)	20.8 (7.6, 34.1)	0.0023
At 14 Weeks								
	N = 723	N = 743	N = 559	N = 637				
OPV 3	84 (12.2)	174 (27.1)	80 (9.8)	328 (55.1)	−2.3 (−7.4, 2.7)	27.9 (19.3, 36.5)	30.2 (20.4, 40.1)	<0.0001
Penta 3	83 (12.1)	174 (27.1)	65 (8.6)	298 (51.6)	−3.6 (−8.3, 1.2)	24.4 (15.5, 33.4)	28.0 (18.0, 38.0)	<0.0001
PCV 3	83 (12.1)	166 (25.8)	65 (8.6)	296 (51.4)	−3.5 (−8.3, 1.3)	25.6 (17.0, 34.2)	29.1 (19.4, 38.8)	<0.0001
IPV 1	167 (22.8)	223 (32.9)	208 (30.0)	440 (70.2)	7.2 (−2.2, 16.7)	37.3 (28.5, 46.1)	30.0 (17.3, 42.8)	<0.0001
At 9 Months								
	N = 605	N = 619	N = 504	N = 534				
Measles 1	132 (20.7)	206 (36.8)	215 (34.0)	408 (75.0)	13.3 (3.9, 22.8)	38.2 (29.7, 46.7)	24.9 (12.2, 37.5)	0.0001
At 15 Months								
	N = 437	N = 458	N = 403	N = 388				
Measles 2	51 (10.6)	105 (25.1)	108 (24.6)	184 (47.9)	14.0 (4.8, 23.2)	22.8 (13.3, 32.3)	8.8 (−4.3, 21.9)	0.1862

A detailed analysis of the characteristics of zero-dose children in all three districts showed that, at baseline, the gender distribution was almost equal with a predominant proportion (88.5%) having mothers with no formal schooling (Table 5). The majority (33.1%) belonged to the middle wealth quintile at baseline and the poor wealth quintile (44%) at endline. The commonest reasons provided by caregivers at baseline for not having these children vaccinated were a fear of side effects (19%) and a lack of faith in the immunization (17.4%). The multiple logistic regression analysis confirmed the odds of a zero-dose child having a mother with no formal education and belonging to the poorest quintile being significantly high (Supplementary Materials, Tables S4 and S6). The same analysis for the NR-RI group showed that the odds were significantly high for these children to belong to the poorest and poor wealth quintiles (Supplementary Materials, Tables S5 and S7).

Table 5. Characteristics of zero-dose children in all three districts.

	Overall			
	Baseline	**Endline**	**% Diff (95% CI)**	***p*-Value**
	N = 869	**N = 60**		
Gender				
Male	440 (49.4)	29 (47.7)	−1.7 (−13.2, 9.7)	0.7675
Female	429 (50.6)	31 (52.3)	1.7 (−9.7, 13.2)	0.7675
Maternal Education				
No formal schooling	790 (88.5)	58 (97.4)	8.9 (3.5, 14.3)	0.0015
Primary	55 (9.3)	1 (0.7)	−8.6 (−12.1, −5.0)	<0.0001
Secondary	14 (1.4)	0 (0.0)		
Intermediate or above	10 (0.8)	1 (2.0)	1.2 (−2.9, 5.2)	0.5729
Wealth Quintile				
Poorest	285 (20.8)	20 (23.5)	2.7 (−14.2, 19.6)	0.7508
Poor	256 (25.6)	26 (44.0)	18.4 (3.1, 33.6)	0.0186
Middle	202 (33.1)	8 (21.1)	−12.0 (−29.0, 5.0)	0.1662
Rich	95 (15.9)	4 (7.8)	−8.1 (−19.0, 2.8)	0.1435
Richest	31 (4.6)	2 (3.6)	−1.0 (−8.5, 6.5)	0.7930
Reason for Not Receiving Immunization				
Place of immunization too far	95 (15.7)	4 (7.1)	−8.5 (−16.9, −0.1)	0.0462
Inconvenient/unknown timing/long wait	47 (6.0)	4 (3.5)	−2.5 (−6.7, 1.8)	0.2492
Parent/caretaker busy	58 (6.2)	4 (8.2)	2.0 (−9.1, 13.1)	0.7231
Child not well	54 (7.1)	2 (2.3)	−4.9 (−9.3, −0.5)	0.0305
Rumors	127 (12.3)	6 (9.2)	−3.1 (−13.3, 7.1)	0.5452
No faith in immunization	141 (17.4)	18 (31.2)	13.9 (−3.9, 31.7)	0.1256
Fear of side effects	205 (19.0)	0 (0.0)		
Vaccinator/vaccine not available	69 (5.6)	1 (3.4)	−2.2 (−9.5, 5.1)	0.5477
Others	5 (0.9)			
Do not know	39 (6.7)	4 (5.9)	−0.8 (−8.0, 6.3)	0.8221

Importantly, an equity analysis showed that the intervention was successful in closing the equity gap for immunization coverage, especially for BCG, OPV 3, and Measles 1, demonstrating that an effective outreach program accompanied by community mobilization was instrumental in reducing equity-related barriers (Figure 2).

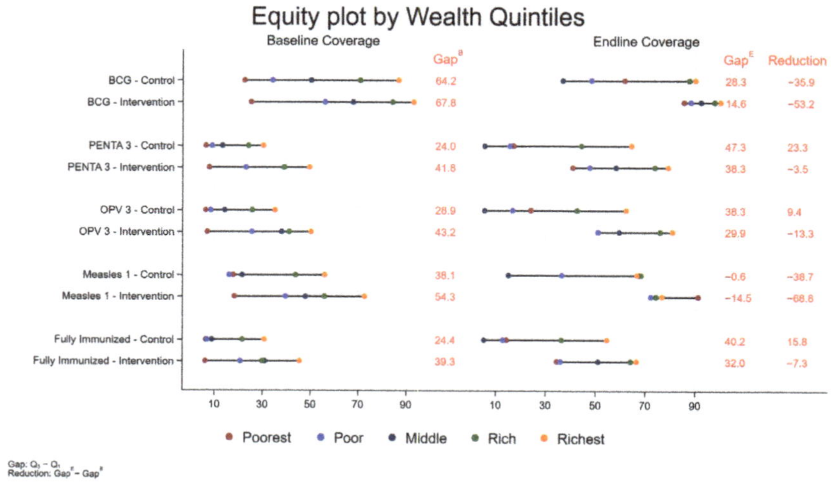

Figure 2. Equity Plot for Coverage of BCG, Penta3, OPV3, Measles1 and Fully Immunized Children (for all three districts).

4. Discussion

The results of our quasi-experimental study demonstrate that the integrated model tested for delivering immunization, health, and nutrition services in conflict-affected high-risk UCs in Pakistan is successful in significantly reducing the proportion of the NR-RI group of children (a subset of zero-dose children), reducing the proportion of zero-dose children, and significantly increasing the proportion of fully immunized children within the intervention areas via mobile health services and community engagement. The activity, in addition to the government-sponsored SIAs, also led to a significant increase in the coverage of all routine EPI vaccines at two conflict-affected intervention sites, with significantly positive impacts on vaccination card ownership and vaccination card retention. This relatively low-cost, simplified intervention was effective in reaching marginalized, at-risk populations and reducing key gaps in childhood immunization and a range of MNCH indicators. The program also included counseling for infant and young child feeding, as well as care seeking for common maternal and child health issues. As previously mentioned, these specific outcomes will be presented and discussed in a separate publication, while the vaccination-related outcomes and behaviors have been reported here.

As the global effort to eradicate polio gears up for the last mile, the focus is increasingly on targeting zero-dose children in the few, restricted areas with a virus transmission in the last two endemic countries: Pakistan and Afghanistan. The Polio Eradication Strategy 2022-2026 emphasizes the interruption of all poliovirus transmission chains by reaching zero-dose children in the seven high-risk, subnational, complex humanitarian areas, which include the Southern KP province in Pakistan [18]. Given the challenging task of reaching zero-dose children, the strategy also recommends an integrated approach to address both community hesitancy and low coverage, as well as to increase the long-term sustainability of the strategy.

The results show that, while the proportion of zero-dose children is reduced in intervention UCs, a similar reduction also occurs in the control UCs. As per the definition, zero-dose children are those who have not received routine immunizations or OPVs during SIAs. In the post-COVID lockdown era, the Government of Pakistan actively implemented SIAs in Balochistan and KP, which targeted children under five years old for OPV administrations, and these would have been implemented across all intervention and control sites. The impact of the SIAs during the study intervention period explains the reduction in zero-dose children in both control and intervention UCs. However, the proportion of the NR-RI group did not reduce in the control UCs while intervention UCs saw a significant reduction, which could potentially be attributable to the mobile health services and community mobilization interventions of *Naunehal*.

The impact of this project underscores the importance of using strategies that strive to "reach the unreached" populations in conflict-affected, underserved locations. This outreach model provides a set of interventions with immunizations integrated with basic maternal and child health services and nutritional counseling. Importantly, the health services being offered enhance the probability of the community interacting with the services and increase the likelihood of community members using immunization services, as have also been the experiences in Nigeria and Afghanistan [19,20]. Offering mobile immunization services in isolation would most likely not evoke the same uptake and response from the community, given the widespread vaccine skepticism and fatigue in these high-risk regions. The idea of a stand-alone "polio program" is presently viewed with suspicion and disdain by many communities; thus, the integration of these activities with other health services can work to build community trust [7]. Nevertheless, the skepticism and misinformation need to be counteracted by health education and counseling.

India was declared polio free in 2014, and in the last stretch of the eradication efforts, the polio program also faced resistance grounded in "fear and fatigue" related to repeated OPV doses [21]. Moreover, it was realized that door-to-door vaccinations, although an effective strategy, did not help alleviate these fears as over-worked and under-resourced health workers were unable to address their concerns and questions. An added strength of the *Naunehal* model was a strong community engagement component, which not only included health information sessions with male and female community members and individual counseling sessions, but also a key focus on engaging with religious and community leaders as an initial step. The program, including mobile health services and private practitioner engagements, was not initiated till there was a complete buy-in from community elders, which in turn inspired trust and motivation from the community members, making them more open to awareness-raising and knowledge-sharing sessions.

The model also reduced the risk of a missed opportunity for vaccination (MOV) where a vaccine-eligible child was aware of the health system but was not vaccinated for a variety of reasons, such as the failure of practitioners to screen him/her, vaccine shortages, or parental resistance [22]. A detailed vaccination coverage survey of all SHRUCs in Pakistan showed that nearly all SHRUCs had a high (>40%) proportion of children who were considered missed opportunities for simultaneous vaccinations (MOSVs) for IPV1, with the proportion being much higher in Balochistan [23]. The *Naunehal* mobile health services were designed in a way that the community was notified in advance of the visit date, and the service was scheduled to return to the same site again to coincide with the next vaccine doses, thus enhancing the convenience for the community and the uptake. Outreach services have proven to be a cost-effective strategy for delivering immunization services; however, the cost can escalate in fragile and remote settings, as has been noted [20,24,25]. Naunehal was implemented using a particularly cost-effective model with an optimal number of targeted, appropriately timed mobile health service visits using essential staff providing immunizations, healthcare services, and nutritional counseling. The added element of community mobilization guaranteed the community was aware and receptive, which ensured the efficient usage of the outreach program, thus minimizing costs.

The strengths of the study include the assessment of the integrated strategy in a real-life, conflict-affected setting with a low-cost model. There exists a noticeable dearth of research assessing the delivery of immunization and health services in conflict-affected settings, and thus this study serves to fill the knowledge gap concerning the implementation and effectiveness of such models, especially in the context of zero-dose children and polio eradication [26,27]. Another strength of the study was the strong engagement of local communities and a close partnership with the government for vaccine provision, personnel training, and facility referrals, which increased the sustainability and cost-effectiveness of the model.

A limitation of the study was that the model was implemented for a limited period and, thus, the sustainability and sustained effect of the program could not be established with the existing data. Additionally, the project encountered several challenges during its implementation. Firstly, navigating the program in an insecure context led to unpredictability where services and movements had to be occasionally suspended in certain areas, and plans adapted accordingly. Secondly, mobile health services and health information sessions were conducted during the challenging, initial waves of COVID-19. The teams followed protocols and worked in close coordination with government partners to avoid any breach of lockdowns or movement restrictions. Thirdly, private medical practitioner engagement could not be fully implemented as planned given, most notably, the lack of resources in private clinics to maintain the vaccine cold chain and the lack of incentives for busy practitioners to take on additional tasks.

5. Conclusions

As the efforts to eradicate polio intensify with experts striving to reach the remaining zero-dose and zero-routine immunization children, this study shows that an integrated model of delivering immunization, health, and nutrition services in combination with community mobilization in conflict-affected, high-risk UCs of Pakistan can reduce the proportion of the NR-RI group of children, a subset of zero-dose children, and increase coverage for all routine vaccines, including OPVs. The results of this pilot project have significant implications for polio eradication, suggesting new strategies for reaching marginalized, at-risk populations. It is advisable to scale up and evaluate this strategy at the population level in other conflict-affected contexts to examine the feasibility and effectiveness of increasing immunization coverage in high-transmission settings, especially for polio.

Supplementary Materials: The following supporting information can be downloaded at: https://www.mdpi.com/article/10.3390/pathogens13030185/s1, Table S1: Peshawar-UC-Level Immunization Coverage at Baseline and Endline for Children Under-Three in Intervention and Control Areas; Table S2: Lakki Marwat-UC-Level Immunization Coverage at Baseline and Endline for Children Under-Three in Intervention and Control Areas; Table S3: Quetta-UC-Level Immunization Coverage at Baseline and Endline for Children Under-Three in Intervention and Control Areas; Table S4: Sociodemographic Factors Associated with Zero-Dose Children based o Logistic Regression for UCs in All Three Districts; Table S5: Sociodemographic Factors Associated with Non-Recipients of Routine Immunization (NR-RI) Children based on Logistic Regression for UCs in All Three Districts; Table S6: Sociodemographic Factors Associated with Zero-Dose Children based on Logistic Regression for UCs in Districts Quetta and Lakki Marwat; Table S7: Sociodemographic Factors Associated with Non-Recipients of Routine Immunization (NR-RI) Children based on Logistic Regression for UCs in Districts Quetta and Lakki Marwat.

Author Contributions: Z.A.B. conceived the study, wrote the protocol along with A.M.K., and secured funding. A.M.K. provided the materials and strategic oversights during the field operations. R.T. oversaw the field operations in Quetta and performed the overall grant management and administration of the project. S.A. and A.A.N. oversaw the field operations in Peshawar and Lakki Marwat. I.A. and M.J. performed the statistical analyses, with contributions from M.I. A.M.K. produced the first draft of the paper with inputs from Z.A.B. and I.A. All authors have read and agreed to the published version of the manuscript.

Funding: This work was supported by Bill and Melinda Gates Foundation, grant number INV-017322.

Institutional Review Board Statement: Ethics approval was obtained from the SickKids Research Ethics Board (#1000072563) and the National Bioethics Committee (#NBC-561) based in Pakistan.

Informed Consent Statement: Informed consent was obtained from all subjects involved in the study.

Data Availability Statement: Data are available on request due to restrictions.

Acknowledgments: This study was funded by the Bill and Melinda Gates Foundation and would not have been possible without the instrumental support of Carl Kirkwood and Anita Zaidi from the Bill and Melinda Gates Foundation. We acknowledge the contributions of Anushka Ataullahjan during the protocol development, project planning, and initial implementation, and that of Tariq Mahmood Chishti in overseeing the field operations in Quetta. We acknowledge the contributions of the Governments of Khyber Pakhtunkhwa and Balochistan and the Provincial Health Directorates in both provinces for their support during the planning and implementation of the project. We would also like to acknowledge the hard work that the health camp teams, field teams, and data management unit provided during the project. Finally, we thank the communities and participants for being a part of this project as the success of this project would not have been possible without their active involvement.

Conflicts of Interest: We declare no competing interests.

References

1. Mbaeyi, C.; Baig, S.; Safdar, R.M.; Khan, Z.; Young, H.; Jorba, J.; Wadood, Z.; Jafari, H.; Alam, M.M.; Franka, R. Progress toward Poliomyelitis Eradication—Pakistan, January 2022–June 2023. *Morb. Mortal. Wkly. Rep.* **2023**, *72*, 880–885. [CrossRef] [PubMed]
2. Centre of Excellence in Women and Child Health—Aga Khan University & Federal Expanded Program on Immunization (EPI). *Third-Party Verification Immunization Coverage Survey (TPVICS)—Survey Report*; Aga Khan University: Karachi, Pakistan, 2022.
3. United Nations Inter-Agency Group for Child Mortality Estimation (UN IGME). *Levels & Trends in Child Mortality Report—Estimates Developed by the United Nations Inter-Agency Group for Child Mortality Estimation*; United Nations Children's Fund (UNICEF): New York, NY, USA, 2023. Available online: https://data.unicef.org/resources/levels-and-trends-in-child-mortality/ (accessed on 5 November 2023).
4. United Nations Children's Fund (UNICEF); World Health Organization (WHO); International Bank for Reconstruction and Development/The World Bank. *Levels and Trends in Child Malnutrition: UNICEF/WHO/World Bank Group Joint Child Malnutrition Estimates: Key Findings of the 2023 Edition*; UNICEF: New York, NY, USA; WHO: Geneva, Switzerland, 2023. Available online: https://www.who.int/publications/i/item/9789240073791 (accessed on 5 November 2023).
5. Owais, A.; Rizvi, A.; Jawwad, M.; Horton, S.; Das, J.K.; Merritt, C.E.; Moreno, R.; Asfaw, A.G.; Rutter, P.; Nguyen, P.H.; et al. Assessing the hidden burden and costs of COVID-19 pandemic in South Asia: Implications for health and well-being of women, children and adolescents. *PLoS Glob. Public Health* **2023**, *3*, e0001567. [CrossRef] [PubMed]
6. Habib, A.; Tabassum, F.; Hussain, I.; Khan, T.; Syed, N.; Shaheen, F.; Soofi, S.B.; Bhutta, Z.A. Exploring knowledge and perceptions of polio disease and its immunization in Polio High-Risk areas of Pakistan. *Vaccines* **2023**, *11*, 1206. [CrossRef] [PubMed]
7. Ataullahjan, A.; Ahsan, H.; Soofi, S.B.; Habib, A.; Bhutta, Z.A. Eradicating polio in Pakistan: A systematic review of programs and policies. *Expert Rev. Vaccines* **2021**, *20*, 661–678. [CrossRef] [PubMed]
8. Gul, A. *WHO: Afghanistan, Pakistan Close to Eradicating Polio*; Voice of America: New York, NY, USA, 2023. Available online: https://www.voanews.com/a/who-afghanistan-pakistan-close-to-eradicating-polio-/7205201.html (accessed on 7 December 2023).
9. Global Polio Eradication Initiative; World Health Organization. *Polio Endgame Strategy 2019–2023: Eradication, Integration, Certification, and Containment*; Global Polio Eradication Initiative; World Health Organization: Geneva, Switzerland, 2017. Available online: https://reliefweb.int/report/world/polio-endgame-strategy-2019-2023-eradication-integration-certification-and-containment?gad_source=1&gclid=CjwKCAiAqY6tBhAtEiwAHeRopbRO0PX7b7WgKR48I2VosT4pv7jhPVmzdXZXCGM7rnZBnXdQylhBJhoCGowQAvD_BwE (accessed on 10 November 2023).
10. Closser, S.; Jooma, R.; Varley, E.; Qayyum, N.; De Sousa Ferreira Guedes Rodrigues, S.; Sarwar, A.; Omidian, P.A. Polio eradication and health systems in Karachi: Vaccine refusals in context. *Glob. Health Commun.* **2015**, *1*, 32–40. [CrossRef]
11. Das, J.K.; Khan, A.; Tabassum, F.; Padhani, Z.A.; Habib, A.; Mirani, M.; Rahman, A.R.; Khan, Z.; Rizvi, A.; Ahmed, I.; et al. The Last Mile—Community Engagement and conditional Incentives to Accelerate polio eradication in Pakistan: Study Protocol for a Quasi-Experimental Trial. *Methods Protoc.* **2023**, *6*, 83. [CrossRef]
12. Kirmani, S.; Saleem, A.F. Impact of COVID-19 pandemic on paediatric services at a referral centre in Pakistan: Lessons from a low-income and middle-income country setting. *Arch. Dis. Child.* **2020**, *106*, 627–628. [CrossRef]
13. Chandir, S.; Siddiqi, D.A.; Setayesh, H.; Khan, A. Impact of COVID-19 lockdown on routine immunisation in Karachi, Pakistan. *Lancet Glob. Health* **2020**, *8*, e1118–e1120. [CrossRef] [PubMed]
14. Rahman, S.U.; Haq, F.U.; Imran, M.; Shah, A.; Bibi, N.; Khurshid, R.; Romman, M.; Gaffar, F.; Khan, M.I. Impact of the COVID-19 lockdown on routine vaccination in Pakistan: A hospital-based study. *Hum. Vaccines Immunother.* **2021**, *17*, 4934–4940. [CrossRef]
15. Habib, A.; Soofi, S.B.; Cousens, S.; Anwar, S.; Haque, N.U.; Ahmed, I.; Ali, N.; Tahir, R.; Bhutta, Z.A. Community engagement and integrated health and polio immunisation campaigns in conflict-affected areas of Pakistan: A cluster randomised controlled trial. *Lancet Glob. Health* **2017**, *5*, e593–e603. [CrossRef] [PubMed]
16. Habib, A.; Soofi, S.; Suhag, Z.; Ahmed, I.; Tahir, R.; Anwar, S.; Nauman, A.A.; Sharif, M.; Islam, M.; Cousens, S.; et al. A holistic strategy of Mother and Child Health Care to improve the coverage of Routine and Polio Immunization in Pakistan, Results from a Large Demonstration Project. *Vaccines* **2024**, *12*, 89. [CrossRef] [PubMed]
17. Ataullahjan, A.; Khan, N.A.; Islam, M.B.; Tahir, R.; Anwar, S.; Ahmed, I.; Nauman, A.; Bhutta, Z.A. NAUNEHAL; Integrated immunization and MNCH interventions: A quasi-experimental study–Protocol. *PLoS ONE* **2023**, *18*, e0287722. [CrossRef] [PubMed]

18. GPEI. *GPEI-2023—Zero-Dose Children in Seven Subnational Consequential Geographies Hold Key to Success*; Global Polio Eradication Initiative; World Health Organization: Geneva, Switzerland, 2023. Available online: https://polioeradication.org/news-post/2023-zero-dose-children-in-seven-subnational-most-consequential-geographies-hold-key-to-success (accessed on 22 December 2023).
19. UNICEF. *The State of the World's Children 2023*; UNICEF: New York, NY, USA, 2023. Available online: https://www.unicef.org/reports/state-worlds-children-2023#SOWC (accessed on 19 December 2023).
20. Edmond, K.; Yousufi, K.; Naziri, M.; Higgins-Steele, A.; Qadir, A.; Sadat, S.M.; Bellows, A.L.; Smith, E.R. Mobile outreach health services for mothers and children in conflict-affected and remote areas: A population-based study from Afghanistan. *Arch. Dis. Child.* **2019**, *105*, 18–25. [CrossRef] [PubMed]
21. Hussain, R.; McGarvey, S.T.; Shahab, T.; Fruzzetti, L. Fatigue and Fear with Shifting Polio Eradication Strategies in India: A Study of Social Resistance to Vaccination. *PLoS ONE* **2012**, *7*, e46274. [CrossRef] [PubMed]
22. World Health Organization. Reducing Missed Opportunities for Vaccination (MOV). 2023. Available online: https://www.who.int/teams/immunization-vaccines-and-biologicals/essential-programme-on-immunization/implementation/reducing-missed-opportunities-for-vaccination (accessed on 29 November 2023).
23. Centre of Excellence in Women and Child Health—The Aga Khan University & Biostat Global Consulting. *2022 Supplementary Immunization Coverage Survey in Super High Risk Union Councils of Pakistan (TPVICS-SHRUCs Round 2)—Survey Report*; Aga Khan University: Karachi, Pakistan, 2023.
24. Carrera, C.; Azrack, A.; Begkoyian, G.; Pfaffmann, J.; Ribaira, E.; O'Connell, T.; Doughty, P.; Aung, K.; Prieto, L.; Rasanathan, K.; et al. The comparative cost-effectiveness of an equity-focused approach to child survival, health, and nutrition: A modelling approach. *Lancet* **2012**, *380*, 1341–1351. [CrossRef] [PubMed]
25. Crocker-Buqué, T.; Edelstein, M.; Mounier-Jack, S. Interventions to reduce inequalities in vaccine uptake in children and adolescents aged <19 years: A systematic review. *J. Epidemiol. Community Health* **2016**, *71*, 87–97. [CrossRef] [PubMed]
26. Amsalu, R.; Firoz, T.; Lange, I.; Tappis, H. Editorial: Maternal Health in Conflict Settings. *Front. Glob. Women's Health* **2022**, *3*, 807257. [CrossRef] [PubMed]
27. Munyuzangabo, M.; Gaffey, M.F.; Khalifa, D.; Als, D.; Ataullahjan, A.; Kamali, M.; Jain, R.; Meteke, S.; Radhakrishnan, A.; Shah, S.; et al. Delivering maternal and neonatal health interventions in conflict settings: A systematic review. *BMJ Glob. Health* **2021**, *5* (Suppl. 1), e003750. [CrossRef] [PubMed]

pathogens

MDPI

Review

Inactivated Poliovirus Vaccine: Recent Developments and the Tortuous Path to Global Acceptance

Roland W. Sutter [1,*], Martin Eisenhawer [2], Natalia A. Molodecky [3], Harish Verma [2] and Hiromasa Okayasu [4]

1 Tamayo Federal Solutions LLC, Virginia Beach, VA 23452, USA
2 Polio Eradication Department, World Health Organization, 1211 Geneva, Switzerland; eisenhawerm@who.int (M.E.); vermah@who.int (H.V.)
3 Polio Surge Capacity Support Program, The Task Force for Global Health, Inc., Decatur, GE 30030, USA; nmolodecky@gmail.com
4 Division of Healthy Environments and Population, Regional Office for the Western Pacific, World Health Organization, Manila 1000, Philippines
* Correspondence: rolandsutter@gmail.com

Abstract: Inactivated poliovirus vaccine (IPV), available since 1955, became the first vaccine to be used to protect against poliomyelitis. While the immunogenicity of IPV to prevent paralytic poliomyelitis continues to be irrefutable, its requirement for strong containment (due to large quantities of live virus used in the manufacturing process), perceived lack of ability to induce intestinal mucosal immunity, high cost and increased complexity to administer compared to oral polio vaccine (OPV), have limited its use in the global efforts to eradicate poliomyelitis. In order to harvest the full potential of IPV, a program of work has been carried out by the Global Polio Eradication Initiative (GPEI) over the past two decades that has focused on: (1) increasing the scientific knowledge base of IPV; (2) translating new insights and evidence into programmatic action; (3) expanding the IPV manufacturing infrastructure for global demand; and (4) continuing to pursue an ambitious research program to develop more immunogenic and safer-to-produce vaccines. While the knowledge base of IPV continues to expand, further research and product development are necessary to ensure that the program priorities are met (e.g., non-infectious production through virus-like particles, non-transmissible vaccine inducing humoral and intestinal mucosal immunity and new methods for house-to-house administration through micro-needle patches and jet injectors), the discussions have largely moved from whether to how to use this vaccine most effectively. In this review, we summarize recent developments on expanding the science base of IPV and provide insight into policy development and the expansion of IPV manufacturing and production, and finally we provide an update on the current priorities.

Keywords: inactivated poliovirus vaccine (IPV); Global Polio Eradication Initiative (GPEI); mucosal immunity; fractional-dose IPV (fIPV)

1. Introduction

In 1988, the World Health Assembly (WHA), the governing body of the World Health Organization (WHO), resolved to eradicate poliomyelitis by the year 2000, and the Global Polio Eradication Initiative (GPEI) was formed [1]. Since the resolution, substantial progress toward eradication has been achieved. However, the eradication target remains elusive [2].

The first vaccine licensed for use against poliovirus was the inactivated poliovirus vaccine (IPV), developed by Jonas Salk, and licensed in the United States in 1955 [3]. Thereafter, IPV was widely used in routine immunization (RI) of infants and children and in campaigns covering all age groups to control poliomyelitis. In the late 1950s, a resurgence of paralytic cases led to concern regarding IPV effectiveness. Subsequently, oral poliovirus vaccine (OPV) was licensed in the United States starting in 1961 and replaced IPV as the vaccine of choice for poliomyelitis prevention. Only two countries (Iceland

and Sweden) never used OPV [4]. Improvements in the potency of IPV by a factor of 10 in the 1960s [5,6] (i.e., enhanced-potency IPV), and progress toward eradication, led to a re-evaluation of IPV use and subsequent re-introduction into RI across North America and Western Europe in the early 2000s. Despite its high efficacy at preventing paralysis, the main limitation of IPV was perceived to be its inability to stop poliovirus from spreading among children.

OPV became the main vaccine of choice for the GPEI due to its ease of use, low cost and ability to induce mucosal immunity, required for preventing transmission [7,8]. Until 2005, when monovalent oral poliovirus vaccine type 1 (mOPV1) and type 3 (mOPV3) were licensed, the GPEI used exclusively trivalent OPV (tOPV), decreasing the number of polio-endemic countries from >125 in 1988 to 6 (Afghanistan, India, Pakistan, Egypt, Nigeria and Niger) [9]. In 2005, Egypt and Niger interrupted endemic transmission, leaving only four polio endemic countries. Despite the tremendous impact of OPV, it was well understood that the use of OPV (comprised of live attenuated Sabin strains) would eventually need to be stopped due to the genetic instability of the Sabin strains. Prolonged replication in an otherwise healthy B-cell deficient vaccinee or circulation in an under-vaccinated population would result in mutation and recombination that ended with the emergence of new polioviruses that were as neurovirulent and transmissible as wild poliovirus (having lost all attenuation mutations) [10]. As long as Sabin strains were introduced into communities, the emerging virus could seed new endemics and epidemic circulation, negating the achievements of the eradication effort, and thus be incompatible with eradication.

In November 2012, the Strategic Advisory Group of Experts (SAGE) on Immunization endorsed the Strategic Plan of Action for Polio Eradication 2013–2018 that called for the withdrawal of Sabin strains from the OPV, starting with Sabin type 2 (OPV2) [11]. OPV2 was selected because indigenous wild poliovirus type 2 (WPV2) was last detected in 1999 in Northern India, and OPV2 continued to cause a predictable burden of vaccine-associated paralytic poliomyelitis (VAPP) [12] that became increasingly unacceptable to parents and health providers. Moreover, outbreaks of type-2 vaccine-derived poliovirus (VDPV2) were reported each year, due to continued OPV2 use in populations with sub-optimal immunity. The GPEI coordinated the global cessation of OPV2 in April 2016 [13].

To mitigate the growing susceptibility gap, the GPEI recommended $\geq$1 dose of IPV to be introduced into RI programs globally in advance of OPV2 withdrawal [11,14]. Figure 1 displays the countries using IPV in 2000, 2016 and 2023. While the majority of countries successfully introduced IPV into RI, due to supply constraints, >43 million children did not receive IPV after OPV2 cessation. In addition, supply constraints limited the use of IPV in outbreak response to cVDPV2 outbreaks, and in 2017, the endorsement for its use in cVDPV2 outbreak response was removed. By 2020, IPV supply constraints were addressed and the GPEI adopted a two-dose IPV schedule for RI [15], in addition to the catch-up IPV vaccination for children that had not received IPV after OPV2 cessation. In 2023, the SAGE restored the recommendation for IPV use in cVDPV2 outbreak response.

To reach a point wherein global technical advisory bodies could recommend IPV first as a risk mitigation tool in 2012 [11] and then as the primary tool for poliomyelitis prevention in 2020 [15] required a massive program of work with IPV, focusing on scientific knowledge, programmatic use, developing safer IPV seed strains and facilitating the expansion of IPV production. This program of work is not yet completed and focuses on non-infectious IPV production, hexavalent vaccine and new administration tools.

In this review, we summarize the recent developments on expanding the science base of IPV and provide insight into policy development and the expansion of IPV manufacturing and production, and finally we provide an update on the current priorities. Thus, we have organized this review into four sections: (1) increasing the scientific knowledge base of IPV; (2) translating new insights and evidence into programmatic action; (3) expanding the IPV supply base for global demand; and (4) continuing to pursue an ambitious research program to develop more immunogenic, easier to administer and safer-to-produce vaccines.

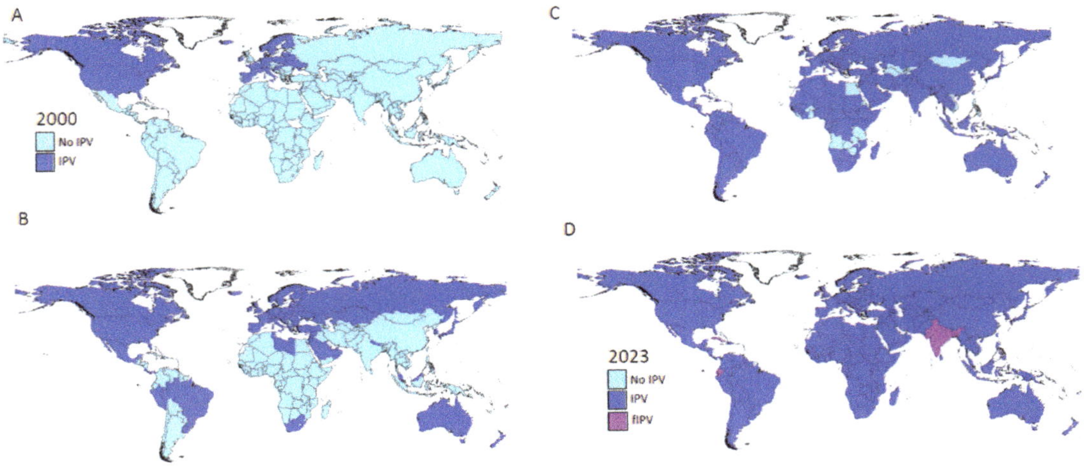

Figure 1. Global map: Countries using IPV/fIPV in routine immunization in: (**A**) 2000; (**B**) 2014; (**C**) 2016; and (**D**) 2023. Source: IPV introduction date: WHO Immunization, (https://immunizationdata.who.int/listing.html?topic=vaccine-intro&location=; accessed on 17 December 2023). fIPV countries [16].

2. Increasing the Scientific Knowledge Base of IPV

This chapter focuses on three critical areas of research: (1) better characterization of IPV-induced or -boosted intestinal mucosal immunity; (2) reduction in the number of IPV doses and antigen content to induce immunity response against poliomyelitis; and (3) understanding IPV's potential in inducing herd immunity.

The first area of the IPV program-of-work was to better characterize its contribution to intestinal mucosal immunity against poliovirus (Figure 2).

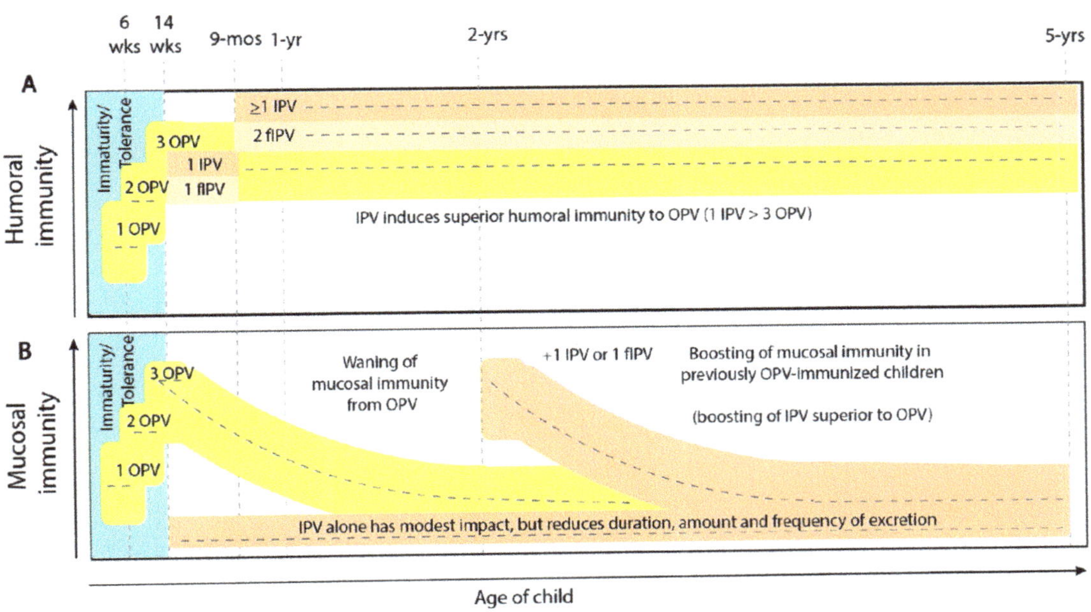

Figure 2. Immunity diagram. (**A**) Humoral immunity. (**B**) Mucosal immunity.

IPV has been shown to not directly induce intestinal mucosal immunity, even with a mucosal adjuvant. Initial attempts to use a mucosal adjuvant (dmLT-double-mutant heat labile E Coli toxin) to induce mucosal immunity after IPV vaccination were unsuccessful [17,18]. IPV does appear to induce pharyngeal mucosal immunity [19], although the evidence is limited.

While IPV on its own in naïve infants does not induce intestinal mucosal immunity, an ever-increasing body of evidence supports that IPV-vaccinated infants excrete poliovirus for significantly shorter periods and with a lower quantity (lower viral titer) after challenge with vaccine virus or natural infection [20] (Table 1). Efforts to quantify this effect suggested a 95% decrease in excreted virus following challenge in IPV vaccinated persons [7,21]. The shorter excretion period was confirmed in Sweden [22] and the decrease in excreted titer in IPV-vaccinated following a tOPV challenge in Cuba [23]. Moreover, a recent study from Bangladesh further demonstrated that the addition of a dose of IPV can decrease the excretion of OPV in a routine schedule [24]. It has been suggested that IPV potentially produces a priming effect leading to faster response. Therefore, while IPV on its own in naïve infants does not stop transmission, it may reduce transmission by inducing a degree of intestinal mucosal immunity, thereby decreasing the amount and duration of viral shedding.

Table 1. IPV vaccine effect on humoral and mucosal immunity.

IPV Effect	Advantages	Geographic Focus	References
Induces humoral immunity	Provides life-long immunity from paralytic poliomyelitis	Globally	Francis [3], Vidor [4]
Closes humoral immunity gaps in previously IPV- or OPV-vaccinated individuals	Prevents paralytic disease after poliovirus exposure	Globally	Vidor [4], Dang [25]
Boosts humoral antibody levels	Can reduce excretion of poliovirus after infection	Globally	Marine [26], Sutter [7]
Generates herd immunity	Less than 100% IPV coverage seem to induce herd immunity	Shown in countries with good hygiene and sanitation–size of effect unknown in high force-of-infection communities, but possibly in Indonesia and Malaysia	Stickle [27], Wahjuhono [28], Snider [29]
Induces pharyngeal mucosal immunity	Reduces oral-to-oral transmission of poliovirus	Mode of transmission more important in industrialized countries	Sutter [7], Onorato [19], Fine [21]
Induces a "modest" degree of mucosal intestinal immunity	Shorter excretion, decrease viral output in stool, and lower frequency → reduction of 95% in excreted poliovirus virions over course of infection	More important in countries with good hygiene and sanitation	Sutter [7], Ghendon [20], Fine [21], Brickley [22], Cuba IPV Collaborative Study Group [23]
Boosts intestinal mucosal immunity in OPV-vaccinated individuals	Reduces fecal-to-oral transmission of poliovirus–from 39 to 76% depending on age	More important in tropical developing countries	John [30], Jafari [31], Snider [24,29], Hird [32], Parker [33], Macklin [34], Gamage [35]
Later administration (age ≥3 mos) overcomes interference of maternally derived antibody	A single dose at 9 mos can lead to almost 100% seroconversion	Globally	Aziz [36], Sharma [37], Anand [38]
Induces priming immune responses in non-responders	A second dose can effectively boost humoral immunity rapidly <7 days	Globally	Resik [39,40], Mohammad [41]

Table 1. *Cont.*

IPV Effect	Advantages	Geographic Focus	References
Priming immune response duration	Demonstrated to persist at least 28 mos	Globally	Sharma [37]
Immunogenicity not affected by tropical enteropathy	IPV immunogenic in populations affected by tropical enteropathy (in contrast to OPV)	More important in tropical developing countries	Saleem [42]
IPV can be administered in house-to-house campaigns	Demonstrated in SIA in Northern Nigeria → may substantially increase coverage	More important in areas with suboptimal health infrastructure	Biya [43]
Fractional-dose IPV (fIPV) can reduce cost of polio immunization schedule or use in campaigns	Two doses of fIPV can induce nearly 100% immunity if given in appropriate schedule but only uses 40% of a full dose of IPV	More important for countries not currently supported by GAVI, such as India	Aziz [36], Sharma [37]
Administration of fIPV with intradermal jet injector Tropis®	Facilitates intradermal administration and results in dose saving	More important in house-to-house campaigns attempting to reach a high proportion of the target population	Bullo [44], Pervaiz [45], Resik [46]
Single-dose IPV vaccine effectiveness close to 90% in Nigeria	Should lead to re-evaluation of strategy to achieve and maintain population immunity in "consequential geographies"	More relevant to tropical areas with suboptimal health infrastructure	Cooper [47]

In contrast to the modest direct impact on intestinal mucosal immunity in naïve infants, IPV has a substantial impact on boosting intestinal mucosal immunity in previously OPV immunized children. Two landmark studies in India demonstrated that IPV could boost intestinal mucosal immunity in OPV-vaccinated children, across age groups from 6-month to 10-year-olds [30,31]. The boosting by IPV on waned mucosal immunity in previously OPV immunized individuals after a bOPV (types 1 + 3) challenge dose was shown to be greater than an additional dose of bOPV. Moreover, a single fractional IPV (fIPV) dose is as effective as a full dose of IPV for boosting previously OPV immunized individuals. This indicates that IPV (and fIPV) can help interrupt transmission in settings with previous OPV use by boosting intestinal mucosal immunity, better than an additional dose of OPV. This is particularly true in age groups >2 years, as these children likely previously received OPV and have waned mucosal immunity (waning estimated at a median rate of 1 year). Thus, in addition to IPV having a direct effect (albeit modest) on intestinal mucosal immunity (through reducing duration, quantity and frequency of excretion), IPV can also boost intestinal mucosal immunity in OPV-vaccinated children. The effect does not appear to be IPV-dose-dependent [48]. The available evidence on IPV mucosal immunity was reviewed [32–34].

The second area explored the limits of how few doses of IPV were needed to induce protection against poliomyelitis. This area of work focused on two aspects: (1) number of doses of IPV; and (2) potency (antigen content) of IPV (fractional-dose IPV, fIPV, i.e., one-fifth of a full IPV dose). To understand these approaches, one has to remember that the original formulation work of IPV was conducted in Northern Europe and North America where it had to overcome the interference of maternally derived antibody against the "wild" poliovirus [4,7]. Swartz demonstrated that a higher-potency IPV could overcome the interference of maternally derived antibody [49]. Our work focused on the reduction in number of IPV doses and on its potency (i.e., fIPV), and was building on the studies conducted earlier in India [50,51]. Many follow-up studies were conducted in subjects that had not received OPV, in Cuba [39,40,46], the Philippines [52], the Netherlands [53], Oman [41], Sri Lanka [35], The Gambia [54], Ecuador [55], India [56], Pakistan [42,44] and Bangladesh [24,36,38,57,58] with vaccines from several manufacturers (Staten Serum Institute, Denmark, Bilthoven Biologicals, the Netherlands, and Sanofi Pasteur, France). These studies demonstrated that two fractional IPV doses given at age 14–16 weeks and 8–9 months could induce high seroconversion rates (above 90%). The India fIPV schedule with doses administered at 6 and 14 weeks was evaluated and compared versus a schedule of 10 and 14 weeks, attempting to answer the question of which is more important, longer interval or older age, at first vaccine administration. A 6- and 14-week schedule was significantly more immunogenic [59].

These studies also demonstrated that most infants who did not seroconvert after IPV were immunologically primed against polioviruses [40,57–59]. Further studies in Bangladesh and Nepal demonstrated that a single dose of IPV induced immunity against type 2 after 28 months in almost 100% of vaccinees (seroconversion and priming), and that a dose of IPV administered at an age of $\geq$9 months immunized almost 100% of vaccinees (seroconversion) while inducing a high titer against poliovirus (type 2) [36,37]. The IPV is effective even in countries where OPV efficacy is negatively affected by tropical enteropathy [59]. This condition somehow interferes with intestinal mucosal barrier integrity [60] and is likely responsible for the poor immunogenicity of OPV in some tropical countries [60–63]. The IPV findings were summarized [32–34,38,64] and strengthened the initial recommendation for a single dose of IPV for risk mitigation after the withdrawal of OPV2 from tOPV [5] (Figure 2).

The third area attempts to answer one important unanswered question. Can exclusive IPV use in RI and SIAs induce herd immunity in high force-of-infection tropical countries? In moderate climate countries, IPV appears to induce herd immunity [57]. Indonesia tried to answer this question in a 5-year IPV-only demonstration project in Yogyakarta Province. Environmental surveillance demonstrated that high IPV coverage in RI prevented the circulation of Sabin poliovirus introduced from adjacent OPV-using provinces [28]. After the demonstration project ended, the province continued to use an all-IPV schedule. No evidence of emergence (or detection) of cVDPV2 has been found, despite an outbreak of cVDPV2 affecting Sumatra and Java (12 AFP cases with cVDPV2) in Indonesia (WHO data as of 21 January 2024)

In addition, after 2016, some tropical countries introduced all-IPV schedules in RI, the most important being Malaysia which reported high coverage with a three-dose IPV schedule (>98% nationwide). Sabah Province, Malaysia, a relatively low IPV coverage province and close to Mindanao, Philippines, experienced cVDPV1 and cVDPV2 outbreaks in 2019 and early 2020 with cVDPV1 and cVDPV2 introduced from the Philippines [29]. The outbreaks were controlled rapidly with two rounds of monovalent type 2 OPV (mOPV2) and two rounds of bOPV. No transmission to other provinces on the Island of Borneo or to the Malayan Peninsula were observed.

3. Translating New Insights and Evidence into Programmatic Action

As a response to the increasing issue with OPV safety, countries investigated new schedules and vaccines to prevent vaccine-associated paralytic poliomyelitis (VAPP) [10]. As polio eradication made rapid progress, the rare cases of VAPP were becoming increasingly unacceptable to parents. The Western Hemisphere was certified free-of-poliomyelitis in 1994 [65]. In 1997, the United States adopted a sequential schedule of two doses of IPV followed by two doses of OPV, and then an all-IPV schedule in 2000 [66]. Other countries followed a similar path or went directly to all-IPV schedules for routine immunization.

In 2012, the SAGE recommended the inclusion of $\geq$1 dose of IPV in all OPV-using countries, primarily for risk mitigation in anticipation of OPV cessation [67]. OPV cessation was implemented in April 2016 in a phased manner, with the withdrawal of Sabin type 2 from the trivalent OPV [11,13]. However, IPV supply constraints required the rationing of IPV to the highest risk countries, and only 4–5 years later, all countries received sufficient

IPV for routine immunization and catch-up vaccination of the 43 million children who had not received a single dose of IPV.

By 2016, approximately 50 countries, categorized primarily as high-income, relied on IPV exclusively for poliomyelitis prevention, many using combination vaccines with IPV–diphtheria–tetanus–pertussis vaccines (IPV-DTP), some of which included Hemophilus type b and Hepatitis B in a hexavalent formulation [Figure 1].

In 2020, after the IPV supply constraints were resolved, the SAGE recommended a second dose of IPV to close remaining immunity gaps, boost titers, and ensure long-term protection against poliovirus type 2 [15]. The first dose of IPV was recommended with the third dose of pentavalent vaccine (DTP, Hemophilus type b, and Hepatitis B) at age 14 weeks in countries using the Expanded Program on Immunization (EPI) schedule. Some countries, primarily on the India Subcontinent (Bangladesh, India, Nepal, Sri Lanka), as well as Cuba and Ecuador, are using or used a two-dose fractional IPV schedule after OPV2 cessation, with doses administered in India at 6 and 14 weeks and with a third dose added to the visit for measles vaccine at 9 months [68]. Responding to the 2020 SAGE recommendation, India now requires three doses of fIPV administered at ages 6 and 14 weeks and 9 months.

In June 2023, GAVI opened a window for eligible countries to apply for support of hexavalent (pentavalent plus IPV) vaccines, the discussions on an appropriate schedule are under way [68]. The hexavalent vaccine, recommended by WHO, must contain the whole-cell pertussis vaccine. To provide the most immunogenicity for all hexavalent components, a four-dose schedule appears to be necessary with doses given at 6, 10, 14 weeks and 12–23 months.

In addition to its role in RI, IPV (and fIPV) has been used in supplementary immunization activities (SIAs) to eradicate type-1 wild poliovirus (WPV1) in endemic countries of Pakistan, Afghanistan and Nigeria (now non-endemic), as a way to close humoral immunity gaps, especially in densely populated areas (Figure 3). Given the benefit of IPV in effectively preventing paralysis and its impact in boosting mucosal immunity in previously OPV-exposed populations, it was initially included as a tool for cVDPV2 outbreak response following OPV2 withdrawal. Due to global shortages of IPV supply, its use was prioritized for WPV1 endemic countries and, from 2017, no longer supported for cVDPV2 outbreak response. Since OPV2 withdrawal, IPV SIAs have been limited in response to cVDPV2, with use in only 14 countries, 4 of which were due to delayed IPV introduction in RI (e.g., Angola, Ghana, Burkina Faso, and Zimbabwe), and 3 were in WPV1 endemic (Pakistan, Afghanistan) or recently endemic countries (Nigeria). Despite the availability of dose-sparing strategies, fIPV SIAs were only conducted in response to aVDPV2s in Hyderabad, India [69] and Hyderabad, Pakistan [45,70].

Now that supply constraints have been addressed, IPV has again been recommended in cVDPV2 outbreak response, to be used in conjunction with OPV2. Most recently, the SAGE recommended that IPV campaigns be considered in areas with difficulties to achieve and maintain high population immunity (consequential geographies) [71]. Additionally, a recent report suggested that it is feasible to administer fIPV in house-to-house campaigns in one of the most difficult areas to eradicate polio in Northern Nigeria [43]. Previous fIPV campaigns using jet injectors demonstrated great success in terms of feasibility, community acceptance and achieved coverage in Cuba and Pakistan [40,42,45,69]. However, questions remain regarding whether to expand fIPV or IPV in campaigns to control poliomyelitis [72,73].

As new scientific information became available, the technical oversight committee of WHO continued to finetune their recommendation for IPV use, clearly demonstrating that IPV has an increasingly larger role to play in inducing immunity and protecting the world's children from poliomyelitis. It is also assumed that IPV will assist in eradicating poliovirus from these populations (Table 1).

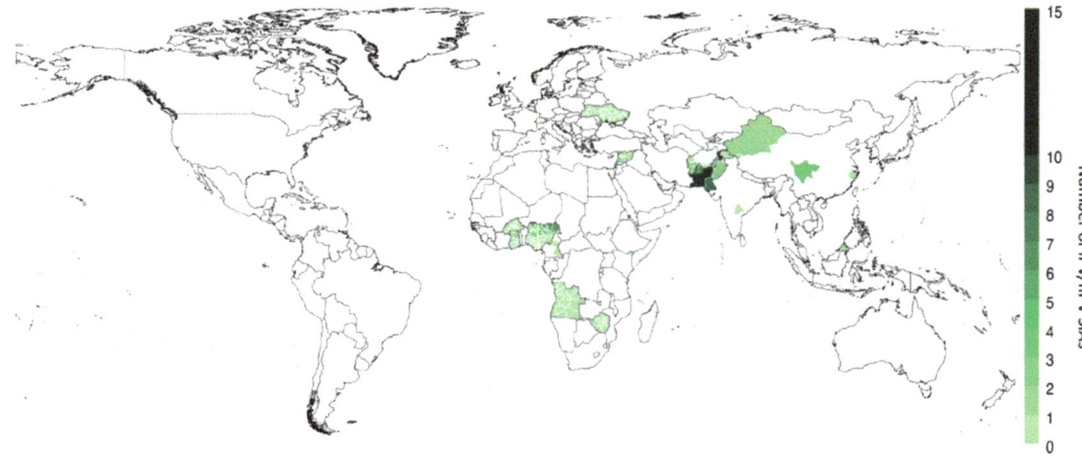

Figure 3. IPV used in campaigns to control cVDPV2 since the switch in 2016.

4. Expanding the IPV Supply Infrastructure for Global Demand

To introduce a new vaccine is a massive undertaking which requires readiness investigation, training of health staff, ensuring adequate cold chain capacity and a public information campaign. It also requires the availability of sufficient vaccines for a stable supply chain [74].

In the case of IPV, the GPEI recognized, as early as 2008, that the existing manufacturing base in Europe and North America was insufficient for the requirements of the developing world. While the traditional manufacturers relied exclusively on wild-type poliovirus serotypes to produce IPV, the containment considerations forced the GPEI to evaluate other options (equally immunogenic, but safer to produce). This directly led to a decision to set up a Sabin-IPV Technology Transfer Project [75].

As is well known, the traditional IPV producers handle massive quantities of wild-type polioviruses during production. The potential for accidental leaks or exposures becomes particularly worrisome in a polio-free world. Therefore, the Global Action Plan IV (GAPIV) on poliovirus containment mandates that all facilities handling the poliovirus, including those for vaccine production, adhere to strict bio-containment guidelines [76]. The plan outlines primary (facility containment), secondary (population immunity) and tertiary (facility location) safeguards. These requirements do, however, restrict the number of IPV producers post-eradication, posing significant obstacles to local manufacturers in developing nations.

Therefore, some manufacturers have shifted toward the production of IPV using the Sabin poliovirus strains, which present fewer biosafety risks. A few producers have successfully demonstrated the viability of this approach. Consequently, Sabin-IPV (S-IPV) has been licensed in various presentations in Japan in 2012, China starting in 2012 (multiple producers) and Korea in 2020 [77,78].

In 2008, the WHA resolved to allow for safer IPV production processes, focusing on affordability and the potential development of S-IPV for lower to middle-income countries [79]. Consequently, a partnership was formed between the WHO and Intravacc (formerly part of the Netherlands Vaccine Institute [NVI]) to facilitate the technology transfer of Sabin IPV production technology.

Intravacc functioned as the central technology transfer hub, providing standard operating procedures (SOPs) for manufacturing and generating GMP materials for Phase I/IIa clinical studies, providing production seed strains, and facilitating technology transfers to manufacturers in the developing world. WHO, on the other hand, conducted clinical studies and led the selection of technology transfer recipients, established the expert advisory panel and aided the pre-qualification and licensure process.

Between 2010 and 2012, the WHO disseminated three calls for expressions of interest to vaccine manufacturers in developing countries, aiming to identify two suitable recipients each year for the S-IPV production technology transfer. Following a rigorous selection process that included a multitude of criteria, six entities were chosen by an independent selection committee. The BMGF funded Intravacc's contribution to the project, while the technology recipients bore the cost of their participation without WHO financial support.

From six producers selected for the S-IPV technology transfer, three achieved national licensure (Sinovac, China; LG Chem, Korea; Beijing Minhai, China) with one (LG Chem) supplying the international market. It required approximately 10 years from first technology transfer selection in 2010 to WHO-prequalification for United Nations purchase. Currently supplied at Euro1.25 per dose in a five-dose formulation to UNICEF, it is the most economical IPV vaccine option [80–82].

Presently, there are 10 WHO-prequalified presentations of IPV from five manufacturers (Sanofi, France; Serum Institute of India [SSI], India; AJ Vaccines, Denmark, Bilthoven Biologicals, Netherlands, and Sanofi Healthcare, India), and four prequalified presentations of S-IPV from three manufacturers (Beijing Institute of Biological Products, China; Sinovac, China; LG Chem, Korea) (Table 2). In addition, one hexavalent vaccine by SII, India containing IPV and whole-cell pertussis vaccine is (and another one by Panacea Biotec, India is expected to be shortly) under evaluation for prequalification The hexavalent base will expand massively in the next 3–5 years as countries are interested to introduce this new vaccine that eliminates injections and protects against six antigens.

Table 2. IPV producers and products with World Health Organization (WHO)-prequalification for United Nations purchase.

Seed Strains	Manufacturers	WHO Pre-Qualification Date	Presentation
Wild poliovirus	Sanofi S.A., Paris, France	9DEC2005 19DEC2014	10-dose IPV DTaP-HBV-Hib-IPV
	Bilthoven Biologicals B.V., Bilthoven, The Netherlands (a subsidiary of SII)	6DEC2010 28NOV2014	1-dose IPV 5-dose IPV
	AJ Vaccines A/S, København, Denmark	23DEC2010 21APR2020	1-dose IPV 5-dose IPV
	Serum Institute of India (SII), Pune, India (IPV from Bilthoven Biologicals B.V.)	28OCT2016 11JUL2019	1 + 2 + 5-dose IPV 10-dose IPV
	Sanofi Healthcare India Private Ltd., India (with IPV from Sanofi S.A., France)	01OCT2018 22APR2022	5-dose IPV 10-dose IPV
Sabin strains	Sinovac Biotec Co., Ltd., Beijing, China §	06JUN2022	Single dose IPV
	LG Chem Ltd., Seoul, Republic of Korea §	01JUN2021 21DEC2020	Single dose IPV 5-dose IPV
	Beijing Institute of Biological Product Co., Ltd., Beijing, China	15FEB2022	Single dose IPV

§ Participants of INTRAVACC/WHO Sabin-IPV technology transfer project.

5. Developing the Next-Generation Polio Vaccine

Currently available IPVs (Salk and Sabin) have a successful manufacturing and regulatory track record and are widely used and accepted, as they are very safe to use in the field, but they have two drawbacks: (1) they require large quantities of live virus in the manufacturing facilities before they are chemically inactivated, which poses a threat should containment of these facilities be breached and, (2) they do not directly induce mucosal immunity and thus, while they efficiently protect those who receive the vaccine, they do not prevent the vaccine recipients from shedding the virus initially, but reduce the proportion of vaccinees excreting, the length of excretion and the titer of virus excreted (Table 1).

The GPEI is thus interested in developing vaccines that are not affected by the drawbacks mentioned, with the highest importance being set on responding to growing containment requirements.

Two major development projects are currently being undertaken:

1. Poliovirus Virus-Like particles (PV VLPs)

This project was launched by WHO in 2010 with the aim of developing PV VLPs as potentially ideal vaccines for the post-eradication era to eventually replace IPVs. Vaccines based on VLPs are already established and successful for other diseases, such as cervical cancer caused by human papillomavirus [83]. WHO contracted a research and development consortium under the lead of the University of Leeds, UK, with this task.

By definition, VLPs are particles that closely resemble viruses, but are non-infectious as they do not contain any viral genetic material. PV VLPs thus do not contain poliovirus RNA. This exempts them from containment requirements, which will only become stricter as the program achieves polio eradication.

Native PV capsid proteins do not form a stable particle in the absence of RNA and thus PV VLPs require genetically modified capsid proteins plus addition of stabilizing elements such as pocket factors [84].

The consortium was able to generate thermostable VLPs that are D-antigenic and have a structure that is indistinguishable from Polio WT virus from a number of expression systems such as plants [85], mammalian cells [86], yeast [87–91] and baculovirus. Preclinical immunogenicity studies of PV VLPs adjuvanted with alum [$Al(OH)_3$] in Wistar rats, the "gold standard" for IPV lot release testing, show similar or better immunogenicity compared to IPV, which is encouraging.

In 2019, WHO published a call for Expression of Interest to find partners for the commercialization of PV VLPs. This call was answered by a large number of interested parties, mainly commercial manufacturers. Following advice of an independent advisory panel, WHO chose some promising applicants with whom collaboration is currently ongoing. The focus is set on yeast and baculovirus as the two expression systems that will most likely allow production of goods at low cost. In addition, the Bill and Melinda Gates Foundation recently issued a request for proposal to selected potential partners for which the final selection is imminent.

The target product profile for PV VLPs, very similar to the one for IPV, calls for PV VLPs as a standalone presentation as well as a component for multivalent vaccines such as hexavalent vaccines. The main use, with an affordable market price as a necessary requirement, is anticipated for RI with a potential for outbreak response as well. The VLPs development is continuing and is now in Phase 1 of clinical development.

In addition, in the quest to develop a poliovirus vaccine presentation that could potentially avoid the need for a cold chain, which would not require highly trained vaccinators as with IM injections and would potentially be dose-sparing (thus cost-effective) and even providing mucosal immunity, the consortium collaborates with the University of Queensland, Australia, to develop microneedle patches (MNPs) with or without the addition of including double-mutant heat-labile enterotoxin of *Escherichia coli* (dmLT) [17,18,92], an adjuvant that has been shown to induce mucosal immunity in other applications.

2. S19 IPV

Following WHO's recommendation for the use of attenuated Sabin strains for IPV production, to avoid or reduce the mentioned risks that Salk and Sabin IPV pose regarding containment, the former National Institute for Biological Standards and Control, UK (NIBSC) now integrated into the Medicines and Healthcare products Regulatory Agency, UK (MHRA) developed a strain (S19) which is hyper-attenuated, genetically stabilized and most probably cannot replicate in people (i.e., S19 cannot replicate at human body temperature) and are also highly restricted in their potential to revert to a neurovirulent form during the manufacturing process. The strain has been shown to be as immunogenic as the current IPV and can be produced on a large scale [93].

S19 strains have obtained a (time-limited) waiver from containment requirements for manufacturing by the Containment Advisory Group (CAG) [94]. This S19 strain is already used for neutralization assays and is replacing the infectious Sabin strains, and S19-based IPV is in development by one manufacturer for a hexavalent presentation which is currently in Phase 1 clinical development and potentially for a standalone adjuvanted presentation.

The WHO SAGE in October 2022 stated "SAGE recognized the importance of clinical research and product development and encouraged accelerated efforts to develop, license and commercialize . . ., VLP and other non-infectiously manufactured IPV-like vaccines, . . .".

The two projects outlined in this section aim to fulfill this guidance. Poliovirus VLPs have just entered Phase 1 of clinical development, but the development is by nature unpredictable as to success and associated timelines, and an optimistic timeline for successful commercialization by manufacturers obtaining national licensure and WHO prequalification could be envisaged by 2028.

VLPs have a theoretical advantage over S19 strains, as by definition they cannot replicate in humans and thus cannot revert to a neurovirulent form, whereas S19 would still need to be proven by studies in humans to have the same properties.

6. Conclusions and Future Perspectives

Much has been learned over the past two decades regarding the efficacy, strategic use for programmatic action and safe production of IPV. Since the 2016 switch from tOPV to bOPV, and the concomitant introduction of $\geq$1 dose of IPV into RI schedules, IPV became a truly global vaccine, benefitting all children regardless of residing in industrialized or developing countries.

IPV has demonstrated versatility. In industrialized countries, most countries use combination pentavalent or hexavalent formulations with IPV [4,95]. In developing countries, countries use stand-alone IPV or fractional-dose IPV. This will change in the next three to five years after GAVI opens a window for support of combination hexavalent vaccines with IPV that use whole-cell pertussis vaccine [68].

For outbreak control, stand-alone IPV and/or fIPV will also be increasingly considered for campaigns use [71]. An evaluation in Northern Nigeria demonstrated the feasibility of fIPV house-to-house campaigns using a needle-free injection device [43]. A recently published case–control study in Nigeria reported a single-dose IPV vaccine effectiveness of almost 90% [47]. This report, the feasibility of house-to-house administration of fIPV [43,45,69], the superior acceptance of an injectable vaccine, particularly fIPV [39,45,56,70] administered with a needle-free device and the recent recommendation of IPV campaign use in consequential geographies [71], suggests that a new strategy to reach and surpass the threshold for herd immunity, especially targeted to difficult areas that may include Northern Nigeria, Eastern Democratic Republic of the Congo (DRC), Somalia and Yemen. In these areas, annual supplemental IPV house-to-house outreach to children <5 years with high coverage (in addition to routine polio vaccine use) could both interrupt cVDPV2 transmission, prevent the emerge of new cVDPVs and most importantly massively reduce the paralytic disease burden. Further innovative thinking is needed to optimize such extended outreach use, especially weighing the cost versus population immunity gain, and increasing quality and coverage (Table 2).

The Sabin-IPV technology transfer project has been successful. At least two manufacturers obtained national licensure, and one manufacturer has obtained WHO-prequalification for supply to United Nations agencies. The entry of LG Chem has disrupted the IPV pricing structure and resulted in massive savings for the global support base (GAVI-supported countries) since 2021 [82].

However, the further development of IPV must eventually result in non-infectious production methods, the cracking of the "holy grail" of non-infectious polio vaccines inducing mucosal immunity, and better methods for administering injectable vaccines in house-to-house campaigns. The development of virus-like particles (VLPs) is encouraging, the S19-based Sabin virus is already used as challenge virus for safer neutralization assays and S19-based IPV may add yet another level of safety for meeting production containment requirements [92,93].

The world has benefitted from two excellent vaccines for polio prevention, IPV and OPV. But neither of these vaccines are perfectly suited for achieving eradication. Whether IPV-induced intestinal mucosal immunity can achieve herd immunity in tropical countries with high force of poliovirus transmission has not been answered conclusively, but findings from Indonesia and Malaysia are encouraging [28,29]. To harvest the full potential of IPV, high vaccination coverage is necessary [95]. OPV use, however, induces mucosal immunity but constantly introduces new live viruses into communities that can mutate and/or recombine to source new endemic and epidemic transmission (i.e., "fighting fire with fire"). This seeding cycle needs to be broken.

Looking into the future, it seems obvious that all infectious poliovirus vaccines must be discontinued to achieve eradication, and that the world must rely solely on non-infectious polio vaccines for maintaining high population immunity. To get to this point, a massive program-of-work will be required, but the rewards will also be massive. Polio eradication will finally be within our grasp.

Author Contributions: Conceptualization, R.W.S., M.E., N.A.M., H.V. and H.O.; methodology, R.W.S., M.E., N.A.M., H.V. and H.O.; software N.A.M.; validation, R.W.S., M.E., N.A.M., H.V. and H.O.; formal analysis, R.W.S., M.E., N.A.M., H.V. and H.O.; investigation, R.W.S., M.E., N.A.M., H.V. and H.O.; data curation, R.W.S., M.E., N.A.M., H.V. and H.O.; writing—original draft preparation, R.W.S., M.E., N.A.M., H.V. and H.O.; writing—review and editing, R.W.S., M.E., N.A.M., H.V. and H.O.; visualization, N.A.M.; supervision, R.W.S.; project administration, R.W.S. All authors have read and agreed to the published version of the manuscript.

Funding: This review received no external funding.

Conflicts of Interest: Roland W. Sutter works as a consultant in Tamayo Federal Solutions LLC, and Natalia A. Molodecky works as a Senior Epidemiologist Consultant at the Task Force for Global Health, Inc. The other authors declare no conflict of interest.

References

1. World Health Assembly. *Global Eradication of Poliomyelitis by the Year 2000. Resolutions of the 41st World Health Assembly;* World Health Organization: Geneva, Switzerland, 1988.
2. Lee, S.E.; Greene, S.A.; Burns, C.C.; Tallis, G.; Wassilak, S.G.F.; Bolu, O. Progress toward poliomyelitis eradication—Worldwide, January 2021–March 2023. *Morb. Mortal. Wkly. Rep.* **2023**, *72*, 517–522. [CrossRef]
3. Francis, T., Jr.; Korns, R.F.; Voight, R.B.; Boisen, M.; Hemphill, F.M.; Napier, J.A.; Tolchinsky, E. An evaluation of the 1954 poliomyelitis vaccine trials. *Am. J. Public Health Nation's Health* **1955**, *45 Pt 2*, 1–63.
4. Vidor, E. Poliovirus Vaccine—Inactivated. In *Plotkin's Vaccines*, 8th ed.; Plotin, S.A., Orenstein, W.A., Offit, P.A., Edwards, K.M., Eds.; Elsevier: Philadelphia, PA, USA, 2018; Volume 48, pp. 841–865.
5. van Wezel, A.L.; van Steenis, G.; van der Marel, P.; Osterhaus, A.D. Inactivated poliovirus vaccine: Current production methods and new developments. *Clin. Infect. Dis.* **1984**, *6* (Suppl. S2), S335–S340. [CrossRef] [PubMed]
6. Böttiger, M.; Larsson, B. Swedish inactivated polio vaccine: Laboratory standardization and clinical experience over a 30-year period. *Biologicals* **1992**, *20*, 267–275. [CrossRef] [PubMed]
7. Sutter, R.W.; Kew, O.M.; Cochi, S.L.; Aylward, R.B. Poliovirus Vaccine—Live. In *Plotkin's Vaccines*, 8th ed.; Plotin, S.A., Orenstein, W.A., Offit, P.A., Edwards, K.M., Eds.; Elsevier: Philadelphia, PA, USA, 2018; Volume 49, pp. 866–917.
8. Bahl, S.; Bhatnagar, P.; Sutter, R.W.; Roesel, S.; Zaffran, M. Global polio eradication—Way ahead. *Indian J. Pediatr.* **2018**, *85*, 124–131. [CrossRef] [PubMed]
9. Global Polio Eradication Initiative. *2005 Annual Report;* World Health Organization: Geneva, Switzerland, 2006; WHO/Polio/06.02.
10. Burns, C.C.; Diop, O.M.; Sutter, R.W.; Kew, O.M. Vaccine-derived polioviruses. *J. Infect. Dis.* **2014**, *210* (Suppl. S1), S283–S293. [CrossRef] [PubMed]
11. Global Polio Eradication Initiative. *Polio Eradication & Endgame Strategic Plan 2013–2018;* World Health Organization: Geneva, Switzerland, 2013.
12. Platt, L.R.; Estívariz, C.F.; Sutter, R.W. Vaccine-associated paralytic poliomyelitis: A review of the epidemiology and estimation of the global burden. *J. Infect. Dis.* **2014**, *210*, S380–S389. [CrossRef] [PubMed]
13. Global Polio Eradication Initiative. Polio endgame & legacy—Implementation, best practices, and lessons learned. *J. Infect. Dis.* **2017**, *216* (Suppl. S1), S1–S379.
14. Thompson, K.M.; Kalkowski, D.A.; Badizagan, K. Looking back at prospective modeling of outbreak response strategies for managing global type 2 oral poliovirus vaccine (OPV2) cessation. *Front. Public Health* **2023**, *11*, 1098419. [CrossRef]
15. World Health Organization. Meeting of the Strategic Advisory Group on Immunization October 2020—Conclusions and recommendations. *Wkly. Epidemiol. Rec.* **2020**, *48*, 585–608.

16. Macklin, G.R.; Mach, O. Fractional dose IPV in polio eradication. *Lancet Infect. Dis.* **2021**, *21*, 1061–1062. [CrossRef]
17. Crothers, J.W.; Ross Colgate, E.; Cowan, K.J.; Dickson, D.M.; Walsh, M.; Carmolli, M.; Wright, P.F.; Norton, E.B.; Kirkpatrick, B.D. Intradermal fractional-dose inactivated polio vaccine (fIPV) adjuvanted with double mutant Enterotoxigenic Escherichia coli heat labile toxin (dmLT) is well-tolerated and augments a systemic immune response to all three poliovirus serotypes in a randomized placebo-controlled trial. *Vaccine* **2022**, *40*, 2705–2713. [CrossRef]
18. Erdem, R.; De Coster, I.; Withanage, K.; Mercer, L.D.; Marchant, A.; Taton, M.; Cools, N.; Lion, E.; Cassels, F.; Higgins, D.; et al. Safety, tolerability, and immunogenicity of inactivated poliovirus vaccine with or without *E. coli* double mutant heat-labile toxin (dmLT) adjuvant in healthy adults; a phase 1 randomized study. *Vaccine* **2023**, *41*, 1657–1667. [CrossRef]
19. Onorato, I.M.; Modlin, J.F.; McBean, A.M.; Thoms, M.L.; Losonsky, G.A.; Bernier, R.H. Mucosal immunity induced by enhance-potency inactivated and oral polio vaccines. *J. Infect. Dis.* **1991**, *163*, 1–6. [CrossRef] [PubMed]
20. Ghendon, Y.U.; Sanakoyeva, I.I. Comparison of resistance of the intestinal tract to poliomyelitis vaccine (Sabin strains) in persons after naturally and experimentally acquired immunity. *Acta Virol.* **1961**, *5*, 265–273.
21. Fine, P.E.; Carneiro, I.A. Transmissibility and persistence of oral polio vaccine viruses: Implications for the global poliomyelitis eradication initiative. *Am. J. Epidemiol.* **1999**, *150*, 1001–1021. [CrossRef] [PubMed]
22. Brickley, E.B.; Connor, R.I.; Wieland-Alter, W.F.; Collett, M.S.; Hartford, M.; Van Der Avoort, H.; Boesch, A.W.; Weiner, J.A.; Ackerman, M.E.; McKinlay, M.A.; et al. Intestinal antibody responses to a live oral poliovirus vaccine challenge among adults previously immunized with inactivated polio vaccine in Sweden. *BMJ Glob. Health* **2019**, *4*, e001613. [CrossRef] [PubMed]
23. Cuba IPV Study Collaborative Group. Randomized, placebo-controlled trial of inactivated poliovirus vaccine in Cuba. *N. Engl. J. Med.* **2007**, *356*, 1536–1544. [CrossRef] [PubMed]
24. Snider, C.J.; Zaman, K.; Wilkinson, A.L.; Binte Aziz, A.; Yunus, M.; Haque, W.; Jones, K.A.V.; Wei, L.; Estivariz, C.F.; Konopka-Anstadt, J.L.; et al. Poliovirus type 1 systemic humoral and intestinal mucosal immunity induced by monovalent oral poliovirus vaccine, fractional inactivated poliovirus vaccine, and bivalent oral poliovirus vaccine: A randomized controlled trial. *Vaccine* **2023**, *41*, 6083–6092. [CrossRef] [PubMed]
25. Dang, T.T.H.; Dang, D.A.; Nguyen, T.T.; Duong, T.H.; Tran, T.T.; Luong, N.T.; Jeyaseelan, V.; Lopez Cavestany, R.; Hendley, W.S.; Mainou, B.A.; et al. Inactivated poliovirus vaccine closing the type 2 immunity gap in Vietnam. *J. Pediatr. Infect. Dis. Soc.* **2022**, *11*, 413–416. [CrossRef]
26. Marine, W.M.; Chin, T.D.; Gravelle, C.R. Limitation of fecal and pharyngeal poliovirus excretion in Salk-vaccinated children. A family study during a type 1 poliomyelitis epidemic. *Am. J. Epidemiol.* **1962**, *76*, 173–195. [CrossRef]
27. Stickle, G. Observed and expected poliomyelitis in the United States, 1958–1961. *Am. J. Public Health Nation's Health* **1964**, *54*, 1222–1229. [CrossRef] [PubMed]
28. Wahjuhono, G.; Revolusiana; Widhiastuti, D.; Sundoro, J.; Mardani, T.; Ratih, W.U.; Sutomo, R.; Safitri, I.; Sampurno, O.D.; Rana, B.; et al. Switch from oral to inactivated poliovirus vaccine in Yogyakarta Province, Indonesia: Summary of coverage, immunity, and environmental surveillance. *J. Infect. Dis.* **2014**, *210* (Suppl. S1), S347–S352. [CrossRef]
29. Snider, C.J.; Boualam, L.; Tallis, G.; Takashima, Y.; Abeyasinghe, R.; Lo, Y.R.; Grabovac, V.; Avagyan, T.; Aslam, S.K.; Eltayeb, A.O.; et al. Concurrent outbreaks of circulating vaccine-derived poliovirus types 1 and 2 affecting the Republic of the Philippines and Malaysia, 2019–2021. *Vaccine* **2023**, *41* (Suppl. S1), A58–A69. [CrossRef]
30. John, J.; Giri, S.; Karthikeyan, A.S.; Iturriza-Gomara, M.; Muliyil, J.; Abraham, A.; Grassly, N.C.; Kang, G. Effect of a single inactivated poliovirus vaccine dose on intestinal immunity against poliovirus in children previously given oral vaccine: An open-label, randomised controlled trial. *Lancet* **2014**, *384*, 1505–1512. [CrossRef]
31. Jafari, H.; Deshpande, J.M.; Sutter, R.W.; Bahl, S.; Verma, H.; Ahmad, M.; Kunwar, A.; Vishwakarma, R.; Agarwal, A.; Jain, S.; et al. Polio eradication. Efficacy of inactivated poliovirus vaccine in India. *Science* **2014**, *345*, 922–925. [CrossRef] [PubMed]
32. Hird, T.R.; Grassly, N.C. Systematic review of mucosal immunity induced by oral and inactivated poliovirus vaccines against virus shedding following oral poliovirus challenge. *PLoS Pathog.* **2012**, *8*, e1002599. [CrossRef] [PubMed]
33. Parker, E.P.; Molodecky, N.A.; Pons-Salort, M.; O'Reilly, K.M.; Grassly, N.C. Impact of inactivated poliovirus vaccine on mucosal immunity: Implications for the polio eradication endgame. *Expert Rev. Vaccines* **2015**, *14*, 1113–1123. [CrossRef] [PubMed]
34. Macklin, G.R.; Grassly, N.C.; Sutter, R.W.; Mach, O.; Bandyopadhyay, A.S.; Edmunds, W.J.; O'Reilly, K.M. Vaccine schedules and the effect on humoral and intestinal immunity against poliovirus: A systematic review and network meta-analysis. *Lancet Infect. Dis.* **2019**, *19*, 1121–1128. [CrossRef]
35. Gamage, D.; Mach, O.; Ginige, S.; Weldon, W.C.; Oberste, M.S.; Jeyaseelan, V.; Sutter, R.W. Poliovirus Type 2 Seroprevalence Following Full- or Fractional-Dose Inactivated Poliovirus Vaccine in the Period After Sabin Type 2 Withdrawal in Sri Lanka. *J. Infect. Dis.* **2019**, *219*, 1887–1892. [CrossRef]
36. Aziz, A.B.; Verma, H.; Jeyaseelan, V.; Yunus, M.; Nowrin, S.; Moore, D.D.; Mainou, B.A.; Mach, O.; Sutter, R.W.; Zaman, K. One Full or Two Fractional Doses of Inactivated Poliovirus Vaccine for Catch-up Vaccination in Older Infants: A Randomized Clinical Trial in Bangladesh. *J. Infect. Dis.* **2022**, *226*, 1319–1326. [CrossRef]
37. Sharma, A.K.; Verma, H.; Estivariz, C.F.; Bajracharaya, L.; Rai, G.; Shah, G.; Sherchand, J.; Jones, K.A.V.; Mainou, B.A.; Chavan, S.; et al. Persistence of immunity following a single dose of inactivated poliovirus vaccine: A phase 4, open label, non-randomised clinical trial. *Lancet Microbe* **2023**, *4*, e923–e930. [CrossRef]
38. Anand, A.; Molodecky, N.A.; Pallansch, M.A.; Sutter, R.W. Immunogenicity to poliovirus type 2 following two doses of fractional intradermal inactivated poliovirus vaccine: A novel dose sparing immunization schedule. *Vaccine* **2017**, *35*, 2993–2998. [CrossRef]

39. Resik, S.; Tejeda, A.; Lago, P.M.; Diaz, M.; Carmenates, A.; Sarmiento, L.; Alemañi, N.; Galindo, B.; Burton, A.; Friede, M.; et al. Randomized controlled clinical trial of fractional doses of inactivated poliovirus vaccine administered intradermally by needle-free device in Cuba. *J. Infect. Dis.* **2010**, *201*, 1344–1352. [CrossRef]
40. Resik, S.; Tejeda, A.; Sutter, R.W.; Diaz, M.; Sarmiento, L.; Alemañi, N.; Garcia, G.; Fonseca, M.; Hung, L.H.; Kahn, A.L.; et al. Priming after a fractional dose of inactivated poliovirus vaccine. *N. Engl. J. Med.* **2013**, *368*, 416–424. [CrossRef]
41. Mohammed, A.J.; AlAwaidy, S.; Bawikar, S.; Kurup, P.J.; Elamir, E.; Shaban, M.M.; Sharif, S.M.; van der Avoort, H.G.; Pallansch, M.A.; Malankar, P.; et al. Fractional doses of inactivated poliovirus vaccine in Oman. *N. Engl. J. Med.* **2010**, *362*, 2351–2359. [CrossRef] [PubMed]
42. Saleem, A.F.; Mach, O.; Yousafzai, M.T.; Khan, A.; Weldon, W.C.; Oberste, M.S.; Sutter, R.W.; Zaidi, A.K.M. Needle adapters for intradermal administration of fractional dose of inactivated poliovirus vaccine: Evaluation of immunogenicity and programmatic feasibility in Pakistan. *Vaccine* **2017**, *35*, 3209–3214. [CrossRef] [PubMed]
43. Biya, O.; Manu, J.I.; Forbi, J.C.; Wa Nganda, G.; Ikwe, H.; Sule, A.; Edukugho, A.; Shehu, A.; Aliyu, N.; Barau, N.D.; et al. Notes from the Field: House-to-House Campaign Administration of Inactivated Poliovirus Vaccine—Sokoto State, Nigeria, November 2022. *MMWR Morb. Mortal. Wkly. Rep.* **2023**, *72*, 1290–1291. [CrossRef] [PubMed]
44. Bullo, U.F.; Mehraj, J.; Raza, S.M.; Rasool, S.; Ansari, N.N.; Shaikh, A.A.; Phul, Z.A.; Memon, S.A.; Baloch, R.I.; Baloch, Z.A.; et al. An experience of mass administration of fractional dose inactivated polio vaccine through intradermal needle-free injectors in Karachi, Sindh, Pakistan. *BMC Public Health* **2021**, *21*, 44. [CrossRef]
45. Pervaiz, A.; Mbaeyi, C.; Baig, M.A.; Burman, A.; Ahmed, J.A.; Akter, S.; Jatoi, F.A.; Mahamud, A.; Asghar, R.J.; Azam, N.; et al. Fractional-dose inactivated poliovirus vaccine campaign—Sindh Province, Pakistan, 2016. *MMWR Morb. Mortal. Wkly. Rep.* **2017**, *66*, 1295–1299. [CrossRef]
46. Resik, S.; Tejeda, A.; Mach, O.; Fonseca, M.; Diaz, M.; Alemany, N.; Garcia, G.; Hung, L.H.; Martinez, Y.; Sutter, R. Immune responses after fractional doses of inactivated poliovirus vaccine using newly developed intradermal jet injectors: A randomized controlled trial in Cuba. *Vaccine* **2015**, *33*, 307–313. [CrossRef]
47. Cooper, L.V.; Erbeto, T.B.; Danzomo, A.A.; Abdullahi, H.W.; Boateng, K.; Adamu, U.S.; Shuaib, F.; Modjirom, N.; Gray, E.J.; Bandyopadhyay, A.S.; et al. Effectiveness of poliovirus vaccines against circulating vaccine-derived type 2 poliomyelitis in Nigeria between 2017 and 2022: A case control study. *Lancet Infect. Dis.* 2024, *online ahead of print*. [CrossRef]
48. Sáez-Llorens, X.; Clemens, R.; Leroux-Roels, G.; Jimeno, J.; Clemens, S.A.; Weldon, W.C.; Oberste, M.S.; Molina, N.; Bandyopadhyay, A.S. Immunogenicity and safety of a novel monovalent high-dose inactivated poliovirus type 2 vaccine in infants: A comparative, observer-blind, randomised, controlled trial. *Lancet Infect. Dis.* **2016**, *16*, 321–330. [CrossRef]
49. Swartz, T.A.; Handsher, R.; Stoeckel, P.; Drucker, J.; Caudrelier, P.; Van Wezel, A.L.; Cohen, H.; Salk, D.; Salk, J. Immunologic memory induced at birth by immunization with inactivated polio vaccine in a reduced schedule. *Eur. J. Epidemiol.* **1989**, *5*, 143–145. [CrossRef]
50. Samuel, B.U.; Cherian, T.; Sridharan, G.; Mukundan, P.; John, T.J. Immune response to intradermally injected inactivated poliovirus vaccine. *Lancet* **1991**, *338*, 343–344. [CrossRef] [PubMed]
51. Nirmal, S.; Cherian, T.; Samuel, B.U.; Rajasingh, J.; Raghupathy, P.; John, T.J. Immune response of infants to fractional doses of intradermally administered inactivated poliovirus vaccine. *Vaccine* **1998**, *16*, 928–931. [CrossRef]
52. Cadorna-Carlos, J.; Vidor, E.; Bonnet, M.-C. Randomized controlled study of fractional doses of inactivated poliovirus vaccine administered intradermally with a needle in the Philippines. *Int. J. Infect. Dis.* **2012**, *16*, e110–e116. [CrossRef]
53. Soonawala, D.; Verdijk, P.; Wijmenga-Monsuur, A.J.; Boog, C.J.; Koedam, P.; Visser, L.G.; Rots, N.Y. Intradermal fractional booster dose of inactivated poliomyelitis vaccine with a jet injector in healthy adults. *Vaccine* **2013**, *31*, 3688–3694. [CrossRef] [PubMed]
54. Bashorun, A.O.; Badjie Hydara, M.; Adigweme, I.; Umesi, A.; Danso, B.; Johnson, N.; Sambou, N.A.; Fofana, S.; Kanu, F.J.; Jeyaseelan, V.; et al. Intradermal administration of fractional doses of the inactivated poliovirus vaccine in a campaign: A pragmatic, open-label, non-inferiority trial in The Gambia. *Lancet Glob. Health* **2022**, *10*, e257–e268. [CrossRef]
55. Trueba, G.; Jeyaseelan, V.; Lopez, L.; Mainou, B.A.; Zhang, Y.; Whittembury, A.; Olmedo Valarezo, A.J.; Baquero, G.; Romero de Aguinaga, R.; Zurita Salinas, L.J.; et al. Achieving high immunogenicity against poliovirus with fractional doses of inactivated poliovirus vaccine in Ecuador-results from a cross-sectional serological survey. *Lancet Reg. Health Am.* **2022**, *11*, 100235. [CrossRef]
56. Ahmad, M.; Verma, H.; Deshpande, J.; Kunwar, A.; Bavdekar, A.; Mahantashetti, N.S.; Krishnamurthy, B.; Jain, M.; Mathew, M.A.; Pawar, S.D.; et al. Immunogenicity of fractional dose inactivated poliovirus vaccine in India. *J. Pediatr. Infect. Dis. Soc.* **2022**, *11*, 60–68. [CrossRef] [PubMed]
57. Snider, C.J.; Zaman, K.; Estivariz, C.F.; Yunus, M.; Weldon, W.C.; Wannemuehler, K.A.; Oberste, M.S.; Pallansch, M.A.; Wassilak, S.G.; Bari, T.I.A.; et al. Immunogenicity of full and fractional dose of inactivated poliovirus vaccine for use in routine immunisation and outbreak response: An open-label, randomised controlled trial. *Lancet* **2019**, *393*, 2624–2634. [CrossRef]
58. Anand, A.; Zaman, K.; Estívariz, C.F.; Yunus, M.; Gary, H.E.; Weldon, W.C.; Bari, T.I.; Steven Oberste, M.; Wassilak, S.G.; Luby, S.P.; et al. Early priming with inactivated poliovirus vaccine (IPV) and intradermal fractional dose IPV administered by a microneedle device: A randomized controlled trial. *Vaccine* **2015**, *33*, 6816–6822. [CrossRef]
59. Louis-Auguste, J.; Kelly, P. Tropical enteropathies. *Curr. Gastroenterol. Rep.* **2017**, *19*, 29. [CrossRef]
60. Patriarca, P.A.; Wright, P.F.; John, T.J. Factors affecting the immunogenicity of oral poliovirus vaccine in developing countries: Review. *Clin. Infect. Dis.* **1991**, *13*, 926–939. [CrossRef]

61. Posey, D.L.; Linkins, R.W.; Oliveria, M.J.; Monteiro, D.; Patriarca, P.A. The effect of diarrhea on oral poliovirus vaccine failure in Brazil. *J. Infect. Dis.* **1997**, *175*, S258–S263. [CrossRef]
62. Hodges, P.; Tembo, M.; Kelly, P. Intestinal Biopsies for the Evaluation of Environmental Enteropathy and Environmental Enteric Dysfunction. *J. Infect. Dis.* **2021**, *224*, S856–S863. [CrossRef]
63. Marie, C.; Ali, A.; Chandwe, K.; Petri, W.A., Jr.; Kelly, P. Pathophysiology of environmental enteric dysfunction and its impact on oral vaccine efficacy. *Mucosal Immunol.* **2018**, *11*, 1290–1298. [CrossRef]
64. Mashunye, T.R.; Ndwandwe, D.E.; Dube, K.R.; Shey, M.; Shelton, M.; Wiysonge, C.S. Fractional dose compared with standard dose inactivated poliovirus vaccine in children: A systematic review and meta-analysis. *Lancet Infect. Dis.* **2021**, *21*, 1161–1174. [CrossRef] [PubMed]
65. de Quadros, C.A.; Hersh, B.S.; Olivé, J.M.; Andrus, J.K.; da Silveira, C.M.; Carrasco, P.A. Eradication of wild poliovirus from the Americas: Acute flaccid paralysis surveillance, 1988–1995. *J. Infect. Dis.* **1997**, *175*, S37–S42. [CrossRef] [PubMed]
66. Prevots, D.R.; Burr, R.K.; Sutter, R.W.; Murphy, T.V.; Advisory Committee on Immunization Practices. Poliomyelitis prevention in the United States. Updated recommendations of the Advisory Committee on Immunization Practices (ACIP). *MMWR Recomm. Rep.* **2000**, *49*, 1–22. [PubMed]
67. World Health Organization. Meeting of the Strategic Advisory Group of Experts on immunization, April 2012—Conclusions and recommendations. *Wkly. Epidemiol. Rec.* **2012**, *87*, 201–216.
68. Global Vaccine Alliance to Deploy Six-in-One Vaccine to Lower-Income Countries, Establish Innovative Mechanisms to Protect against Future Epidemic Threats. Available online: https://www.gavi.org/news/media-room/global-vaccine-alliance-deploy-six-one-vaccine-lower-income-countries (accessed on 1 January 2024).
69. Bahl, S.; Verma, H.; Bhatnagar, P.; Haldar, P.; Satapathy, A.; Kumar, K.N.; Horton, J.; Estivariz, C.F.; Anand, A.; Sutter, R. Fractional-dose inactivated poliovirus vaccine immunization campaign—Telangana State, India, June 2016. *MMWR Morb. Mortal. Wkly. Rep.* **2016**, *65*, 859–863. [CrossRef]
70. Daly, C.; Molodecky, N.A.; Sreevatsava, M.; Belayneh, A.D.; Chandio, S.A.; Partridge, J.; Shaikh, A.; Laghari, M.; Agbor, J.; Safdar, R.M.; et al. Needle-free injectors for mass administration of fractional dose inactivated poliovirus vaccine in Karachi, Pakistan: A survey of caregiver and vaccinator acceptability. *Vaccine* **2020**, *38*, 1893–1898. [CrossRef]
71. World Health Organization. Meeting of the Strategic Advisory Group of Experts on Immunization, March 2023: Conclusions and recommendations. *Wkly. Epidemiol. Rec.* **2023**, *98*, 239–256.
72. Estivariz, C.F.; Kovacs, S.D.; Mach, O. Review of use of inactivated poliovirus vaccine in campaigns to control type 2 circulating vaccine derived poliovirus (cVDPV) outbreaks. *Vaccine* **2023**, *41*, A113–A121. [CrossRef]
73. Bandyopadhyay, A.S.; Lopez Cavestany, R.; Blake, I.M.; Macklin, G.; Cooper, L.; Grassly, N.; Nery, A.L.M.D.S.; Mach, O. Use of inactivated poliovirus vaccine for poliovirus outbreak response. *Lancet Infect. Dis.* 2023, *online ahead of print*. [CrossRef]
74. World Health Organization. Introduction of New Vaccines. Available online: https://www.who.int/teams/immunization-vaccines-and-biologicals/essential-programme-on-immunization/implementation/introduction-of-new-vaccines (accessed on 1 January 2024).
75. Okayasu, H.; Sutter, R.W.; Jafari, H.S.; Takane, M.; Aylward, R.B. Affordable inactivated poliovirus vaccine: Strategies and progress. *J. Infect. Dis.* **2014**, *210*, S459–S464. [CrossRef]
76. World Health Organization. *WHO Action Plan for Poliovirus Containment*, 4th ed.; World Health Organization: Geneva, Switzerland, 2022. Available online: https://polioeradication.org/wp-content/uploads/2022/07/WHO-Global-Action-Plan-for-Poliovirus-Containment-GAPIV.pdf (accessed on 1 January 2024).
77. Shimizu, H. Development and introduction of inactivated poliovirus vaccines derived from Sabin strains in Japan. *Vaccine* **2016**, *34*, 1975–1985. [CrossRef]
78. Available online: https://www.thelancet.com/cms/10.1016/j.lanwpc.2021.100133/attachment/8c660f65-c236-4b2e-a8ba-1f6a42983adc/mmc4.pdf (accessed on 1 January 2024).
79. World Health Assembly. Resolutions and Decisions. WHA61.1. Poliomyelitis: Mechanism for management of potential risks to eradication. In Proceedings of the Sixty-First World Health Assembly, Geneva, Switzerland, 19–24 May 2008; pp. 1–2.
80. Sutter, R.W.; Okayasu, H.; Kieny, M.P. Next generation inactivated poliovirus vaccine: The future has arrived. *Clin. Infect. Dis.* **2017**, *64*, 1326–1327. [CrossRef]
81. Okayasu, H.; Sein, C.; Hamidi, A.; Bakker, W.A.; Sutter, R.W. Development of inactivated poliovirus vaccine from Sabin strains: A progress report. *Biologicals* **2016**, *44*, 581–587. [CrossRef] [PubMed]
82. United Nations Children's Fund. Available online: https://www.unicef.org/supply/media/17981/file/IPV-vaccine-prices-17-07-2023.pdf (accessed on 1 January 2024).
83. Cheng, L.; Wang, Y.; Du, J. Human Papillomavirus Vaccines: An Updated Review. *Vaccines* **2020**, *8*, 391. [CrossRef]
84. Fox, H.; Knowlson, S.; Minor, P.D.; Macadam, A.J. Genetically Thermo-Stabilised, Immunogenic Poliovirus Empty Capsids; a Strategy for Non-replicating Vaccines. *PLoS Pathog.* **2017**, *13*, e1006117. [CrossRef]
85. Marsian, J.; Fox, H.; Bahar, M.W.; Kotecha, A.; Fry, E.E.; Stuart, D.I.; Macadam, A.J.; Rowlands, D.J.; Lomonossoff, G.P. Plant-made polio type 3 stabilized VLPs—A candidate synthetic polio vaccine. *Nat. Commun.* **2017**, *8*, 245. [CrossRef]
86. Bahar, M.W.; Porta, C.; Fox, H.; Macadam, A.J.; Fry, E.E.; Stuart, D.I. Mammalian expression of virus-like particles as a proof of principle for next generation polio vaccines. *npj Vaccines* **2021**, *6*, 5. [CrossRef]

87. Bahar, M.W.; Nasta, V.; Fox, H.; Sherry, L.; Grehan, K.; Porta, C.; Macadam, A.J.; Stonehouse, N.J.; Rowlands, D.J.; Fry, E.E.; et al. A conserved glutathione binding site in poliovirus is a target for antivirals and vaccine stabilisation. *Commun. Biol.* **2022**, *5*, 1293. [CrossRef]
88. Adeyemi, O.O.; Nicol, C.; Stonehouse, N.J.; Rowlands, D.J. Increasing type 1 poliovirus capsid stability by thermal selection. *J. Virol.* **2017**, *91*, e01586-16. [CrossRef]
89. Sherry, L.; Grehan, K.; Snowden, J.S.; Knight, M.L.; Adeyemi, O.O.; Rowlands, D.J.; Stonehouse, N.J. Comparative molecular biology approaches for the production of Poliovirus Virus-Like Particles using *Pichia pastoris*. *mSphere* **2020**, *5*, e00838-19. [CrossRef] [PubMed]
90. Sherry, L.; Grehan, K.; Swanson, J.J.; Bahar, M.W.; Porta, C.; Fry, E.E.; Stuart, D.I.; Rowlands, D.J.; Stonehouse, N.J. Production and characterisation of stabilised PV-3 Virus-like Particles using *Pichia pastoris*. *Viruses* **2022**, *14*, 2159. [CrossRef] [PubMed]
91. Sherry, L.; Swanson, J.J.; Grehan, K.; Xu, H.; Uchida, M.; Jones, I.M.; Stonehouse, N.J.; Rowlands, D.J. Protease-independent production of Poliovirus Virus-like Particles in Pichia pastoris: Implications for efficient vaccine development and Insights into capsid assembly. *Microbiol. Spectr.* **2023**, *11*, e0430022. [CrossRef]
92. Clements, J.D.; Norton, E.B. The Mucosal Vaccine Adjuvant LT(R192G/L211A) or dmLT. *mSphere* **2018**, *3*, e00215-18. [CrossRef] [PubMed]
93. Knowlson, S.; Burlison, J.; Giles, E.; Fox, H.; Macadam, A.J.; Minor, P.D. New strains intended for the production of Inactivated Polio Vaccine at low-containment after eradication. *PLoS Pathog.* **2015**, *11*, e1005316. [CrossRef] [PubMed]
94. World Health Organization. CAG-TC3-20180630-EN.pdf. Available online: https://polioeradication.org/ (accessed on 1 January 2024).
95. World Health Organization. Polio vaccines: WHO position paper—June 2022. *Wkly. Epidemiol. Rec.* **2022**, *97*, 277–300.

pathogens

MDPI

Review

Novel Oral Polio Vaccine Type 2 Use for Polio Outbreak Response: A Global Effort for a Global Health Emergency

Feyrouz Damji Kurji [1], Ananda Sankar Bandyopadhyay [2,*], Simona Zipursky [2], Laura V. Cooper [3], Chris Gast [4], Margaret Toher [4], Ralf Clemens [5], Sue Ann Costa Clemens [6], Rayasam Prasad [2] and Adriansjah Azhari [7]

1 FDK Consulting, LLC, Watford WD17 1HP, UK; feyrouz@fdkconsult.com
2 Bill & Melinda Gates Foundation, Seattle, WA 98109, USA; simona.zipursky@gatesfoundation.org (S.Z.); ray.prasad@gatesfoundation.org (R.P.)
3 MRC Centre for Global Infectious Disease Analysis, School of Public Health, Imperial College London, London SW7 2BX, UK; l.cooper@imperial.ac.uk
4 Center for Vaccine Innovation and Access, PATH, Seattle, WA 98121, USA; cgast@path.org (C.G.); mtoher@path.org (M.T.)
5 International Vaccine Institute IVI, Seoul 08826, Republic of Korea
6 Institute for Global Health, Siena University, 53100 Siena, Italy; sueannclemens@outlook.com
7 PT Bio Farma, Kota Bandung 40161, Indonesia; adriansjah@biofarma.co.id
* Correspondence: ananda.bandyopadhyay@gatesfoundation.org

Abstract: A sharp rise in circulating vaccine-derived poliovirus type 2 (cVDPV2) outbreaks in the years following the cessation of routine use of poliovirus type 2-containing oral polio vaccine and the trend of seeding new emergences with suboptimal vaccination response during the same time-period led to the accelerated development of the novel oral polio vaccine type 2 (nOPV2), a vaccine with enhanced genetic stability and lower likelihood of reversion to neuroparalytic variants compared to its Sabin counterpart. In November 2020, nOPV2 became the first vaccine to be granted an Emergency Use Listing (EUL) by the World Health Organization (WHO) Prequalification Team (PQT), allowing close to a billion doses to be used by countries within three years after its first rollout and leading to full licensure and WHO prequalification (PQ) in December 2023. The nOPV2 development process exemplifies how scientific advances and innovative tools can be applied to combat global health emergencies in an urgent and adaptive way, building on a collaborative effort among scientific, regulatory and implementation partners and policymakers across the globe.

Keywords: poliovirus; novel oral poliovirus vaccine; emergency use listing; WHO prequalification; vaccine; public health emergency of international concern

1. Introduction

The novel oral polio vaccine type 2 (nOPV2) was the first vaccine to be granted an Emergency Use Listing (EUL) by the World Health Organization (WHO) Prequalification Team (PQT) in November 2020, leading eventually to full licensure by the Indonesian regulatory authority (Badan POM) and WHO prequalification (PQ) in December 2023 [1]. The first successful use of a unique clinical development and regulatory pathway and the subsequent massive rollout of nOPV2 have had a meaningful impact on the global polio eradication effort: use of the vaccine under the EUL from March 2021 to December 2023 allowed for the administration of approximately one billion doses of nOPV2 across 35 countries [1]. Throughout this period, the enhanced genetic stability of nOPV2 was demonstrated, a key feature of its design, compared with Sabin oral polio vaccine (OPV).

OPVs induce primary intestinal mucosal immunity to reduce replication of polioviruses in the gut when subsequently exposed to the virus, making their use in outbreak scenarios an important tool in halting poliovirus transmission. However, in rare circumstances, OPV strains can revert to virulence, causing paralysis in vaccine recipients and close contacts, a phenomenon known as vaccine-associated paralytic poliomyelitis (VAPP). Moreover, OPVs can revert following replication in the human gut and lose key attenuating mutations in the process, leading to the generation of vaccine-derived polioviruses (VDPVs). In areas with persistently low vaccination coverage, such revertant OPV strains can propagate from person to person and generate circulating vaccine-derived polioviruses (cVDPVs), which have regained the transmissibility properties of wild polioviruses and thus can cause outbreaks of paralytic disease. Outbreaks from wild polioviruses and cVDPVs are indistinguishable. The determining factors of the scale and impact of polio outbreaks are affected by differences in the underlying factors in the sub-populations where outbreaks occur, such as background immunity, population density, and the status of sanitation and hygiene. In addition, based on the primary serotype associated with the polio outbreak, the proportion of paralytic cases might vary, with type 1 being the most paralytic strain and type 2 the least [2]. Wild type 2 and wild type 3 polioviruses were certified to be eradicated in 2015 and 2019, respectively, once indigenous transmission of these viruses had been interrupted globally, according to criteria followed by the global certification committee for polio eradication.

The strategy of responding to cVDPV type 2 (cVDPV2)—the leading cause of cVDPV outbreaks globally—with Sabin OPV type 2 (OPV2), in monovalent (mOPV2) or trivalent (tOPV) formulations, has been largely successful in stopping transmission; however, due to the inherent genetic instability of Sabin strains and waning population immunity following the global cessation of the routine use of OPV2 since April 2016, an increasing number of new cVDPV2 outbreaks are attributable to OPV2 use [3]. While inactivated poliovirus vaccine (IPV) used in routine immunization and occasionally in outbreak response protects against paralytic disease from type 2 polioviruses, it provides limited primary intestinal mucosal immunity necessary to stop outbreaks of cVDPV2 [4,5]. Therefore, the idea of an OPV with enhanced genetic stability at key primary attenuation sites and with lower risk of reversion to paralytic and outbreak-inducing forms has long been considered a potential game changer for achieving and sustaining eradication of all forms of polioviruses.

2. nOPV2 Development

Early work for nOPV2 development began in 2011 with a scientific consortium convened by the Bill & Melinda Gates Foundation (BMGF) to address the risk of cVDPV and VAPP associated with the use of Sabin OPVs. The primary objective of the consortium was to develop a genetically modified vaccine that is as effective immunologically and as affordable as the Sabin OPV but has lower risk of reversion to neurovirulent forms, with an aim to minimize the risk of VAPP and to limit the rate of seeding of new outbreaks of cVDPV. Researchers from the National Institute for Biological Standards and Controls (NIBSC) in the United Kingdom, the US Centers for Disease Control and Prevention (US CDC), the US Food and Drug Administration (US FDA), and the University of California at San Francisco (UCSF) were the primary constituents of the consortium that collaborated to design, produce, and test several novel OPV strains in a variety of pre-clinical studies.

To increase the genetic stability of the vaccine, modifications were made to targeted sites on the vaccine strain's genome. Some of the final, key modifications are listed in Figure 1, depicting the rationale behind the changes in selected nOPV2 candidates [6,7].

The vaccine was designed to preserve its fitness and immunogenicity. Individual genetic modifications contributed to the genetic stability and attenuation of the vaccine. In addition, their combination prevented detectable reversion to neurovirulence by reducing the capacity of the virus to acquire mutations that increase replication fitness in neuronal tissues [6].

In September 2015, wild poliovirus type 2 (WPV2) was certified as eradicated, leading to the withdrawal of OPV2 from routine immunization programs in April 2016. Following this, the use, study, and production of all type 2 polioviruses had to be completed under WHO Global Action Plan (GAP) III containment guidelines, which imposed restrictions such as limiting the handling and storing of polioviruses to only poliovirus-essential facilities [8]. Based on the GAP III restrictions and given that the nOPV2 candidates were not available for clinical evaluation before April 2016, additional measures were needed to study nOPV2 candidates. Anticipating these complexities, prior to the cessation of routine use of OPV2, several organizations from around the world partnered to rapidly plan and implement studies with Sabin OPVs, which would serve as historical control trials once nOPV2 preclinical development was complete. Primary study partners for phase I–II clinical trials included the University of Antwerp, Fighting Infectious Disease in Emerging Countries (FIDEC), Vaxtrials, CEVAXIN, International Centre for Diarrhoeal Disease Research, Bangladesh (icddr,b), and Assign, among others. Lab partners for sample evaluation included the US CDC, ViroClinics, and Dartmouth College [9]. An independent Data and Safety Monitoring Board (DSMB), with representation from global experts from different fields, monitored the safety findings of the EUL-informing studies. PATH sponsored the phase III clinical trial, partnering with Medical Research Council (MRC) Unit—The Gambia, and assisted with regulatory interactions, dossier preparation and coordination of the integrated product development efforts [10].

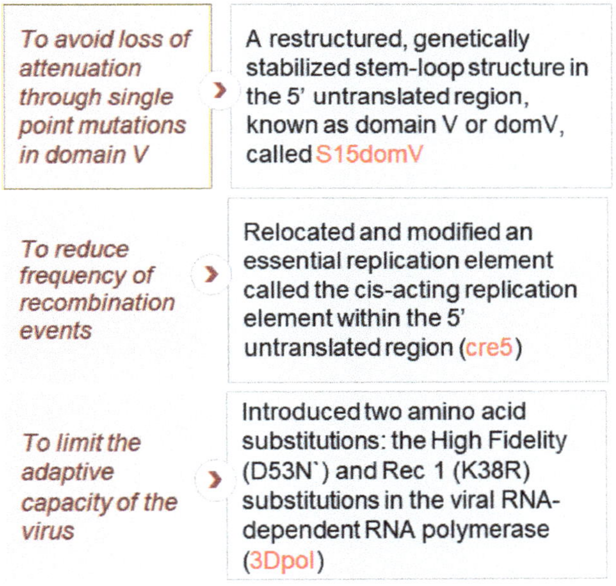

Figure 1. Modifications made to the Sabin Oral Polio Vaccine Type 2 virus genome to design novel Oral Polio Vaccine Type 2.

To comply with policy and regulatory requirements in the years following the global cessation of OPV and to avoid any accidental environmental release, the first-in-human study with nOPV2 was conducted in a fully contained, purpose-built facility named Poliopolis in Antwerp, Belgium, thereby ensuring that all biological samples potentially containing vaccine virus could be contained for subsequent decontamination [11]. This purpose-built unit was created through a collaborative effort across clinical and administrative staff at the University of Antwerp along with the local municipality and government as well as global stakeholders. The subsequent clinical trials with nOPV2 in Belgium and Panama that were conducted outside of contained settings closely mimicked the historical OPV2 control trials, as they were conducted at the same sites with the same investigators using the same protocol and procedures as the prior historic control studies with OPV2 [12–14]. This strategy was agreed upon with the relevant regulatory authorities prior to the initiation of the studies. Sites and countries were selected based on the feasibility of conducting the OPV studies in a timeframe relevant for developing a response tool for a Public Health Emergency of International Concern (PHEIC) and on assessment of a minimal risk of exposure of study volunteers to local poliovirus transmission, among other factors, to generate robust immunogenicity data. The regulatory authorities of the countries where clinical trials of nOPV2 were conducted played a key role in enabling the use of the study vaccines and related requirements for data collection, surveillance, and monitoring. Data from the phase I and phase II clinical studies in Belgium and Panama contributed to the selection of one of the two initially evaluated nOPV2 candidates and informed the eventual regulatory pathway [12–14].

3. Regulatory Pathway

In January 2020, the WHO published the EUL procedure, replacing the former Emergency Use Assessment and Listing (EUAL), which had been established in response to the Ebola outbreak of 2014–2016. The purpose of the EUL is to streamline access to unlicensed products through a risk-based assessment during public health emergencies [15]. The issuance of a WHO EUL is contingent on the vaccine first receiving an emergency use authorization (EUA) from the regulatory agency of record, usually the country in which the vaccine is produced. For nOPV2, which is manufactured by PT Bio Farma, the relevant regulatory agency is Badan POM (BPOM) in Indonesia.

In order to be eligible for an EUL, there are several criteria that must be met, including that the disease that the product is intended to treat or prevent is serious or life threatening, with the potential for outbreaks, epidemics, or pandemics, and that the existing products have not been able to eradicate or prevent the outbreaks. Given the sharp increase in cVDPV2 cases and outbreaks in 2019 and the risk of seeding additional outbreaks with continued OPV2 use in suboptimal quality response campaigns, nOPV2 was identified as a prime candidate for the EUL pathway. Further, without an EUL, nOPV2 would not be available for use until at least 2023–2024, following the availability of phase III clinical trial data for review of a marketing authorization and PQ dossier.

A dossier for an EUA and EUL was submitted to BPOM and the WHO, respectively, on 28 February 2020; an EUA was granted by BPOM on 12 November 2020, and an EUL was granted by the WHO on 13 November 2020, approximately three years from the time the first-in-human study was completed with nOPV2. nOPV2 was the first vaccine ever to receive EUL authorization.

Obtaining the EUL ahead of the completion of the phase III clinical study allowed nearly one billion doses of nOPV2 to be used over a span of nearly three years before the WHO prequalification of the vaccine. Following the completion of the phase III clinical trial at the MRC Unit—The Gambia, a dossier for marketing authorization and prequalification was submitted to BPOM and the WHO, respectively, in March 2023. nOPV2 was licensed in Indonesia on 23 December 2023, and on 27 December 2023, nOPV2 was prequalified by the WHO [1].

4. Policy Framework

In February 2020, the WHO Executive Board issued a decision that called on the WHO Director-General (DG) to accelerate the assessment and rollout of nOPV2 [16]. This decision urged Member States to implement an expedited process for national approval of the importation and use of vaccines to respond to polio outbreaks, including nOPV2, on the basis of its anticipated EUL authorization, which included careful and rigorous analysis of available quality, safety and efficacy data. This decision paved the way for prioritization of nOPV2 review under the EUL pathway and was a powerful tool for advocating for countries to prepare proactively for nOPV2 use in case of need.

Engagement with the Strategic Advisory Group of Experts to the WHO (SAGE) provided the policy framework for nOPV2 development. Early on, as the EUL pathway was being advanced, the Global Polio Eradication Initiative (GPEI) sought SAGE's endorsement of a phased rollout framework. The development of this framework (Figure 2) became a key feature of the risk mitigation approach under the EUL: the vaccine was first used under an 'Initial Use' phase, where countries had to meet a more stringent set of readiness verification requirements, followed by a 'Wider Use' phase, with fewer requirements.

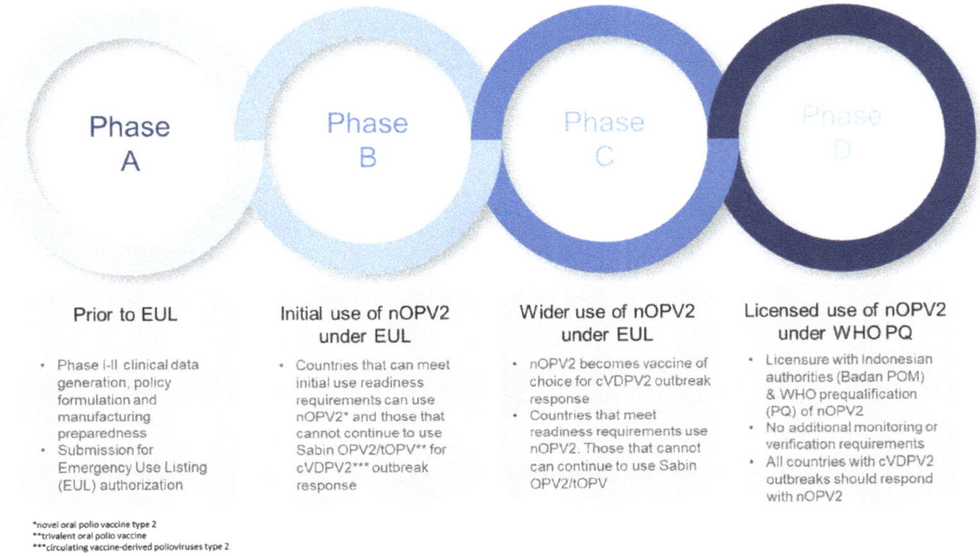

Figure 2. nOPV2 usage framework (endorsed by the Strategic Advisory Group of Experts to the WHO).

While a range of additional data on genetic stability and effectiveness were collected and analysis was done to comply with EUL commitments, the determining factor for the recommendation to move beyond initial use was the absence of any concerning signals emerging from the analysis of safety data. SAGE made its recommendation on the basis of nOPV2 meeting safety milestones as assessed by a dedicated nOPV2 subcommittee established by the Global Advisory Committee on Vaccine Safety (GACVS).

More broadly, the independent review and guidance by SAGE were important for national acceptance and independent technical validation of the roll-out approach. Based on the available data and analysis, SAGE issued recommendations regarding nOPV2 use, which included endorsement for the clinical development of nOPV2, guidance on policies of nOPV2 use, and advice on phases of use under the EUL. SAGE also reviewed clinical and epidemiologic data and provided guidance on issues such as vaccine choice (nOPV2 vs. mOPV2 or tOPV), co-administration of nOPV2 with IPV, other parenterally administered childhood vaccines and interventions, and other OPV vaccines. Importantly, SAGE reiterated the importance of timely and high-quality campaign responses for vaccines to be most effective as outbreak response tools.

Under the EUL, governments of countries using nOPV2 chose to do so based on their own decision-making criteria; both national regulatory approval and documentation of a national decision (i.e., from a National Immunization Technical Advisory Group or the Ministry of Health) was required to be submitted as part of the readiness verification process. Regional and national decision making was supported by global guidance as well as the provision of regularly updated technical data and analysis. Thirty-five countries used nOPV2 during the EUL period (Figure 3). The majority of nOPV2 doses were used in Nigeria (approximately 500 million), followed by the Democratic Republic of the Congo (DRC) (approximately 68 million) [1].

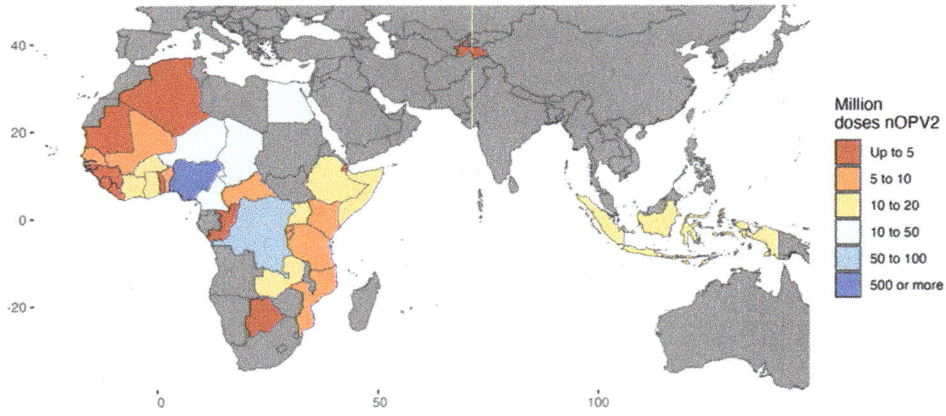

Figure 3. Scale of novel Oral Polio Vaccine Type 2 use for outbreak response under Emergency Use Listing authorization (between 1 March 2021 and 31 December 2023).

5. Country Readiness for Deployment and De-Risking Supply

As with all OPV type 2 vaccines following the global switch in April 2016, nOPV2 is only available through a global stockpile under the oversight and release authority of the WHO DG. Given the monitoring requirements of the EUL, countries had to be verified for readiness to use nOPV2 prior to the DG's release of the vaccine; those who did not meet these requirements could instead use OPV2, which was also available in the global stockpile. In the initial use phase, countries had to meet 25 readiness verification requirements across the seven areas referenced below, including meeting baseline thresholds for surveillance system performance. In its wider-use phase, there were no surveillance thresholds to meet, and the number of readiness requirements decreased to 16 across the same seven areas:

Coordination
Approvals (regulatory and national decision making)
Cold Chain and Vaccine Management (VM)
Surveillance
Safety
Advocacy, Communications, and Social Mobilization (ACSM)
Laboratories

5.1. Country Readiness

Countries were supported through the verification process jointly by WHO and UNICEF regional offices and nOPV2 regional (and, in some cases, country) focal points as well as a global readiness verification team. National Regulatory Authorities (NRAs) in countries where nOPV2 was used also contributed to the review of the vaccine and subsequent use of data under the EUL. The verification of requirements was conducted by GPEI subject matter experts and took place at both global and regional levels, depending on the requirement, and was overseen and coordinated at a global level. Countries were verified for nOPV2 use after all requirements were met. Verification was a one-time occurrence; once a country received verification, it could request nOPV2 during its EUL phase as needed in the future, without needing to go through the readiness verification process again.

Communications materials were developed to create a common understanding of nOPV2 development, processes, requirements, and rollout and provide technical content for those planning for and using the vaccine, with the intent of aligning technical and external communications. Multilingual guidance was developed to explain the process in general as well as to implement activities in each specific technical area. Materials were available for a range of stakeholders—from technical staff to ministers—in all key languages and were updated regularly. All information was available on a dedicated nOPV2 page within the GPEI website, including links to nOPV2-related SAGE and GACVS meeting summaries and recommendations, advocacy tools, and summaries of clinical development. GPEI partners held regular webinars and published an internal bulletin at a two-monthly interval, to share the latest findings for key GPEI staff. The WHO and UNICEF engaged at regional and country levels to support country decision making and planning for the use of nOPV2.

5.2. De-Risking Supply

One important element of preparation for nOPV2 use was early planning for supply of the vaccine. PT Bio Farma's initial production was achieved through direct funding from the Gates Foundation for "at-risk" production of millions of doses. This forward-thinking action was critical in ensuring that the vaccine was available as soon as the EUL was granted, through a United Nations Children's Fund (UNICEF) tender on behalf of GPEI for services to produce drug substances and finished products, including storing and managing a global stockpile. The manufacturer of nOPV2, PT Bio Farma, was responsible for producing and supplying all nOPV2 for the EUL period. To bolster the stability of the nOPV2 supply, a second manufacturer was subsequently identified, and as of early 2024, the process for review of the dossier for WHO prequalification of the second supplier was initiated. Despite the early planning and implementation of contingency measures around supply, there have been disruptions in global supplies of the vaccine due to a variety of reasons, which include supply chain challenges during the COVID-19 pandemic, occasional technical issues at the manufacturing facility, and increasing demand for the vaccine given the expansion of cVDPV2 outbreaks. A consistent and adequate supply of the vaccine remains a critical priority of the program to decisively interrupt ongoing cVDPV2 outbreaks.

6. Surveillance and Risk Mitigation

An EUL requires enhanced post-deployment monitoring of the vaccine. If quality or safety issues are identified during field use, or data gaps make monitoring results unreliable, the EUL procedure allows for the WHO to revoke the EUL recommendation. For nOPV2, these commitments included ongoing monitoring and assessment of the vaccine's safety, genetic stability, and effectiveness, along with ensuring country systems were ready to detect and respond to any unanticipated findings. These commitments were outlined in the risk management plan (RMP), which was submitted to and accepted by Indonesian regulators and the WHO PQ as part of the EUL review process. While monitoring requirements vary by vaccine, unique factors to the nOPV2 EUL risk–benefit analysis included the fact that there was already a licensed polio vaccine (Sabin OPV2) to target type 2 outbreaks, that the vaccine would be used only for outbreak response (limited lead times to set up additional surveillance, i.e., sentinel surveillance sites), and that the countries most likely to use the vaccine were often those with complex field-level challenges (i.e., DRC, Nigeria, Yemen).

One of the key benefits for which nOPV2 was designed is its enhanced genetic stability compared with Sabin OPV2. Therefore, a key commitment under the EUL was to conduct intensive genetic stability analysis, including whole genome sequencing of isolates, which were reviewed on a regular basis, with findings summarized in initial monthly and subsequent quarterly reports. Samples evaluated in this pipeline came from the stool specimens of acute flaccid paralysis (AFP) cases and their contacts as well as environmental surveillance and also from cases of primary immunodeficiency involving long-term excretion of nOPV2. The whole genome sequencing was conducted by laboratories within GPEI's Global Polio Laboratory Network (GPLN). A classification scheme was developed to categorize the results of the whole genome sequencing of isolates with respect to their relative level of concern regarding virulence [17].

Assays specific to the detection of nOPV2 were developed well in advance of nOPV2 use, and training was conducted at labs within the GPLN. To manage the number of poliovirus type 2 (PV2) isolates being sent to whole genome sequencing labs, a prioritization framework was put into place. Laboratory partners performed critical testing and analysis across a range of areas. The US CDC supported preclinical and clinical testing and analysis in support of nOPV2 studies. Once the EUL was in place, the US CDC, NIBSC, Institut Pasteur, and the Dutch National Institute for Public Health and the Environment (RIVM) performed whole genome sequencing on field isolates. The US CDC and NIBSC led the genetic characterization analysis and reporting effort, which was critical for compliance with EUL requirements and for understanding the new vaccine's genetic characteristics in field use. These results were reviewed and discussed in a dedicated expert subgroup within the GPEI. Membership included PATH and a range of subject-matter experts in addition to GPEI partner agencies, who supported these efforts by providing context from the clinical development as well as recommendations for regulatory reporting.

Countries planning to use nOPV2 under an EUL were required to meet additional safety monitoring requirements and submit their data for consolidation at the global level, to ensure no concerning signals were missed. The GACVS Subcommittee on nOPV2 safety conducted periodic reviews of the safety data and analysis provided by countries using nOPV2 in order to provide an independent assessment of safety data emerging from countries during the EUL period. Through these reviews, the committee determined the presence or absence of any safety red flags and provided regular updates to both the full GACVS and SAGE, with summary reports published on the GPEI nOPV2 webpage.

Prior to the rollout of nOPV2, a number of possible conditions, designated as adverse events of special interest (AESIs), were identified, which constituted "safety signals" (Figure 4). To detect these, all countries using nOPV2 in the initial phases had to conduct active AESI surveillance as well as the standard adverse events following immunization (AEFI) surveillance. Over time, as the safety profile of nOPV2 became better characterized, it was noted by the GACVS that AFP surveillance formed the backbone of safety surveillance, as it captured conditions that were most likely to be related to AESIs from nOPV2 [18]. As such, in February 2022, the GACVS Subcommittee on nOPV2 Safety updated its guidance to note that active AESI surveillance [18] for nOPV2 safety was recommended but not required for countries without sufficient technical capacity and human resources to implement the active AESI protocol, thereby paving the way for additional countries to access the vaccine.

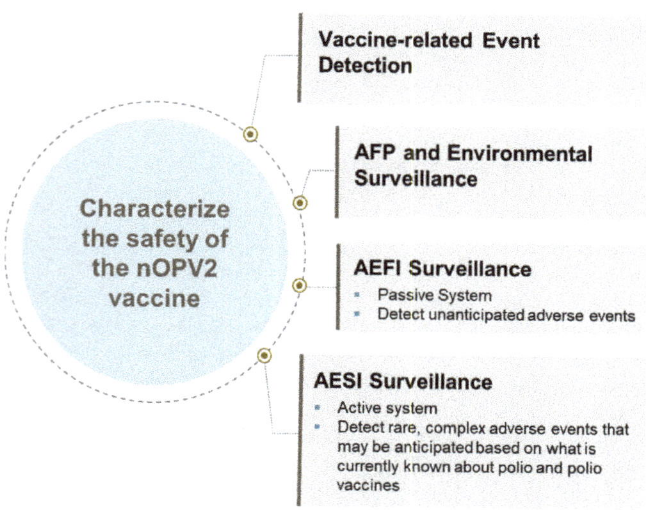

Figure 4. Safety monitoring framework.

As the manufacturer of nOPV2, PT Bio Farma held accountability for meeting requirements for deployment under the EUL, and now under the PQ. Given the unique and complex nature of the commitments required under the EUL, the GPEI has supported PT Bio Farma in the funding, coordination, and implementation of these activities. In November 2019, the GPEI established a time-limited working group, the 'nOPV Working Group' (nOPV WG), to support PT Bio Farma in developing and implementing a monitoring plan to comply with requirements for the anticipated use of nOPV2 for outbreak response (Figure 5). The Working Group included representatives from all GPEI partners in its core group and established expert subgroups to guide key areas of work that would need to be implemented under the unique EUL conditions. Where technical groups already existed under the GPEI, the Working Group drew on the expertise of liaisons to these groups rather than establishing duplicative subgroups. The nOPV WG will sunset in 2024 based on the end of EUL use of the vaccine and the transition to being a WHO pre-qualified vaccine in December 2023.

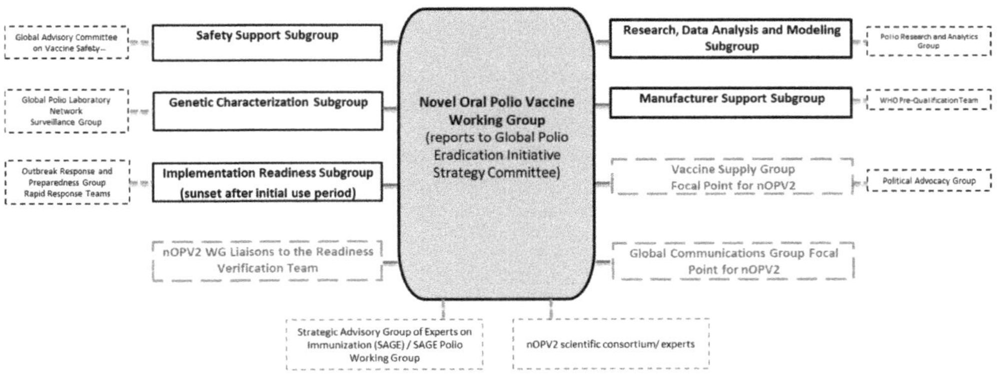

Figure 5. Novel Oral Polio Vaccine Working Group of Global Polio Eradication Initiative.

7. Assessment of Vaccine Effectiveness

The EUL for nOPV2 also required generating an evidence base regarding nOPV2 effectiveness in outbreak control. Evaluation of effectiveness in geographic regions eligible for outbreak response with nOPV2 presented significant challenges, given the lack of infrastructure in certain geographies to execute traditional vaccine effectiveness assessment studies. nOPV2 effectiveness in the field was assessed through multiple analytic methods: (1) interrupted time-series analysis, (2) time-Susceptible-Infectious-Recovered (tSIR) model-based analysis [19], and (3) a case–control study [20]. Because of their differing methodologies, each study required different types of data to assess different measures of nOPV2 effectiveness when used in outbreak response campaigns. Together, the results of these studies provided an understanding of the effectiveness of nOPV2 in the field during the EUL period.

The objective of nOPV2 development was to enhance the genetic stability of the existing vaccine while maintaining comparable effectiveness and safety to OPV2. Field and clinical data continue to support the enhanced genetic stability of nOPV2. Most nOPV2 isolates from AFP and environmental surveillance following supplementary immunization activities (SIAs) analyzed through whole genome sequencing indicate no or minimal changes in the genetic structure of nOPV2, while approximately 3% (as of September 2023) showed evidence of losing key stabilizing genetic modifications at domain V of the vaccine virus genome, compared with an expected 75% for mOPV2 [21]. A subset of these reverted strains led to 13 new cVDPV2 emergences, impacting 14 countries, as of February 2024. While any new emergence of cVDPV2 is a matter of serious concern, modelling assessment suggests that the risk of seeding cVDPV2 emergences following SIAs with nOPV2 is substantially reduced relative to SIAs with Sabin OPV2 [22]. Moreover, the primary mechanism of nOPV2 to revert to neurovirulent cVDPV2 strains, as demonstrated from the field data, is through a double recombination pathway that necessitates concurrent enterovirus infection in the gut, whereas with OPV2, single recombination events and point mutations can also lead to the generation of neurovirulent strains.

Data from field use and clinical trials support the hypothesis that nOPV2 would have similar immunogenicity and effectiveness to OPV2. Although findings of reduced immunogenicity of nOPV2 in young children when co-administered with bOPV indicated that nOPV2 may be less robust to competition with other enteroviruses in the gut [23], a study in the Gambia demonstrated excellent seroconversion in infants and young children (63% post-dose 1 in infants seronegative at baseline [n = 499], 65% in children [n = 66]), at levels comparable to those observed in an mOPV2 trial in a similar setting in Mozambique (68% in children seronegative at baseline [n = 75]) [10,24]. In addition, two in-depth studies comparing mOPV2 and nOPV2 effectiveness in Nigeria, which experienced a large cVDPV2 outbreak in 2021 and used the most nOPV2 of any country, found no significant difference between the two vaccines used in outbreak response campaigns [19,20]. Both nOPV2 and OPV2 campaigns were found to be highly effective in reducing transmission of cVDPV2. As noted, results from nOPV2 use in the field are consistent with the comparable individual immunogenicity of nOPV2 and mOPV2 found in clinical trials. More broadly, surveillance data suggest there is no substantial difference in the number of SIAs required to interrupt cVDPV2 transmission between nOPV2 and mOPV2 (Figure 6), with a few countries such as DRC and Nigeria requiring three or more SIAs to interrupt transmission irrespective of vaccine choice, and most countries achieving interruption with fewer than three SIAs.

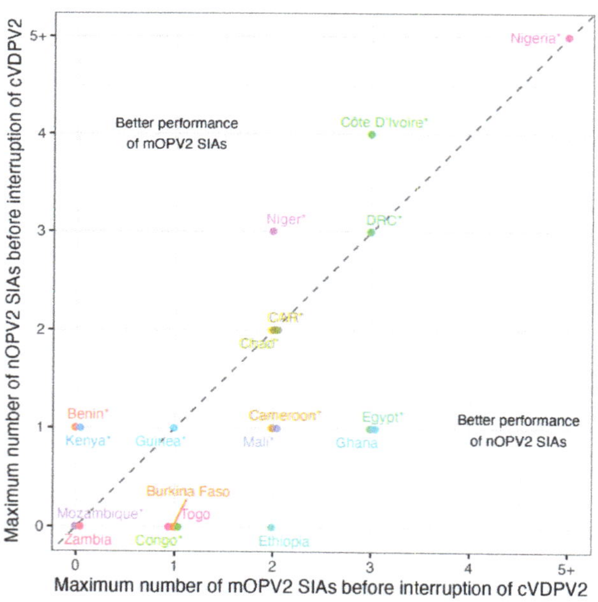

Figure 6. Maximum number of monovalent oral polio vaccine type 2 (mOPV2) or novel oral polio vaccine type 2 (nOPV2) supplementary immunization activities (SIAs) before interruption of circulating vaccine-derived polioviruses type 2 (cVDPV2) transmission in 19 countries that have used both vaccines (excluding Somalia, which also used trivalent oral polio vaccine (tOPV)). Interruption of transmission is defined as 180 days with no detection of cVDPV2 in poliomyelitis cases or environmental surveillance. Data were downloaded on 5 Feb 2024 from the Polio Information System [25]. Asterisks (*) indicate countries where the most recent detection is within 180 days of the most recent surveillance data, so interruption cannot yet be confirmed.

8. Conclusions

The ultimate goal of the global polio eradication initiative is a world free from all forms of polioviruses. The development of nOPV2 is a significant advancement toward this audacious goal. Building on breakthroughs in genetic and vaccine science, and bringing together clinical, regulatory, and implementation partners, the nOPV2 development and rollout journey (Figure 7) is a shining example of a global collaboration to confront a public health emergency of international concern (PHEIC). Innovations in the clinical development of polio vaccines, such as conducting a phase I clinical trial in fully contained conditions, were matched with critical thinking on designing of the studies and development of novel assays to evaluate key study endpoints such as neurovirulence while maintaining the feasibility of the study population size. With countries from four out of six WHO regions joining the clinical development effort, it was a massive undertaking to generate data from different parts of the world with age groups ranging from adults to neonates, while effort was maintained to minimize interference on study endpoints from passive environmental exposure by avoiding trial sites in areas with ongoing polio outbreaks or with campaign use of OPVs [26]. Forward-looking decisions were taken on the manufacturing front to frontload production, with at-risk scaling up of production facilities at PT Bio Farma and with real-world innovations such as using a 50-dose vial to expand the availability of doses instead of the standard 20- or 10-dose vials. Consistent and planned communications with policymakers such as SAGE and independent expert groups such as GACVS ensured regular evaluation of the clinical and field data to inform and fine-tune use policies.

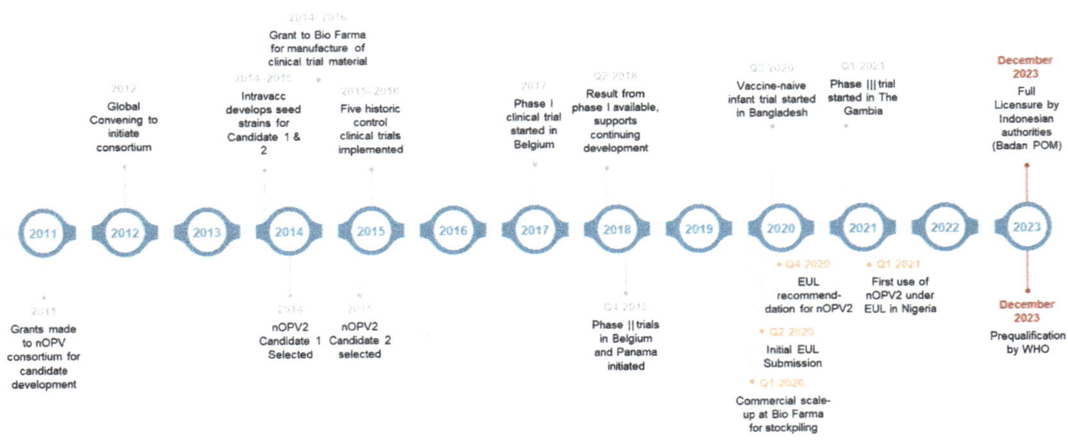

Figure 7. nOPV2: From idea generation to field use [adapted from 9].

However, advances on the innovation front alone will be insufficient to achieve complete eradication. The critical importance of timely, high-quality outbreak response and sufficient vaccination coverage remain central to the strategy for global eradication of all forms of polioviruses. The urgency and ambition that underpinned nOPV2 development allowed for it to be the first vaccine approved under the EUL pathway with close to a billion doses used by countries in less than three years from its first use. In the coming years, in addition to strengthening essential immunization coverage of two or more doses of IPV, considerations for the use of nOPV2 in broader, preventative campaigns or select use in routine immunization schedules in specific settings may have to be evaluated if cVDPV2 circulation persists. Finally, it will really be the act of reaching every child in underserved communities with sufficient frequency and urgency to stop the transmission of vaccine-derived polioviruses from all corners of the earth. The overall development effort should also pave the way for accelerated and adaptive pathways for introducing critical response tools for other public health emergencies of international concern. Affordability of these tools for scaled-up production and accessibility to vulnerable populations for immunization response will continue to hold the key for a meaningful public health impact, much like what we have seen with the polio eradication effort and nOPV2 experience.

Author Contributions: Conceptualization, A.S.B.; resources, F.D.K.; data curation, F.D.K., A.S.B. and L.V.C.; writing—original draft, F.D.K. and A.S.B.; writing—review and editing, F.D.K., A.S.B., S.Z., L.V.C., C.G., M.T., R.C., S.A.C.C., R.P. and A.A.; visualization, F.D.K. and L.V.C.; supervision, A.S.B. and S.Z. All authors have read and agreed to the published version of the manuscript.

Funding: This review article received no external funding.

Institutional Review Board Statement: Not applicable.

Informed Consent Statement: Not applicable.

Data Availability Statement: All data used in the article available through GPEI resources or published materials.

Acknowledgments: We acknowledge GPEI's nOPV Working Group Subgroup Leads and Liaisons, including Grace Macklin (WHO), Corey Peak (Bill & Melinda Gates Foundation), Cara C. Burns (CDC), Javier Martin (NIBSC), Ann Ottosen (UNICEF), Ian Lewis (UNICEF), Rissa Durham (Bill & Melinda Gates Foundation), Peter Dull (Bill & Melinda Gates Foundation), Harish Verma (WHO), Martin Eisenhawer (WHO), Joseph Swan (WHO), and the GPEI's nOPV Core Working Group, including Steven Oberste (CDC), Stephen Sosler (Gavi, the Vaccine Alliance), Concepcion Estivariz (CDC), Ondrej Mach (WHO), and Tunji Funsho (Rotary International). We thank Amy Weiner at the Bill & Melinda Gates Foundation for coordinating the initial work with the nOPV2 scientific consortium. We are grateful to John Konz, PATH, for helpful comments on the paper. We acknowledge the important role played by the nOPV2 clinical trial sponsors, clinical development and laboratory partners, and the nOPV2 scientific consortium. We thank colleagues at the polio, vaccine development, integrated development, and discovery and translational sciences teams at the Bill & Melinda Gates Foundation, GPEI task teams, WHO regional and country focal persons, the Global Polio Laboratory Network (GPLN), and the GPEI Strategy Committee. We thank Keith Veitch (keithveitch communications) for the assistance with manuscript formatting and editing.

Conflicts of Interest: The authors declare no conflicts of interest.

List of Acronyms and Abbreviations

AESIs	Adverse Events of Special Interest
AFP	Acute Flaccid Paralysis
bOPV	Bivalent Oral Polio Vaccine
BPOM	Badan POM (Indonesian Regulatory Authority)
cVDPV	Circulating Vaccine-derived Poliovirus
cVDPV2	Circulating Vaccine-derived Poliovirus type 2
DG	Director-General (of WHO)
DRC	Democratic Republic of the Congo
EUA	Emergency Use Authorization
EUAL	Emergency Use Assessment and Listing
EUL	Emergency Use Listing
GACVS	Global Advisory Committee on Vaccine Safety
GAP	Global Action Plan
GPEI	Global Polio Eradication Initiative
GPLN	Global Polio Laboratory Network
IPV	Inactivated Poliovirus Vaccine
mOPV2	Monovalent Oral Polio Vaccine type 2
MRC	Medical Research Council
NIBSC	National Institute for Biological Standards and Controls
nOPV	Novel Oral Polio Vaccine
nOPV2	Novel Oral Polio Vaccine type 2
nOPV WG	Novel Oral Polio Vaccine Working Group

OPV	Oral Polio Vaccine
OPV2	Oral Polio Vaccine type 2
PQ	Prequalification
PQT	Prequalification Team
SAGE	Strategic Advisory Group of Experts to the WHO
SIAs	Supplementary Immunization Activities
tOPV	Trivalent Oral Polio Vaccine
UNICEF	United Nations Children's Fund
US CDC	US Centers for Disease Control and Prevention
VAPP	Vaccine-associated Paralytic Poliomyelitis
VDPV	Vaccine-derived Poliovirus
WHO	World Health Organization
WPV2	Wild Poliovirus type 2

References

1. Bandyopadhyay, A.S.; Cooper, L.V.; Zipursky, S. One billion doses and WHO prequalification of nOPV2: Implications for the global polio situation and beyond. *PLoS Glob. Public Health* **2024**, *4*, e0002920. [CrossRef] [PubMed]
2. Nathanson, N.; Kew, O.M. From emergence to eradication: The epidemiology of poliomyelitis deconstructed. *Am. J. Epidemiol.* **2010**, *172*, 1213–1229. [CrossRef] [PubMed]
3. Macklin, G.R.; O'Reilly, K.M.; Grassly, N.C.; Edmunds, W.J.; Mach, O.; Krishnan, R.S.G.; Voorman, A.; Vertfeuille, J.F.; Abdelwahab, J.; Gumede, N.; et al. Evolving epidemiology of poliovirus serotype 2 following withdrawal of the serotype 2 oral poliovirus vaccine. *Science* **2020**, *368*, 401–405. [CrossRef] [PubMed]
4. Bandyopadhyay, A.S.; Rocio Lopez Cavestany, R.C.; Blake, I.M.; Macklin, G.; Cooper, L.; Grassly, N.; dos Santos Nery, A.L.M.; Mach, O. Use of inactivated poliovirus vaccine for poliovirus outbreak response. *Lancet Infect. Dis.* **2023**. [CrossRef] [PubMed]
5. Macklin, G.R.; Grassly, N.C.; Sutter, R.W.; Mach, O.; Bandyopadhyay, A.S.; Edmunds, W.J.; O'Reilly, K.M. Vaccine schedules and the effect on humoral and intestinal immunity against poliovirus: A systematic review and network meta-analysis. *Lancet Infect. Dis.* **2019**, *19*, 1121–1128. [CrossRef] [PubMed]
6. Yeh, M.T.; Bujaki, E.; Dolan, P.T.; Smith, M.; Wahid, R.; Konz, J.; Weiner, A.J.; Bandyopadhyay, A.S.; Van Damme, P.; De Coster, I.; et al. Engineering the live-attenuated polio vaccine to prevent reversion to virulence. *Cell Host Microbe* **2020**, *27*, 736–751.e8. [CrossRef] [PubMed]
7. Konopka-Anstadt, J.L.; Campagnoli, R.; Vincent, A.; Shaw, J.; Wei, L.; Wynn, N.T.; Smithee, S.E.; Bujaki, E.; Yeh, M.T.; Laassri, M.; et al. Development of a new oral poliovirus vaccine for the eradication end game using codon deoptimization. *NPJ Vaccines* **2020**, *5*, 26. [CrossRef] [PubMed]
8. WHO-GAP III. WHO Global Action Plan to Minimize Poliovirus Facility-Associated Risk after Type-Specific Eradication of Wild Polioviruses and Sequential Cessation of Oral Polio Vaccine Use. Available online: https://polioeradication.org/wp-content/uploads/2016/12/GAPIII_2014.pdf (accessed on 20 March 2024).
9. Macklin, G.R.; Peak, C.; Eisenhawer, M.; Kurji, F.; Mach, O.; Konz, J.; Gast, C.; Bachtiar, N.S.; Bandyopadhyay, A.S.; Zipursky, S. nOPV2 Working Group. Enabling accelerated vaccine roll-out for Public Health Emergencies of International Concern: Novel Oral Polio Vaccine type 2 Experience. *Vaccine* **2023**, *41* (Suppl. 1), A122–A127. [CrossRef] [PubMed]
10. Ochoge, M.; Futa, A.C.; Umesi, A.; Affleck, L.; Kotei, L.; Daffeh, B.; Saidy-Jah, E.; Njie, A.; Oyadiran, O.; Edem, B.; et al. Safety of the novel oral polio vaccine type 2 (nOPV2) in infants and young children aged 1 to <5 years and lot-to-lot consistency of the immune response to nOPV2 infants in The Gambia: A phase 3, double-blind, randomized controlled trial. *Lancet* **2024**. [CrossRef]
11. Van Damme, P.; De Coster, I.; Revets, H.; Bandyopadhyay, A.S. Poliopolis. *Lancet* **2019**, *394*, 115. [CrossRef] [PubMed]
12. Van Damme, P.; De Coster, I.; Bandyopadhyay, A.S.; Revets, H.; Withanage, K.; De Smedt, P.; Suykens, L.; Oberste, M.S.; Weldon, W.C.; Costa-Clemens, S.A.; et al. Safety and immunogenicity of two novel live attenuated monovalent (serotype 2) oral poliovirus vaccines in healthy adults: A double-blind, single-centre phase 1 study. *Lancet* **2019**, *394*, 148–158. [CrossRef] [PubMed]
13. De Coster, I.; Leroux-Roels, I.; Bandyopadhyay, A.S.; Gast, C.; Withanage, K.; Steenackers, K.; De Smedt, P.; Aerssens, A.; Leroux-Roels, G.; Oberste, M.S.; et al. Safety and immunogenicity of two novel type 2 oral poliovirus vaccine candidates compared with a monovalent type 2 oral poliovirus vaccine in healthy adults: Two clinical trials. *Lancet* **2021**, *397*, 39–50. [CrossRef] [PubMed]
14. Sáez-Llorens, X.; Bandyopadhyay, A.S.; Gast, C.; De Leion, T.; DeAntonio, R.; Jimeno, J.; Caballero, M.I.; Aquirre, G.; Oberste, M.S.; Weldon, W.C.; et al. Safety and immunogenicity of two novel type 2 oral poliovirus vaccine candidates compared with a monovalent type 2 oral poliovirus vaccine in children and infants: Two clinical trials. *Lancet* **2021**, *397*, 27–38. [CrossRef] [PubMed]
15. WHO. Regulation and Prequalification: Emergency Use Listing. Available online: https://www.who.int/teams/regulation-prequalification/eul (accessed on 16 February 2024).
16. WHO. Polio Eradication. 7 February 2020. EB146(11). Available online: https://apps.who.int/gb/ebwha/pdf_files/EB146/B146(11)-en.pdf (accessed on 16 February 2024).

17. Martin, J.; Burns, C.C.; Jorba, J.; Shulman, L.M.; Macadam, A.; Klapsa, D.; Majumdar, M.; Bullows, J.; Frolov, A.; Mate, R.; et al. Genetic characterization of novel oral polio vaccine type 2 viruses during initial use phase under Emergency Use Listing—Worldwide, March–October 2021. *MMWR. Morb. Mortal. Wkly. Rep.* **2022**, *71*, 786–790. [CrossRef] [PubMed]
18. Global Advisory Committee on Vaccine Safety Sub-Committee on nOPV2 Safety. Summary Note for the Record (21 February 2022). Available online: https://polioeradication.org/wp-content/uploads/2022/03/GACVS-sub-committee-on-nOPV2-Report-20220221.pdf (accessed on 16 February 2024).
19. Voorman, A.; Lyons, H.; Shuab, F.; Adamu, U.S.; Korir, C.; Erbeto, T.; Bandyopadhyay, A.S.; Okiror, S. Evaluation of novel oral polio vaccine type 2 SIA impact in a large outbreak of circulating vaccine-derived poliovirus in Nigeria. *J. Infect. Dis.* **2024**, *229*, 805–812. [CrossRef] [PubMed]
20. Cooper, L.V.; Erbeto, T.B.; Danzomo, A.A.; Abdullahi, H.W.; Boateng, K.; Adamu, U.S.; Shuaib, F.; Modjirom, N.; Gray, E.J.; Bandyopadhyay, A.S.; et al. Effectiveness of poliovirus vaccines against circulating vaccine-derived type 2 poliomyelitis in Nigeria between 2017 and 2022: A case-control study. *Lancet Infect. Dis.* **2024**, *24*, 427–436. [CrossRef] [PubMed]
21. Famulare, M.; Chang, S.; Iber, J.; Zhao, K.; Adeniji, J.A.; Bukbuk, D.; Baba, M.; Behrend, M.; Burns, C.C.; Oberste, M.S. Sabin vaccine reversion in the field: A comprehensive analysis of Sabin-like poliovirus isolates in Nigeria. *J. Virol.* **2015**, *90*, 317–331. [CrossRef] [PubMed]
22. Peak, C.; Lyons, H.; Voorman, A.; Cooper, L.; Hawes, K.; Bandyopadhyay, A. Monitoring the risk of type-2 circulating vaccine-derived poliovirus emergence during roll-out of type-2 novel oral polio vaccine. In Proceedings of the 9th International Conference on Infectious Disease Dynamics: P2.029, Bologna, Italy, 28 November–1 December 2023. Available online: https://ssrn.com/abstract=4654922 (accessed on 16 February 2024).
23. Wilkinson, A.L.; Zaman, K.; Hoque, M.; Estivariz, C.F.; Burns, C.C.; Konopka-Anstadt, J.L.; Mainou, B.A.; Kovacs, S.D.; An, Q.; Lickness, J.S.; et al. Immunogenicity of novel oral poliovirus vaccine type 2 administered concomitantly with bivalent oral poliovirus vaccine: An open-label, non-inferiority, randomised, controlled trial. *Lancet Infect. Dis.* **2023**, *23*, 1062–1071. [CrossRef] [PubMed]
24. de Deus, N.; Capitine, I.P.U.; Bauhofer, A.F.L.; Marques, S.; Cassocera, M.; Chissaque, A.; Bero, D.M.; Langa, J.P.; Padama, F.M.; Jeyaseelan, V.; et al. Immunogenicity of reduced-dose monovalent type 2 oral poliovirus vaccine in Mocuba, Mozambique. *J. Infect. Dis.* **2022**, *226*, 292–298. [CrossRef] [PubMed]
25. World Health Organization. Polio Information System. Available online: https://extranet.who.int/polis/public/CaseCount.aspx (accessed on 14 February 2024).
26. Bandyopadhyay, A.S.; Zipursky, S. nOPV2 development as a global effort for polio outbreak response. *Lancet Glob. Health* **2023**, *11*, e1695. [CrossRef] [PubMed]

pathogens

MDPI

Review

The Last Mile in Polio Eradication: Program Challenges and Perseverance

Rocio Lopez Cavestany *, Martin Eisenhawer, Ousmane M. Diop, Harish Verma, Arshad Quddus and Ondrej Mach

Polio Eradication, World Health Organization, 1202 Geneva, Switzerland; eisenhawerm@who.int (M.E.); diopo@who.int (O.M.D.); vermah@who.int (H.V.); quddusa@who.int (A.Q.); macho@who.int (O.M.)
* Correspondence: lopezro@who.int

Abstract: As the Global Polio Eradication Initiative (GPEI) strategizes towards the final steps of eradication, routine immunization schedules evolve, and high-quality vaccination campaigns and surveillance systems remain essential. New tools are consistently being developed, such as the novel oral poliovirus vaccine to combat outbreaks more sustainably, as well as non-infectiously manufactured vaccines such as virus-like particle vaccines to eliminate the risk of resurgence of polio on the eve of a polio-free world. As the GPEI inches towards eradication, re-strategizing in the face of evolving challenges and preparing for unknown risks in the post-certification era are critical.

Keywords: poliomyelitis; Global Polio Eradication Initiative; outbreak response; immunization; vaccine-derived poliovirus

1. Introduction

From the earliest believed documentation of polio c. the 1400s BC through a depiction on an Egyptian stele, it was not until the mid-19th century that the first systematic investigation of polio was conducted. The first records of large-scale polio epidemics began appearing in North America and Europe; only in the mid 20th century was it possible to confirm global poliovirus spread, which killed or paralyzed over half a million people every year [1].

The development of polio vaccination in the 1950s and 1960s was a turning point to begin controlling transmission and reducing the burden of disease. The inactivated poliovirus vaccine (IPV), containing formalin-killed virus, was developed by US physician Jonas Salk and licensed for use in 1955. Shortly after, the oral poliovirus vaccine (OPV), containing live-attenuated poliovirus, was developed by Polish American microbiologist Albert Sabin. IPV and OPV induce a strong humoral response capable of protecting the vaccinated individual; however, only the latter has an established role in inducing mucosal intestinal immunity, which is essential to block viral transmission, making it a necessary tool for eradication [2]. Each vaccine type has its own unique set of advantages and limitations; both continue to play an essential role in polio eradication to this day.

The impact of immunization was immediate; however, there was a geographical disparity in vaccine choice. Countries adopting IPV were largely confined to high-income settings due to the cost, required skill, and hygiene measures associated with injectable vaccines. Easily administered and accessible, OPV was the ideal candidate for use in lower-income settings for routine immunization or outbreak control. Independent of vaccine choice, the prevalence of low vaccination coverage in low-income and high-risk settings created a widening health divide, with the burden of disease shifting to areas in Africa and Asia with weak health and hygiene infrastructure.

Polio eradication later led by the Global Polio Eradication Initiative (GPEI) was launched in 1988 with the aim to eradicate poliomyelitis caused by poliovirus by 2000. This motivation followed smallpox eradication, one of the greatest successes in public health history, paving the way for polio as the second candidate for eradication. The

GPEI coordinates global, regional, and country-level interdisciplinary actions towards eradication of polioviruses. The partnership is led by six agencies (the WHO, CDC, Rotary, BMGF, Gavi, and UNICEF) working closely with countries, donors, foundations, NGOs, research partners, and vaccine manufacturers. The GPEI strategy includes strengthening routine immunization (RI), implementing supplementary immunization activities (SIAs) at different scales for large outbreaks or local emergences, and rapid detection and response to transmission via clinical (acute flaccid paralysis, AFP) and environmental surveillance (ES) [3]. This review discusses the status of polio eradication, the latest advancements, and the next (and final) steps needed to achieve eradication. We also discuss what a polio-free world would look like and whether polio vaccination can—or should—ever be stopped once eradication is achieved.

2. Current Status of Polio Eradication

2.1. Global Polio Epidemiology

Since the start of the global polio eradication program in 1988, there has been a >99% reduction in polio cases caused by Wild Polioviruses (WPVs) (from >350,000 to just 12 WPV cases in two countries in 2023) and 20 million paralysis cases prevented attributed to vaccination [4,5]. Two out of the three WPV serotypes have been certified as eradicated namely WPV2 in 2015 and WPV3 in 2019, with the last detections in 1999 in India and 2012 in Nigeria, respectively [6,7]. There are only two endemic countries left with WPV1 transmission, namely Afghanistan and Pakistan. Nigeria was the latest former endemic country, with the last WPV1 case reported in 2016 [8,9].

WPV is not the only poliovirus that can cause paralytic poliomyelitis. On rare occasions, the live-attenuated polioviruses from OPV can mutate, circulate in populations with inadequate immunization levels for an extended period, and revert into circulating vaccine-derived polioviruses (cVDPVs) capable of inducing paralysis and causing outbreaks [10]. Clinically and epidemiologically, WPV and cVDPV are indistinguishable. Both readily transmit in poorly immunized communities, cause paralytic outbreaks, and require the same level of programmatic response. Since 2012, paralytic poliomyelitis cases caused by cVDPV have surpassed those caused by WPV. Poliovirus transmission, both by WPV and cVDPV, has been declared as a Public Health Emergency of International Concern (PHEIC) since 2014 [11]. Polio is the longest-standing PHEIC and the only one declared by the World Health Organization at present (January 2024).

In 2023, there were 12 paralytic cases caused by WPV1 globally and 491 paralytic cases caused by cVDPV (133 by type 1, 373 by type 2, and 0 by type 3) (Figure 1) [4,12]. A timeline of global WPV and cVDPV AFP case counts in the last 10 years is depicted in Figure 2.

WPV1 cases have been largely restricted to one epidemiological block centered along the Pakistan–Afghanistan border with only two genetic clusters (YB3A and YB3C); several historic endemic reservoirs are no longer endemic, including Khyber–Peshawar and the Quetta Block [13]. In 2021, there was a WPV1 circulation in Malawi and Mozambique after importation of the virus from Pakistan. A multi-country vaccination and surveillance response successfully stopped the transmission, and the outbreak has since been contained, with the last detection in August 2022. This is a stark reminder that although the prevalence of endemicity has markedly diminished, the presence of transmission anywhere implies a persistent global risk of importation.

WPV2 had been certified as eradicated in 2015, and OPV2 use was resulting in cVDPV2 cases, setting the stage for tOPV withdrawal [14]. As such, in 2016, there was a globally synchronized switch in routine immunization schedules, replacing trivalent OPV (tOPV) with bivalent OPV (bOPV, containing live Sabin poliovirus serotypes 1 and 3) as part of a phased withdrawal of all Sabin strains from OPV, starting with type 2. Although successfully implemented, the inability to quickly and effectively respond to post-switch cVDPV2 outbreaks and IPV shortages creating a widening type 2 immunity gap resulted in a steep increase in cVDPV2 cases in 2020–2022, the effects of which are still present to date [15].

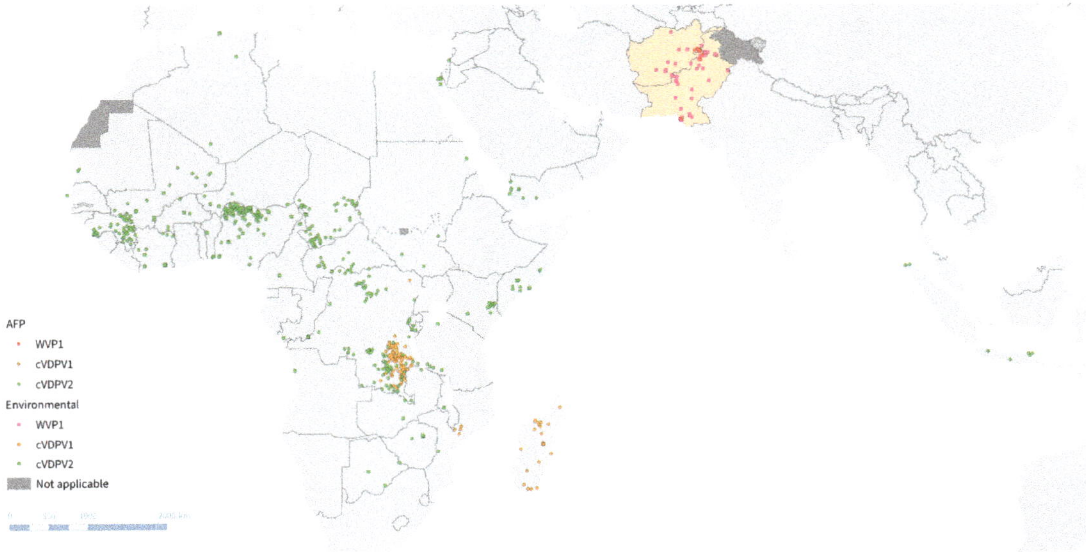

Figure 1. 2023 global overview of positive poliovirus isolates, including types 1, 2, and 3 wild poliovirus (WPV) and circulating vaccine-derived poliovirus (cVDPV). Clinical acute flaccid paralysis (AFP) and environmental surveillance (ES) poliovirus detections are depicted. On the left, there is a per-country list of the latest detections of AFP and ES. Data source: from WHO HQ as of 27 February 2024.; figure adapted from internal WHO HQ figures; map creation 5 April 2024; map produced by WHO GIS Centre for Health, DNA/DDI. Disclaimer: The designations employed and the presentation of the material in this publication do not imply the expression of any opinion whatsoever on the part of the WHO concerning the legal status of any country, territory, city, or area or of its authorities or concerning the delimitation of its frontiers or boundaries. Dotted and dashed lines on maps represent approximate border lines for which there may not yet be full agreement.

Until 2021, the majority of the global cVDPV2 burden was in Nigeria; in 2023, eastern DRC, northwestern Nigeria, northern Yemen, and south–central Somalia accounted for >80% of the caseload. These have been referred to as 'consequential geographies', identified as continuous drivers of cVDPV emergence and transmission. cVDPV2 was recently detected in regions where poliovirus transmission had long ago been eliminated. There were genetically linked cVDPV2 detections in the UK, Israel, Canada, and the USA [16]. These outbreaks, however, did not progress, and only one paralytic case was detected. The remaining cVDPV2 detections were from environmental samples.

Recent successes in the control of transmission have been due to high-quality SIAs and intensified efforts to access zero-dose or underimmunized children in hard-to-reach or conflict settings. However, the gains are fragile and easily reversible when program quality is not maintained. Even small pockets of transmission can have global implications and slow the final steps towards eradication.

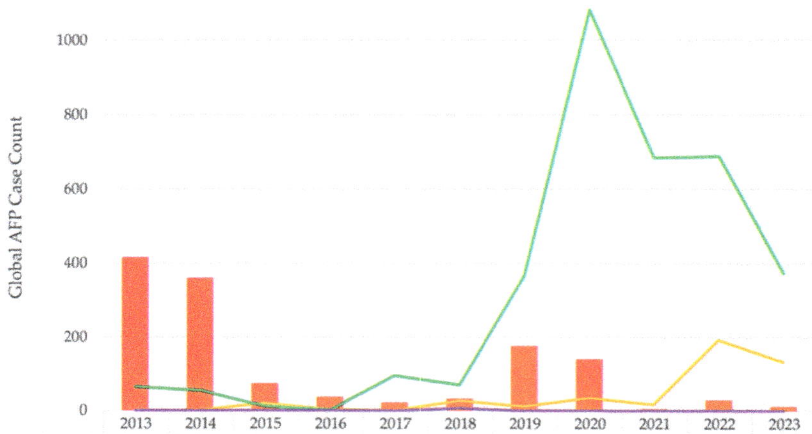

	2013	2014	2015	2016	2017	2018	2019	2020	2021	2022	2023
WPV1	416	359	74	37	22	33	176	140	6	30	12
cVDPV1	0	1	20	3	0	27	12	35	17	193	133
cVDPV2	65	55	12	2	96	71	367	1082	685	689	373
cVDPV3	1	0	0	0	0	7	0	0	0	1	0

Figure 2. Case count of global clinical AFP poliovirus cases in the past decade (2013–2023) including WPV1 and cVDPV types 1, 2, and 3. Data from WHO HQ as of 27 February 2024. Abbreviations: cVDPV, circulating vaccine-derived poliovirus; WPV, wild-type poliovirus; AFP, acute flaccid paralysis.

2.2. Poliovirus Surveillance

The gold standard for detecting poliovirus is through acute flaccid paralysis (AFP) surveillance supplemented by environmental surveillance of sewage samples, the latter of which is capable of detecting early indicators of silent transmission in a population (i.e., non-paralytic cases). Genomic sequencing analyses determine genetic relationships among polioviruses identified in stool and ES specimens. All collected samples are tested in WHO-accredited laboratories belonging to the Global Polio Laboratory Network (GPLN).

Ensuring high-quality surveillance through sensitivity and timeliness indicators is critical for outbreak detection and rapid activation of national and program-level responses. The Global Polio Surveillance Action Plan 2022–2024 sets a target of 35 days from paralysis onset or collection of a sewage sample to the notification of a polio detection. However, at present, this target is barely met, mainly due to delays in field-to-lab and inter-laboratory shipment of biological samples [17]. Countries with polio laboratories that can complete all procedures in-house are able to meet this target more easily, as is the case in Pakistan, for example.

The COVID-19 pandemic negatively affected both AFP and ES surveillance systems [18,19]. However, these were improved in 2021, and by the end of 2022, nearly 80% of priority countries experiencing or at high risk of polio transmission met national AFP targets, and the number of ES sites increased by 31% [20]. Recently, the USA and UK have also increased the number of ES sites due to cVDPV2 detections in 2022 [21,22]. Genetic sequencing allowed for identification of the link between poliovirus detections in the USA, UK, Canada, and Israel.

2.3. Challenges and the Current GPEI Polio Eradication Strategy

The current GPEI framework is based on the Polio Eradication Strategy 2022–2026, Delivering on a Promise [3]. The two main goals highlighted in the strategy are (1) permanently interrupting WPV1 transmission in endemic countries and (2) stopping cVDPV transmission and preventing outbreaks in non-endemic countries, both by the end of 2023, with the aim of reaching eradication by 2026. The Independent Monitoring Board (IMB), a panel of external advisors promoting program accountability, analyzed current program performance and the remaining challenges and concluded that goal one is off-track and goal two will be missed for the end of 2023 [23]. The GPEI has amended timelines and forecasts that certification of WPV1 will continue to be achieved in 2026 and that cVDPV2 transmission will be interrupted in 2025 [24].

Geopolitical risks directly impact eradication efforts, particularly through conflict, insecurity, and inaccessibility; these are present in the endemic reservoirs and 'consequential geographies' [23]. The deteriorating acute humanitarian crisis in Afghanistan and rising insecurity alongside political instability in Pakistan pose formidable challenges. Although vaccination activities and accessibility in Afghanistan are at their best since 2018, house-to-house vaccination campaigns have been forbidden in southern and northeastern regions of Afghanistan by the Taliban; this could have influenced the recent re-emergence of transmission in Kandahar for the first time in two years [13].

Poliovirus serotype co-circulation increases the complexity of outbreak response in terms of vaccine choice and implementation; eastern DRC has been a strong focal point of cVDPV1 and cVDPV2 co-circulation. In addition to DRC, there are pockets of persistently missed children due to inaccessibility, notably in northwestern Nigeria, south–central Somalia, and the Mehsud Belt in Pakistan. In northern Yemen, there has been an explosive outbreak of VDPV since limited immunization activities have been possible since late 2022. There have been over 200 boycotts of polio vaccination campaigns in Khyber–Pakhtunkhwa, Pakistan. These are only some examples of the formidable challenges that affect global polio eradication efforts; the GPEI continuously reviews and reformats program activities and priorities according to the evolving landscape.

As previously mentioned, the COVID-19 pandemic has significantly affected the polio program. Routine childhood immunization programs, vaccination campaigns (>60 polio SIAs were suspended), and surveillance systems (with gaps and detection lags) were severely disrupted.

3. Closing in on Poliovirus Eradication

3.1. Evolving Routine Immunization Schedules

The Strategic Advisory Group of Experts on Immunization (SAGE) is a committee established to advise the WHO on global policies and strategies for vaccines and immunization. As previously mentioned, to eliminate the risk of Sabin type 2-containing vaccines, the SAGE recommended the synchronized withdrawal of tOPV from RI schedules and replacement with bOPV [14]. This meant that only types 1 and 3 antigens were administered via OPV through RI. As such, the SAGE recommended that at least 1 dose of IPV be introduced to bridge the type 2 immunity gap; the recommendation was then extended in November 2020 to at least two doses of IPV [25–27]. As of May 2019, all countries have at least one dose of IPV in their RI schedules. However, 41 countries have yet to introduce the second dose, primarily in Africa.

Due to the delay in IPV manufacturing scale-up after 'the switch', several birth cohorts remained naïve to type 2 poliovirus. As a dose- and cost-sparing method, fractional-dose IPV (fIPV) was recommended by SAGE as a viable option for countries to implement in their national immunization guidelines [28]. Clinical trials demonstrate superior immunogenicity of two fIPV doses over one full dose of IPV [29,30]. There are six countries that currently use off-label fIPV administered intradermally in their RI schedules, namely Bangladesh, Cuba, Ecuador, India, Sri Lanka, and Nepal. Serological assessments from Cuba, Ecuador and India demonstrated high immunogenicity of their fIPV immunization schedules [29,31,32].

As countries become polio-free, are at reduced risk of importation and transmission, and have high and homogenous RI coverage and good sanitation, there is a shift in RI schedules from using OPV to IPV only. There are 67 countries that have IPV-only RI schedules—primarily industrialized countries (Figure 3) [33]. The use of OPV is incompatible with complete poliovirus eradication, as it contains live virus; therefore, plans are being made for complete cessation of OPV use in RI. bOPV cessation is planned to be implemented one year after certification of eradication of WPV1, provided all (yet-to-be-determined) pre-requisites are met.

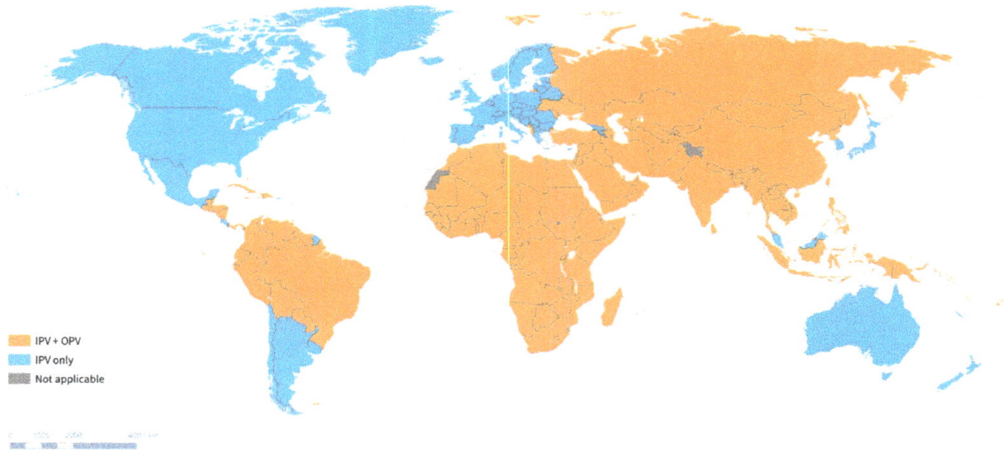

Figure 3. Routine polio immunization schedules of countries using inactivated poliovirus vaccines (IPVs) or IPVs plus oral poliovirus vaccines (OPVs) administered sequentially. Data source: WHO as of December 2023; map creation date 05 April 2024; map production by WHO GIS Centre for Health, DNA/DDI. Disclaimer: The designations employed and the presentation of the material in this publication do not imply the expression of any opinion whatsoever on the part of WHO concerning the legal status of any country, territory, city, or area or of its authorities or concerning the delimitation of its frontiers or boundaries. Dotted and dashed lines on maps represent approximate border lines for which there may not yet be full agreement.

Most of the countries using IPV-only RI schedules are using combination vaccines instead of standalone IPV—in most cases, pentavalent or hexavalent vaccines with an acellular pertussis component. Gavi, The Vaccine Alliance, besides their ongoing support for standalone IPV, approved the addition of a whole-cell pertussis hexavalent (wP-Hexavalent) vaccine to its portfolio in June 2023, making it more accessible globally [34]. The wP-Hexavalent vaccine contains six antigens, including the full dose IPV and the pentavalent vaccine antigens, including diphtheria, tetanus, pertussis, hepatitis B, and haemophilus influenza type b. Benefits of a hexavalent vaccine include a reduced number of injections in the RI schedule and higher sustainable IPV coverage. SAGE recommended a 3–4 dose schedule to accelerate and secure polio eradication [35]. The official launch of the hexavalent program was on 1 December 2023, and the first introduction of wP-Hexavalent in any country is expected in mid-2024 [34]. Gradually, more countries are expected to adopt wP-Hexavalent vaccines fulfilling the Gavi criteria, prioritization, and demand–supply dynamics.

3.2. New Tools and Strategies: Outbreak Response

Between 2010 and 'the switch' in 2016, there were 318 cVDPV2 cases in 15 countries; since OPV2 withdrawal in RI, there has been a ~10-fold increase to 3129 cVDPV2 cases in 41 countries. The majority have been attributed to seedings of VDPV2 following mOPV2 use [36].

nOPV2 is a genetically modified version of mOPV2 designed to increase the genetic stability of the vaccine virus and thereby reduce the chance of reversion to a neurovirulent phenotype, all while maintaining comparable immunogenicity [37]. In November 2020, the WHO Prequalification program recommended nOPV2 for cVDPV2 outbreak response under Emergency Use Listing (EUL) [38]. nOPV2 was the first-ever vaccine to receive an EUL, paving the way for other emergency vaccines. Since the start of the rollout in March 2021, nearly one billion doses of nOPV2 have been administered in 35 countries to date, as of January 2024. nOPV2 manufactured by BioFarma, Indonesia obtained full WHO prequalification in December 2023, making it the first vaccine to reach licensure after having been granted an EUL [39].

Field data demonstrate that nOPV2 retains its enhanced genetic stability with a substantially lower rate of reversion and risk of cVDPV2 emergence compared to Sabin OPV2. In fact, the number of recorded global cVDPV2 emergences has decreased markedly since nOPV2 implementation (Figure 4, [40]). By the end 2023, there had been 11 cVDPV2 emergences linked to nOPV2 use—4 originating in DRC, 2 in CAR, 1 in Nigeria, 1 in Egypt, 1 in Botswana, 1 in Cameroon, and 1 in Zimbabwe [41,42]. Modelling suggests that if nOPV2 seeded new emergences at the same rate as Sabin OPV2, 58.4 cVDPV2 nOPV2-derived emergences would be expected, given the total volume of nOPV2 doses used in AFRO (as of 17 November 2023). This results in an estimated 82% reduction in risk of the emergence of cVDPV2 with nOPV2 use compared to Sabin OPV2 [41]. The SAGE recently recommended that the second round of nOPV2 in outbreak response be implemented in a shorter timeframe of 1–4 weeks to ensure timeliness and reduce the risk of emergence [43].

For more efficient outbreak response, SAGE also recommends that IPV (full or fractional dose) be added to OPV in campaigns in areas with persistent poliovirus transmission to more efficiently close the humoral immunity gap and boost mucosal immunity [44].

3.3. New Tools and Strategies: Surveillance and Timeliness of Detection

Once a stool or environmental sample is collected for analysis, there is a critical period until the confirmation of a poliovirus isolate, including transport to the laboratory and analysis of the sample.

The current algorithm used to identify poliovirus from stool specimens and environmental samples involves viral isolation and molecular characterization of the isolates. Sample analysis in the laboratory can take 2–3 weeks, on average, from sample receipt to final sequencing results. The steps in the standard process involve cell culturing for virus isolation, intertypic differentiation by quantitative PCR, and Sanger sequencing to distinguish between vaccine, vaccine-derived, and wild-type polioviruses.

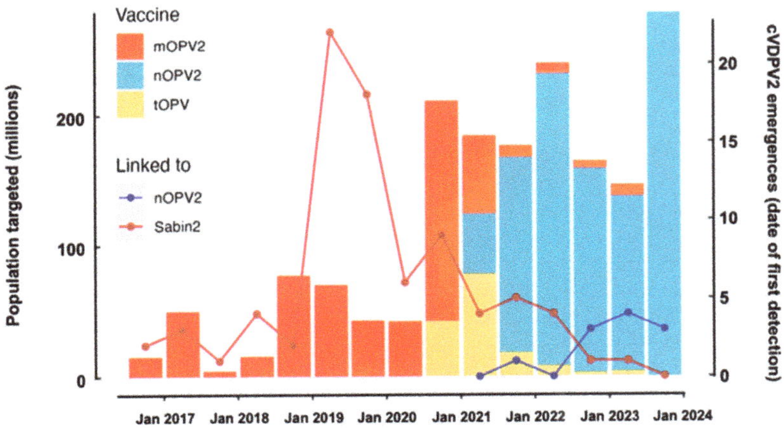

Figure 4. Emergences of cVDPV2 in 2016–2023 after the tOPV-to-bOPV switch linked to OPV use. The figure depicts the use of Sabin OPV (mOPV2 and tOPV) for outbreak response and the introduction of nOPV2 in March 2021. The data are from 1 July 2016, to 31 December 2023. Figure from Bandyopadhyay et al., 2024 [40]. Abbreviations: cVDPV2, type 2 circulating vaccine-derived poliovirus; tOPV, trivalent oral poliovirus vaccine; bOPV, bivalent oral poliovirus vaccine; mOPV2, type 2 monovalent oral poliovirus vaccine; nOPV2, novel type 2 oral poliovirus vaccine.

There are two alternative direct detection technologies currently being assessed, namely (i) direct detection with intratypic differentiation (DD-ITD) and (ii) direct detection nanopore sequencing (DDNS) [45,46]. These methods are faster and safer alternatives compared to standard cell culture regarding containment-related risks associated with growing live viruses. Using direct detection methods aims for increased timeliness in outbreak detection and response. Both DD-ITD and DDNS are being parallel-tested against the current recommended method in several GPLN laboratories, and data are regularly reviewed to assess if the methods meet all evaluation criteria. A decision for implementation into routine use is expected in 2024–2025 after full validation by the GPLN.

While the speed of obtaining laboratory results would be improved by utilizing direct detection methods, an additional impediment to timely case reporting lies within the logistics infrastructure, with sample/isolate transport as the key driver for delays. Village Reach has recently started implementing a program in 15 high-risk countries for poliovirus transmission in Africa to reduce the sample-to-lab transport times via direct engagement with local governments and partners to create tailored plans [47]. The initiative began in 2022 and a positive impact is already noticeable, especially in countries without national laboratory capacity.

4. Preparing for a Polio-Free World

4.1. Challenges and the GPEI Post-Certification Strategy

The polio Post-Certification Strategy outlines the global technical standards and activities (e.g., containment, vaccination, and surveillance) needed to sustain a polio-free world after global certification of wild poliovirus eradication [48]. The primary risks of a potential resurgence of polio in the post-certification era are the continued use of OPVs, accidental release of poliovirus from a laboratory or vaccine manufacturing facility, and the chronic excretion of VDPVs by persons with primary immunodeficiency (iVDPVs). In addition, bioterrorism involving poliovirus engineering and release is also considered a risk.

Today, live poliovirus is present in four sites, namely humans, the environment, within OPV, or held in designated research or vaccine production facilities. Even when transmission of poliovirus and OPV use is stopped, there is still poliovirus within these facilities, which creates a risk of (intentional or accidental) release into the environment and the re-establishment of transmission. This has happened in the past. Most recently, in the Netherlands, a WPV3 isolate was detected in sewage water originating from an industrial plant; however, no transmission was established [49]. As such, laboratories, vaccine production sites, or any other facility that handles or stores poliovirus must adhere to strict containment guidelines and biosafety requirements. The WHO Global Actional Plan for Poliovirus Containment, recently updated in July 2022 (GAPIV), is the chief reference document for poliovirus containment measures [50].

Finally, a less understood risk is that of iVDPVs (VDPVs chronically excreted by persons with certain forms of primary immunodeficiencies [PID]). When OPV is accidentally administered to an immunodeficient individual, there is a risk of prolonged virus excretion, potentially initiating an outbreak (note that no iVDPV-related outbreaks have been conclusively attributed to iVDPV excretors to date). The SAGE recommended that a specialized surveillance system for PID patients and iVDPV be integrated into routine polio environmental and AFP surveillance [51]. Thus far, PID surveillance is being implemented in twelve countries as pilot initiatives, research projects, or related to nOPV2 EUL requirements [17]. Additionally, there are several R&D projects to pursue effective antiviral drugs to reduce excretion and risk of paralysis in iVDPV-infected PID patients, including V-7404 and pocapavir as potential candidates led by the Poliovirus Antivirals Initiative (PAI) [52]. Identification and management of iVDPV are essential in the post-certification era, as it could be the only persistent reservoir (aside from manufacturing facilities) of poliovirus after eradication and OPV withdrawal.

Current manufacturing of IPV vaccines requires the use of large quantities of live poliovirus (either WPV for production of conventional IPV or Sabin poliovirus for production of sIPV). Efforts are being made to produce IPV in a process that will not involve the use of live poliovirus. A virus-like particle (VLP) platform for the production of IPV-like vaccines is being developed, with CanSino, China ready to start in-human clinical trials and multiple other candidates in the preclinical phase [53,54]. The goal is to have a VLP product on the market in late 2020s. In addition to polio VLPs and following the WHO's recommendation to produce IPVs using attenuated strains, IPV is being developed using S19 virus strains developed by MHRA (formerly NIBSC, UK). The S19 strain has been modified so that it is unlikely to replicate in humans, so it has obtained a containment waiver [55]. Currently, an S19 hexavalent vaccine from Biological E, India is in phase I clinical study.

4.2. Polio Vaccination in the Post-Certification Era

Current SAGE recommendations call for continuation of vaccinations with IPV for at least 10 years after the last poliovirus type is certified as eradicated and indefinitely in countries hosting facilities handling live polioviruses [56]. It is, however, anticipated that some countries, especially those using hexavalent vaccines, will continue to immunize their populations against polio indefinitely.

5. Concluding Remarks

The historical narrative and persisting work towards polio eradication underscore the challenges, failures, and successes of this tremendous global effort. Since there is no cure for poliomyelitis, the strategic delivery of polio vaccination through all its forms (routine immunization programs, supplementary polio campaigns, injectables, oral administration, etc.) is the most effective method to achieve eradication. Moreover, research and development with respect to novel tools, including diagnostic methods, vaccines, antivirals, and outreach initiatives, are essential for rapid notification of outbreaks and sustainable vaccination.

There are many unforeseen challenges in the polio endgame. Geopolitical risks directly impact eradication efforts, particularly through conflict, insecurity, and inaccessibility of certain populations. Poliovirus serotype co-circulation increases the complexity of outbreak response, and competing public health priorities require available resources to be shared. Nonetheless, historically endemic reservoirs of WPV1 are disappearing, and the genetic diversity is markedly reduced to just two chains of transmission in one epidemiological block. Surveillance indicators and vaccination coverage have steadily recovered and surpassed pre-COVID-19 pandemic levels.

The eradication endgame is incredibly complex, and successes are fragile. Eradicating the final chains of WPV1 and cVDPV transmission and preventing more children from becoming paralyzed by poliovirus will require renewed financial and political commitments from governments, donors, multilateral organizations, and local communities from across the world.

Author Contributions: Conceptualization, O.M. and R.L.C.; writing—original draft preparation, R.L.C.; writing—review and editing, R.L.C., M.E., O.M.D., H.V., A.Q. and O.M. All authors have read and agreed to the published version of the manuscript.

Funding: This research received no external funding.

Conflicts of Interest: The authors declare no conflicts of interest.

References

1. History of the Polio Vaccine. Available online: https://www.who.int/news-room/spotlight/history-of-vaccination/history-of-polio-vaccination?topicsurvey=ht7j2q)&gclid=CjwKCAiAhJWsBhAaEiwAmrNyq96p4otvLmTvsY_CT9YnLuQo-9VdI3OTAlb5SQaKrl8Wlq-WGGasARoCBYoQAvD_BwE (accessed on 22 December 2023).
2. Hird, T.R.; Grassly, N.C. Systematic review of mucosal immunity induced by oral and inactivated poliovirus vaccines against virus shedding following oral poliovirus challenge. *PLoS Pathog.* **2012**, *8*, e1002599. [CrossRef] [PubMed]
3. GPEI Polio Eradication Strategy 2022–2026: Delivering on a Promise. Available online: https://polioeradication.org/wp-content/uploads/2021/10/9789240031937-eng.pdf (accessed on 6 January 2021).

4. Global Wild Poliovirus 2017–2023—Data in WHO HQ as of 19 December 2023. Available online: https://polioeradication.org/polio-today/polio-now/wild-poliovirus-list/ (accessed on 22 December 2023).
5. Global Polio Eradication. Available online: https://www.cdc.gov/polio/global-polio-eradication.html (accessed on 14 December 2023).
6. Global Eradication of Wild Poliovirus Type 2 Declared. Available online: https://polioeradication.org/news-post/global-eradication-of-wild-poliovirus-type-2-declared/ (accessed on 6 December 2023).
7. Global Certification of Eradication of Indigenous Wild Poliovirus Type 3. Available online: https://www.cdc.gov/globalhealth/immunization/stories/global-certification-of-eradication-of-indigenous-wild-poliovirus-type-3.html (accessed on 6 December 2023).
8. WHO. Global Wild Poliovirus 2015–2020. Available online: https://polioeradication.org/wp-content/uploads/2020/12/weekly-polio-analyses-WPV-20201222.pdf (accessed on 22 December 2023).
9. WHO AFRO. *Polio Eradication: Africa Regional Certification Commission begins Verification Visit to Nigeria*; WHO AFRO: Abuja, Nigeria, 2019.
10. GPEI; WHO. Variant Poliovirus (cVDPV). Available online: https://polioeradication.org/polio-today/polio-prevention/the-virus/variant-poliovirus-cvdpv/ (accessed on 5 April 2024).
11. World Health Organization. *Statement of the Thirty-Sixth Meeting of the Polio IHR Emergency Committee*; World Health Organization: Geneva, Switzerland, 2023.
12. Global Circulating Vaccine-Derived Poliovirus (cVDPV)—Data in WHO HQ as of 19 December 2023. Available online: https://polioeradication.org/this-week/variant-poliovirus-cvdpv/ (accessed on 22 December 2023).
13. Bjork, A.; Akbar, I.; Chaudhury, S.; Wadood, M.Z.; Ather, F.; Jorba, J.; Martinez, M. Progress Toward Poliomyelitis Eradication—Afghanistan, January 2022–June 2023. *MMWR Morb. Mortal. Wkly. Rep.* **2023**, *72*, 1020–1026. [CrossRef] [PubMed]
14. Sutter, R.W.; Platt, L.; Mach, O.; Jafari, H.; Aylward, R. The new polio eradication end game: Rationale and supporting evidence. *J. Infect. Dis.* **2014**, *210*, S434–S438. [CrossRef] [PubMed]
15. Sutter, R.W.; Cochi, S.L. Inactivated Poliovirus Vaccine Supply Shortage: Is There Light at the End of the Tunnel? *J. Infect. Dis.* **2019**, *220*, 1545–1546. [CrossRef] [PubMed]
16. Lee, S.; Greene, S.; Burns, C.C.; Tallis, G.; Wassilak, S.; Bolu, O. Progress Toward Poliomyelitis Eradication—Worldwide, January 2021–March 2023. *MMWR Morb. Mortal. Wkly. Rep.* **2023**, *72*, 517–522. [CrossRef] [PubMed]
17. World Health Organization. *Global Polio Surveillance Action Plan 2022–2024*; World Health Organization: Geneva, Switzerland, 2022.
18. Tuma, J.; Wilkinson, A.L.; Diop, O.M.; Jorba, J.; Gardner, T.; Snider, C.J.; Anand, A.; Ahmed, J. Surveillance to Track Progress Toward Polio Eradication—Worldwide, 2019–2020. *MMWR Morb. Mortal. Wkly. Rep.* **2021**, *70*, 667–673. [CrossRef]
19. Zomahoun, D.; Burman, A.; Snider, C.J.; Chauvin, C.; Gardner, T.; Lickness, J.S.; Ahmed, J.A.; Diop, O.M.; Gerber, S.; Anand, A. Impact of COVID-19 Pandemic on Global Poliovirus Surveillance. *MMWR Morb. Mortal. Wkly. Rep.* **2020**, *69*, 1648–1652. [CrossRef] [PubMed]
20. Stehling-Ariza, T.; Wilkinson, A.L.; Diop, O.M.; Jorba, J.; Asghar, H.; Avagnan, T.; Grabovac, V.; Johnson, T.; Joshi, S.; Kfutwah, A.; et al. Surveillance to Track Progress toward Poliomyelitis Eradication—Worldwide, 2021–2022. *MMWR Morb. Mortal. Wkly. Rep.* **2023**, *72*, 613–620. [CrossRef] [PubMed]
21. Kuehn, B.M. CDC to Expand Wastewater Testing for Poliovirus. *JAMA* **2023**, *329*, 116–117. [CrossRef]
22. Expansion of Polio Sewage Surveillance to Areas Outside London. UK Health Security Agency: Health and Social Care, Public Health. Published 2 September 2022. Available online: https://www.gov.uk/government/news/expansion-of-polio-sewage-surveillance-to-areas-outside-london#:~:text=We%20are%20now%20expanding%20the,areas%20as%20the%20need%20arises (accessed on 5 April 2024).
23. Independent Monitoring Board: Global Polio Eradication Initiative. *Closing in on Zero: Adapting to Complexity and Risk on the Path to End Polio*; World Health Organization: Geneva, Switzerland, 2023.
24. World Health Organization. *Polio Eradication Strategy: GPEI Response to the Midterm Review*; World Health Organization: Geneva, Switzerland, 2023.
25. Immunization Systems Management Group of the Global Polio Eradication Initiative. Introduction of Inactivated Poliovirus Vaccine and Switch from Trivalent to Bivalent Oral Poliovirus Vaccine—Worldwide, 2013–2016. *MMWR Morb. Mortal. Wkly. Rep.* **2015**, *64*, 699–702.
26. World Health Organization. Meeting of the Strategic Advisory Group of Experts on Immunization, November 2012—Conclusions and Recommendations. *Wkly. Epidemiol. Rec.* **2013**, *88*, 1–16.
27. WHO. Meeting of the Strategic Advisory Group of Experts on Immunization, October 2020—Conclusions and recommendations. *Wkly. Epidemiol. Rec.* **2020**, *95*, 585–608.
28. World Health Organization. *15th Meeting of the SAGE Polio Working Group—Conclusions and Recommendations*; World Health Organization: Geneva, Switzerland, 2018.
29. Ahmad, M.; Verma, H.; Deshpande, J.; Kunwar, A.; Bavdekar, A.; Mahantashetti, N.S.; Krishnamurthy, B.; Jain, M.; Mathew, M.A.; Pawar, S.D.; et al. Immunogenicity of Fractional Dose Inactivated Poliovirus Vaccine in India. *J. Pediatr. Infect. Dis. Soc.* **2022**, *11*, 60–68. [CrossRef]
30. Anand, A.; Molodecky, N.A.; Pallansch, M.A.; Sutter, R. Immunogenicity to poliovirus type 2 following two doses of fractional intradermal inactivated poliovirus vaccine: A novel dose sparing immunization schedule. *Vaccine* **2017**, *35*, 2993–2998. [CrossRef] [PubMed]

31. Trueba, G.; Jeyaseelan, V.; Lopez, L.; Mainou, B.A.; Zhang, Y.; Whittembury, A.; Olmedo Valarezo, A.; Baquero, G.; Romero de Aguinaga, R.; Zurita Salinas, L.; et al. Achieving high immunogenicity against poliovirus with fractional doses of inactivated poliovirus vaccine in Ecuador-results from a cross-sectional serological survey. *Lancet Reg. Health Am.* **2022**, *11*, 100235. [CrossRef] [PubMed]
32. Resik, S.; Mach, O.; Tejeda, A.; Jeyaseelan, V.; Fonseca, M.; Diaz, M.; Alemany, N.; Hung, L.H.; Aleman, Y.; Mesa, I.; et al. Immunogenicity of Intramuscular Fractional Dose of Inactivated Poliovirus Vaccine. *J. Infect. Dis.* **2020**, *221*, 895–901. [CrossRef]
33. WHO Immunization Data Portal. Available online: https://immunizationdata.who.int/ (accessed on 18 December 2023).
34. Hexavalent Vaccine Programme Information. Available online: https://www.gavi.org/our-support/guidelines/hexavalent-vaccine-programme-information (accessed on 31 January 2024).
35. WHO. Polio vaccines: WHO position paper—June 2022. *Wkly. Epidemiol. Rec.* **2022**, *97*, 277–300.
36. Macklin, G.R.; Goel, A.; Mach, O.; Tallis, G.; Ahmed, J.; O'Reilly, K.M.; Grassly, N.C.; Diop, O.M. Epidemiology of type 2 vaccine-derived poliovirus outbreaks between 2016 and 2020. *Vaccine* **2023**, *41*, A19–A24. [CrossRef]
37. Yeh, M.T.; Bujaki, E.; Dolan, P.T.; Smith, M.; Wahid, R.; Konz, J.; Weiner, A.J.; Bandyopadhyay, A.; Van Damme, P.; De Coster, I.; et al. Engineering the Live-Attenuated Polio Vaccine to Prevent Reversion to Virulence. *Cell Host Microbe* **2020**, *27*, 736–751. [CrossRef]
38. Macklin, G.; Peak, C.; Eisenhawer, M.; Kurji, F.; Mach, O.; Konz, J.; Gast, C.; Bachtiar, N.S.; Bandyopadhyay, A.; Zipursky, S. Enabling accelerated vaccine roll-out for Public Health Emergencies of International Concern (PHEICs): Novel Oral Polio Vaccine type 2 (nOPV2) experience. *Vaccine* **2023**, *41*, A122–A127. [CrossRef]
39. GPEI Press Release on nOPV2 Prequalification. Available online: https://polioeradication.org/news-post/gpei-press-release-on-nopv2-prequalification/ (accessed on 5 April 2024).
40. Bandyopadhyay, A.; Cooper, L.; Zipursky, S. One billion doses and WHO Prequalification of nOPV2: Implications for the global polio situation and beyond. *PLoS Glob. Public Health* **2024**, *4*, e0002920. [CrossRef] [PubMed]
41. Peak, C.M.; Lyons, H.; Cooper, L.V.; Voorman, A.; Hawes, K.; Bandyopadhyay, A. Monitoring Risk of Type-2 Circulating Vaccine-Derived Poliovirus Emergence during Roll-Out of Type-2 Novel Oral Polio Vaccine. In Proceedings of the 9th International Conference on Infectious Disease Dynamics, Bologna, Italy, 28 November–1 December 2023.
42. Davlantes, E.; Jorba, J.; Henderson, E.; Bullard, K.; Deka, M.A.; Kfutwah, A.; Martin, J.; Bessaud, M.; Shulman, L.; Diop, O.M.; et al. Notes from the Field: Circulating Vaccine-Derived Poliovirus Type 2 Emergences Linked to Novel Oral Poliovirus Vaccine Type 2 Use—Six African Countries, 2021–2023. *MMWR Morb. Mortal. Wkly. Rep.* **2023**, *72*, 1041–1042. [CrossRef] [PubMed]
43. WHO. Meeting of the Strategic Advisory Group of Experts on Immunization, September 2023: Conclusions and recommendations. *Wkly. Epidemiol. Rec.* **2023**, *95*, 599–620.
44. Bandyopadhyay, A.; Lopez Cavestany, R.; Blake, I.; Macklin, G.; Cooper, L.V.; Grassly, N.; Melquiades dos Santos Nery, A.; Mach, O. Use of inactivated poliovirus vaccine for poliovirus outbreak response. *Lancet Infect. Dis.* 2023, *online ahead of print*. [CrossRef]
45. Shaw, A.G.; Majumdar, M.; Troman, C.; O'Toole, Á.; Benny, B.; Abraham, D.; Praharaj, I.; Kang, G.; Sharif, S.; Alam, M.M.; et al. Rapid and Sensitive Direct Detection and Identification of Poliovirus from Stool and Environmental Surveillance Samples by Use of Nanopore Sequencing. *J. Clin. Microbiol.* **2020**, *58*, e00920. [CrossRef]
46. Harrington, C.; Sun, H.; Jeffries-Miles, S.; Gerloff, N.; Mandelbaum, M.; Pang, H.; Collins, N.; Burns, C.C.; Vega, E. Culture-Independent Detection of Poliovirus in Stool Samples by Direct RNA Extraction. *Microbiol. Spectr.* **2021**, *9*, e0066821. [CrossRef]
47. Lab Sample Transport for Polio Eradication. Available online: https://www.villagereach.org/project/polio-laboratory-sample-transport/ (accessed on 19 December 2023).
48. WHO; GPEI. Polio Post-Certification Strategy. Available online: http://polioeradication.org/polio-today/preparing-for-a-polio-free-world/transition-planning/polio-post-certification-strategy (accessed on 10 May 2023).
49. Duizer, E.; Ruijs, W.L.M.; Hintaran, A.D.P.; Hafkamp, M.C.; van der Veer, M.; te Wierik, M.J. Wild poliovirus type 3 (WPV3)-shedding event following detection in environmental surveillance of poliovirus essential facilities, The Netherlands, November 2022 to January 2023. *Eurosurveillance* **2023**, *28*, 2300049. [CrossRef]
50. World Health Organization. *WHO Global Action Plan for Poliovirus Containment*; World Health Organization: Geneva, Switzerland, 2023.
51. WHO. Meeting of the Strategic Advisory Group of Experts on immunization, October 2016—Conclusions and recommendations. *Wkly. Epidemiol. Rec.* **2016**, *91*, 561–584.
52. Polio Antivirals Initiative. Available online: https://www.taskforce.org/polio-antivirals-initiative/ (accessed on 19 December 2023).
53. Sherry, L.; Swanson, J.J.; Grehan, K.; Xu, H.; Uchida, M.; Jones, I.M.; Stonehouse, N.J.; Rowlands, D.J. Protease-Independent Production of Poliovirus Virus-like Particles in Pichia pastoris: Implications for Efficient Vaccine Development and Insights into Capsid Assembly. *Microbiol. Spectr.* **2023**, *11*, e0430022. [CrossRef]
54. A Study to Evaluate the Safety and Immunogenicity of Recombinant Trivalent Poliomyelitis Vaccine (Sf-RVN Cell) in Healthy Adults, CanSino Biologics Inc. 2024. Available online: https://classic.clinicaltrials.gov/ct2/show/NCT06101173 (accessed on 5 April 2024).

55. World Health Organization: Containment Advisory Group on Novel Poliovirus Strains. Report: CAG TC2 on Novel Poliovirus Strains. Available online: https://polioeradication.org/wp-content/uploads/2018/05/containment-advisory-group-novel-poliovirus-strains-8-march-2018-20180518.pdf (accessed on 8 March 2018).
56. WHO. Meeting of the Strategic Advisory Group of Experts on immunization, April 2017—Conclusions and recommendations. *Wkly. Epidemiol. Rec.* **2017**, *92*, 301–320.

pathogens

MDPI

Project Report

Polio Surge Capacity Support Program Contributions to Building Country Capacities in Support of Polio Outbreak Preparedness and Response: Lessons Learned and Remaining Challenges

Fikru Abebe [1], Victor Anochieboh Eboh [1], Mesfin Belew Weldetsadik [1], Ibrahima Kone [1], Tessema Assegid Kebede [1], Paul Thomas Harries [2] and Veh Kesse Fabien Diomande [1,*]

1 Polio Surge Capacity Support Program, Center for Vaccine Equity (CVE), The Task Force for Global Health (TFGH), Decatur, GA 30030, USA; fabebe@taskforce.org (F.A.); veboh@taskforce.org (V.A.E.); mweldetsadik@taskforce.org (M.B.W.); kibrahima_consultant@taskforce.org (I.K.); tkebede-consultant@taskforce.org (T.A.K.)

2 Global Security Department (GSD), The Task Force for Global Health (TFGH), Decatur, GA 30030, USA; gsd@taskforce.org

* Correspondence: fdiomande@taskforce.org

Abstract: Despite coordinated efforts at global level, through the Global Polio Eradication Initiative (GPEI), poliomyelitis disease (Polio) is still a major public health issue. The wild poliovirus type-1 (WPV1) is still endemic in Afghanistan and Pakistan, and new circulations of the WPV1 were confirmed in southeast Africa in 2021, in Malawi and Mozambique. The circulating vaccine derived polioviruses (cVDPV) are also causing outbreaks worldwide. The Task Force for Global Health (TFGH)'s Polio Surge Capacity Support Program, established in 2019, is an effort to reinforce the existing partnership with the GPEI to strengthen countries' capacities for polio outbreak preparedness and response. In four years, its coordinated efforts with GPEI partners have resulted in a remarkable improvement in the early detection of poliovirus circulation and reducing the missed children gaps in many countries. However, these encouraging results cannot hide an increasingly complex programmatic environment with numerous funding and operational challenges.

Keywords: poliovirus; partnership; surveillance; campaign; vaccine; children

1. Introduction

The Global Polio Eradication Initiative (GPEI) has successfully reduced the poliomyelitis disease (Polio) burden globally by more than 99% worldwide [1,2]. The Polio Eradication End Game Strategic Plans (2013–2018 and 2019–2023) and the Polio Eradication Strategy 2022–2026 are aimed at eradicating Wild Poliovirus type-1 (WPV1) globally, as well as circulating Vaccine Derived Poliovirus type-2 (cVDPV2) simultaneously [3,4]. Only one serotype of wild poliovirus is still circulating and is endemic in Afghanistan and Pakistan [5]. In 2021, outbreaks of WPV1 were confirmed in southeast Africa (Malawi and Mozambique) [6,7]. In addition to WPV1, circulating Vaccine Derived Polioviruses (cVDPVs) continue to cause multiple outbreaks worldwide since 2000 [5,7]. The global poliovirus outbreak situation remains concerning despite efforts undertaken for the early detection of poliovirus circulation through strengthening country surveillance systems and reinforcing population immunity against the poliovirus through routine immunization services and supplemental immunization activities (SIA). In 2023, 1057 poliovirus positive samples were detected from Acute Flaccid Paralysis (AFP) cases and/or environmental samples worldwide (Africa, Asia, the Middle East, Europe, and America). Among them, 162 were WPV1 and 895 were circulating Vaccine Derived Poliovirus type-1 (cVDPV1) and cVDPV2 [8].

In 2019, the Task Force for Global Health (TFGH)'s Center for Vaccine Equity (CVE) and the US Centers for Disease Control and Prevention (CDC)'s Polio Eradication Branch

(PEB) established the Polio Surge Capacity Support Program in partnership with the GPEI to develop and implement activities to strengthen the early detection and confirmation of poliovirus circulation, improve the performance and coverage of immunization services, reach under-immunized populations, strengthen the reach and quality of SIA, tailor strategies for high-risk areas and populations, and increase the demand for polio vaccination.

2. Support to Polio Outbreak Countries

The TFGH's Polio Surge Capacity Support Program works closely with the US CDC and all GPEI partners at the country level through a collaborative platform to provide needed technical support to polio outbreak countries in support of their outbreak preparedness and response: country Ministry of Health, World Health Organization (WHO), United Nations International Children's Emergency Fund (UNICEF), Bill and Melinda Gate Foundation (BMGF), and ROTARY. This includes a review of surveillance and immunization program data (SIA and routine immunization) to identify high-risk program areas, priority countries, and sub-national consequential geographies for surge support and capacity building. Technical support to polio outbreak countries follows GPEI Standard Operating Procedures (SOPs) [9] and provides training, monitoring of activities, and supervision and coaching of actors at all levels. Program areas targeted for support include:

- Coordination of the response at the country polio Emergency Operating Centers (EOCs)
- Strengthening of the surveillance systems
- Polio campaign preparation, implementation, and evaluation
- Outbreak response assessments, including defining the number of missed children and special populations (refugees, internally displaced populations, and populations living in security-compromised areas).

Over the past four years, the Polio Surge Capacity Support Program has performed 64 deployments of senior epidemiologists and local contractors in 16 polio outbreak countries in Africa, representing a cumulative 16 deployments per year and a total cumulative 167 months (almost 14 years) of fieldwork. Among the outbreak countries supported, five countries were classified as high-security risk at the time of deployments: Somalia, Ethiopia, Nigeria, South Sudan, and the Democratic Republic of Congo (DRC).

3. Security Risks and Mitigation Measures

Many polio outbreak countries being supported are at the highest security risk due to political unrest, terrorism, etc. Also, some countries with overall low or medium security risks could have pockets of high-risk areas at the sub-national level. Reaching all of the communities to bring them immunization and surveillance services and reaching all of the eligible children for polio vaccination, including those living in security-compromised areas, is a program priority. The deployments of Surge teams in high-security risk countries or security-compromised areas are performed through a detailed and careful security review and assessment by the TFGH Global Security Director (GSD). Security clearance for the deployment of the Surge team comes with security mitigation measures, which include the following activities and processes:

- All trips are entered into the Concur Travel system, and reports are generated for the TFGH Leadership and GSD.
- Travelers receive a guidance document including information on travel risks and reminders.
- The GSD assesses every trip, with higher-risk locations receiving increased scrutiny.
- Countries are risk assessed using Healix Sentinel (TFGH travel insurance provider), which uses a five (5) tier rating system (extreme, high, moderate, low, or minimal), and the US State Department Travel Advisory country risk rating system, which uses a four-tier system (Level: 4 Do Not Travel Level; 3 Reconsider Travel Level; 2 Exercise Increased Caution Level; and 1 Exercise Normal Precautions).
- Travelers are offered a pre-travel briefing before they travel.

- A three-day in-person Hostile Environment Awareness Training (HEAT) workshop is provided to the polio Surge staff.
- GSD has access to the Risk and Strategic Management Corps, within the SIGMA 7 (RSM/SIGMA 7) system provided by Intelligence Fusion, which provides a database of incidents recorded in different locations worldwide.
- GSD monitors TFGH staff using the Healix Sentinel mapping system.
- For higher-risk destinations, there is an additional layer where the traveler opens a WhatsApp Group, including the Program Leadership and GSD.
- GSD regularly contacts long-term deployed contractors and staff to discuss their safety and security.

4. Achievements

Over the past four years, the Polio Surge Capacity Support Program, in close coordination with the US CDC PEB team and the GPEI partners, has assessed and prioritized technical support requests from polio outbreak countries and provided in-country human resource capacities where needed, with the recruitment and increased engagement of local contractors in Liberia, Senegal, Somalia, Ethiopia, Kenya, Malawi, Tanzania, and Zambia. Where needed, the program has also reinforced in-country human resource capacity with the deployments of senior epidemiologists in Ghana, Sierra Leone, Senegal, Gambia, Somalia, Djibouti, Ethiopia, Kenya, Tanzania, Zambia, Malawi, DRC, and Nigeria.

The collaborative efforts between the Polio Surge Capacity Support Program and the US CDC PEB, in close coordination with GPEI partners, have enabled improvement of the early detection of poliovirus circulation in many countries, and contributed to the outbreak countries' efforts to reach and vaccinate cumulatively over two hundred million children against polio over the past four years in sixteen countries in Africa. These remarkable results are illustrated by the trend in the reduction in missed children for polio vaccination in SIAs during the Southeast Africa outbreak response from 2022 to 2023 in Malawi (Figure 1). Similar trends in progressively reducing the number of missed children have also been observed in several supported outbreak countries, such as Djibouti, Somalia, Tanzania, Zambia, and the DRC.

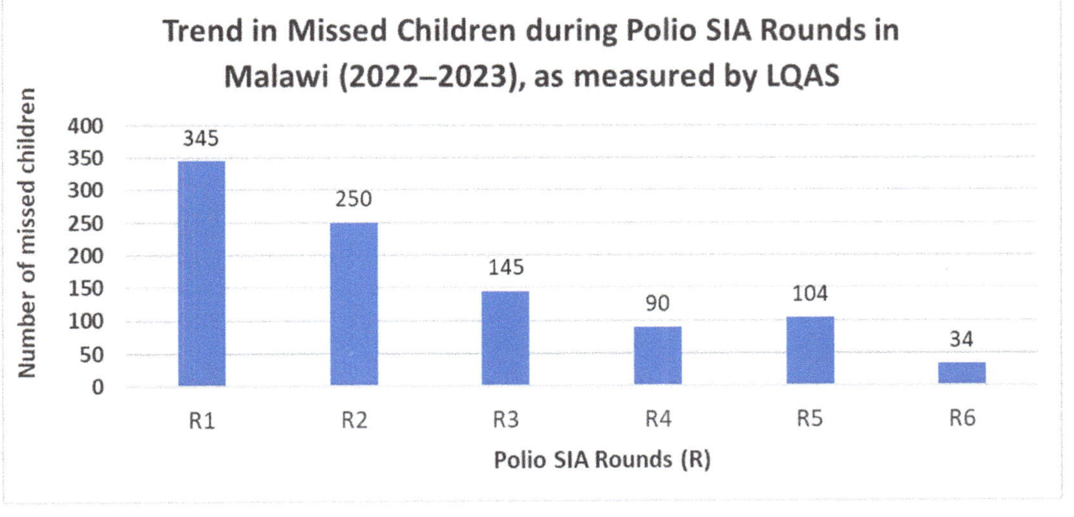

Figure 1. Trends in missed children during Polio SIA in Malawi (2022–2023), as measured by LQAS. Notes: SIA—supplementary immunization activities; LQAS—lot quality assurance sampling.

5. Growing Program Complexity with Persistent Challenges

Program complexity has grown and is related to several internal and external factors that negatively impact the program's effectiveness at reaching all the communities and eligible children for polio vaccination and surveillance activities. The major persistent challenges are the following:

- The lack of sufficient funding to address countries' growing technical assistance needs is a result of insufficient government contributions to polio outbreak response and the reduction of the funding stream at a global level. To address funding gaps, the Polio Surge Capacity Support Program regularly conducts prioritization exercises in close coordination with the CDC and other GPEI partners to determine a list of high-priority countries to be supported for outbreak preparedness and response: countries with a circulation of WPV. These "wide-spreader" countries are defined as countries with factors heightening the risk of widespread of poliovirus (poor disease surveillance leading to undetected transmission, growing vaccine hesitancy, large proportion of unvaccinated populations, important population movements, etc.) and countries with no recent experience with polio outbreak responses. The program resources are then redirected to the highest priority countries, leaving other priority countries without support to sustain previous gains against polio (the early detection of poliovirus circulation and sustaining population immunity against poliovirus). The lack of sufficient funding to address countries' needs for outbreak preparedness and response represents a serious threat to polio eradication efforts.
- The observed limited vaccine supplies of the novel Oral Polio Vaccine type-2 (nOPV2) [10], as documented in many country outbreak response situation reports (SitReps), is impacting polio campaign schedules, resulting in a delay in the implementation and a reduction in the rounds of the campaigns. The lack of sufficient vaccines to address country needs represents a major challenge in increasing population immunity to prevent continuing the transmission of VDPV2.
- Inadequate country-level engagement: The country-level engagement for polio outbreak response by national authorities at all levels is still inadequate in most outbreak countries, mainly related to competing public priorities and other post-COVID-19 pandemic socio-economic priorities. This leads to poor ownership, the absence of an accountability framework, a lack of supportive supervision during SIAs and surveillance activities, and late disbursement of resources at operational levels. Poor engagement and lack of ownership represent a major challenge in reaching all communities and eligible children for polio vaccination.
- The lack of adequate funding and poor engagement of national authorities for polio outbreak response contribute to persistent operational constraints and inadequate program performance. This results in late detection and laboratory confirmation of poliovirus circulations, late deployments of human resources to outbreak countries, late disbursement of funds to operational levels, delays in service delivery, lack of adequate microplanning, weak cross-border collaborations, and lack of effective measures to track and address persistent rumors against vaccination and/or vaccine hesitancies.
- The underlying growing burden of epidemic diseases in developing countries, the post-COVID-19 socio-economic impacts, and the impact of emerging military crises worldwide on the global economy are major factors influencing leadership decision-making not to prioritize disease outbreak preparedness and response, including polio.
- As described above, the need for adequate resources to simultaneously address the growing public health and development needs is a major challenge for disease epidemic preparedness and response. This context of competing public health emergencies and priorities is fueling weak country-level engagement and ownership and poor government contributions to the funding of polio outbreak response. Most of the polio outbreak countries are still facing multiple public health emergencies at the same time (measles, cholera, viral hemorrhagic fever outbreaks, natural disasters, etc.). Inaccu-

rate population figures, due to the lack of reliable census data, worsen this situation and affect the quality of the planning of activities and the accuracy of coverage results.

- Growing security risks in many countries has resulted in political instability, leading to poor engagement and commitment of local authorities. The resulting conflict exacerbates access issues due to population movements (refugees, internally displaced populations (IDPs)), wide geographies and difficult terrain resulting in chronically missed children, poor vaccination coverage, continued circulation of poliovirus, and spreading of outbreaks.
- Chronically missed children for vaccination: The interactions between the multiple factors above described lead to the late detection of poliovirus circulation, resulting in the late and poor planning and implementation of polio outbreak preparedness and responses in many countries. The persistent poor SIA quality in many outbreak settings and the existence of many pockets of underserved populations (insecurity, difficult terrains, displaced populations, and populations with persistent rumors against vaccination and/or vaccine hesitancies) are the main contributing factors to the chronically missed children for vaccination that is observed.

6. Conclusions

The Polio Surge Capacity Support Program collaborative platform with the US CDC and GPEI partners for polio outbreak preparedness and response is providing a unique opportunity for the routine review of country technical assistance needs, program performance review, and ability to provide technical assistance needs in the context of available resources. This collaborative platform continues to effectively support polio outbreak countries in improving the early detection of poliovirus circulation and narrowing the missed children's gaps. The above-described growing program complexity and challenges require increased resources and strong measures to allow for the effective eradication of polio outbreaks. Among these measures, priority should be provided to strongly advocating GPEI partners and member states in order to continue to mobilize more resources for polio eradication, especially to strengthen the mobilization of local resources by member states to complement GPEI efforts. Urgent attention should also be provided to review the identified emerging program challenges, as described above, and to determine realistic and country-specific action plans to address them.

Author Contributions: Conceptualization, V.K.F.D., F.A., V.A.E., M.B.W., I.K., T.A.K. and P.T.H.; methodology, V.K.F.D., F.A., V.A.E., M.B.W., I.K., T.A.K. and P.T.H.; validation, V.K.F.D.; data curation, F.A. and V.K.F.D.; writing—original draft preparation, V.K.F.D.; writing—review and editing, V.K.F.D., F.A., V.A.E., M.B.W., I.K., T.A.K. and P.T.H.; visualization, F.A. and V.K.F.D.; supervision, V.K.F.D.; project administration, V.K.F.D. All authors have read and agreed to the published version of the manuscript.

Funding: The TFGH's Polio Surge Capacity Support Program is funded by the US CDC through a Cooperative Agreement. This manuscript is a project report. It does not require any additional project funding.

Data Availability Statement: Restrictions apply to the availability of these data. Data were obtained from the Situation Reports of outbreak countries, and are available from the authors with the permission of countries.

Acknowledgments: The authors are grateful to Mahamadou Dao, Monica Grier, Pamela Jenkins, and Lorna Cameron, who contributed to the deployments of the Polio Surge team members to outbreak countries. The findings and conclusions of this report are those of the authors, and do not necessarily represent the official position of TFGH and the polio eradication initiative partners.

Conflicts of Interest: The authors declare no conflict of interest.

References

1. Sutter, R.W.; Tangermann, R.H.; Aylward, R.B.; Cochi, S.L. Poliomyelitis eradication: Progress, challenges for the end game, and preparation for the post-eradication era. *Infect. Dis. Clin. N. Am.* **2001**, *15*, 41–64. [CrossRef] [PubMed]
2. Cochi, S.L.; Freeman, A.; Guirguis, S.; Jafari, H.; Aylward, B. Global Polio Eradication Initiative: Lesson learned and legacy. *J. Infect. Dis.* **2014**, *210* (Suppl. S1), S540–S546. [CrossRef] [PubMed]
3. Sutter, R.W.; Platt, L.; Mach, O.; Jafari, H.; Aylward, R.B. The new polio eradication end game: Rationale and supporting evidence. *J. Infect. Dis.* **2014**, *210* (Suppl. S1), S434–S438. [CrossRef] [PubMed]
4. Global Polio Eradication Initiative. *Polio Eradication Strategy 2022–2026*; World Health Organization: Geneva, Switzerland, 2021.
5. Bigouette, J.P. Progress Toward Polio Eradication—Worldwide, January 2019—June 2021. *Morb. Mortal. Wkly. Rep.* **2021**, *70*, 1129–1135. [CrossRef] [PubMed]
6. Davlantes, E. Update on Wild Poliovirus Type 1 Outbreak—Southeastern Africa, 2021–2022. *Morb. Mortal. Wkly. Rep.* **2023**, *14*, 72. [CrossRef] [PubMed]
7. Lee, S.E. Progress Toward Poliomyelitis Eradication—Worldwide, January 2021–March 2023. *Morb Mortal Wkly Rep.* **2023**, *72*, 517–522. [CrossRef] [PubMed]
8. GPEI Global Circulating Vaccine Derived Polio Virus (cVDPV). Available online: https://polioeradication.org/wp-content/uploads/2024/04/weekly-polio-analyses-cVDPV-20240423.pdf (accessed on 28 December 2023).
9. Global Polio Eradication Initiative. *Standard Operating Procedures, Responding to a Poliovirus Event or Outbreak*; Version 3.1; World Health Organization: Geneva, Switzerland, 2020.
10. Kalkowska, D.A.; Wassilak, S.G.; Pallansch, M.A.; Burns, C.C.; Wiesen, E.; Durry, E.; Badizadegan, K.; Thompson, K.M. Outbreak response strategies with type 2—Containing oral poliovirus vaccines. *Vaccine* **2023**, *41* (Suppl. S1), A142–A152. [CrossRef] [PubMed]

pathogens

MDPI

Review

Review of Poliovirus Transmission and Economic Modeling to Support Global Polio Eradication: 2020–2024

Kimberly M. Thompson * and Kamran Badizadegan

Kid Risk, Inc., Orlando, FL 32819, USA; kb@kidrisk.org
* Correspondence: kimt@kidrisk.org

Abstract: Continued investment in the development and application of mathematical models of poliovirus transmission, economics, and risks leads to their use in support of polio endgame strategy development and risk management policies. This study complements an earlier review covering the period 2000–2019 and discusses the evolution of studies published since 2020 by modeling groups supported by the Global Polio Eradication Initiative (GPEI) partners and others. We systematically review modeling papers published in English in peer-reviewed journals from 2020–2024.25 that focus on poliovirus transmission and health economic analyses. In spite of the long-anticipated end of poliovirus transmission and the GPEI sunset, which would lead to the end of its support for modeling, we find that the number of modeling groups supported by GPEI partners doubled and the rate of their publications increased. Modeling continued to play a role in supporting GPEI and national/regional policies, but changes in polio eradication governance, decentralized management and decision-making, and increased heterogeneity in modeling approaches and findings decreased the overall impact of modeling results. Meanwhile, the failure of the 2016 globally coordinated cessation of type 2 oral poliovirus vaccine use for preventive immunization and the introduction of new poliovirus vaccines and formulation, increased the complexity and uncertainty of poliovirus transmission and economic models and policy recommendations during this time.

Keywords: polio; eradication; modeling; policy; decision

1. Introduction

The over 100 publications related to polio eradication modeling since 2020 [1–102] provide an indication of ongoing challenges in the quest to achieve the 1988 World Health Assembly (WHA) resolution to eradicate paralytic poliomyelitis ("polio") [103]. The WHA target of achieving polio eradication by the year 2000 led a small group of core partners to establish the Global Polio Eradication Initiative (GPEI) to provide, mobilize, and coordinate the necessary planning, financial, and technical resources [104]. Although early action plans expected the achievement of polio eradication as a result of national efforts to strengthen their routine polio immunization programs and global improvements in surveillance, the strategies for meeting the year 2000 target also included immunization campaigns [105]. Over time, operational challenges and the complexity of polio eradication became increasingly apparent, with successive target deadlines for various objectives repeatedly missed [104]. Shortly before 2000, policymakers began to recognize the potential role of using insights from dynamic poliovirus transmission (e.g., [106–109]) and static health economics (e.g., [110]) modeling to support decision-making for the polio eradication endgame. These early studies helped to motivate the GPEI core partners to formally engage independent modeling groups to provide policy and decision insights, as discussed in a prior systematic review of poliovirus transmission and health economic modeling studies published in English from 2000 to 2019 [1].

Recognizing the importance of facilitating access for modelers to national, regional, and global data, the GPEI core partners developed a data sharing agreement to support polio modeling groups [1]. The prior review of 2000–2019 included documentation of all polio-related publications by the three independent modeling groups supported by GPEI core partners under the data sharing agreement as of 2019 [1]. Since 2019, however, the polio modeling landscape has evolved and expanded. While two groups, Kid Risk, Inc. (KRI, Orlando, FL, USA) and Imperial College (IC, London, UK), continued to perform independent modeling with support from GPEI partners, in 2020, the third modeling group included in the prior review [1], the Institute for Disease Modeling (IDM, Seattle, WA, USA), became part of the Bill and Melinda Gates Foundation (BMGF). With this transition, IDM modeling went fully under the operational control of an influential GPEI core partner that presumably could rely on internal modeling results for decision-making without external peer review. In addition, with personnel moves and the expansion of the GPEI data sharing agreement to allow each core partner to support more than one independent modeling group, several other groups also became GPEI-partner-supported polio modeling groups. These include the London School of Hygiene and Tropical Medicine (LSHTM), the South African Centre for Epidemiological Modelling and Analysis (SACEMA), and the Georgia Institute of Technology (GIT). In addition to studies by GPEI-supported polio modeling groups (henceforth "modeling groups"), the literature continues to include some poliovirus transmission and economic modeling studies published by others.

The complexity of modeling poliovirus transmission remains a challenge due to the presence of three distinct poliovirus serotypes (i.e., types 1, 2, and 3) and numerous strains of live polioviruses (LPVs), including wild polioviruses (WPVs), live attenuated oral poliovirus vaccines (OPVs), and OPV-related strains. OPV-related strains include vaccine-derived polioviruses (VDPVs) that can result in outbreaks of circulating VDPVs (cVDPVs, also referred to as "variant" polioviruses), if OPV-related viruses transmit in populations with low immunization coverage. The GPEI reports cases of WPVs and cVDPVs weekly, but not other strains. However, other OPV-related strains, including immunodeficiency-associated VDPVs (iVDPVs), which occur rarely in individuals with primary immunodeficiencies, represent an important concern for eradication because immunodeficient patients can become prolonged or chronic poliovirus excreters and potentially act as a local source for re-introduction in an otherwise polio-free population. OPV-related risks also include rare cases of vaccine-associated paralytic polio (VAPP) that can occur in OPV recipients or their close contacts.

Additional challenges arise from the complex historical use of inactivated poliovirus vaccines (IPV) and OPV, including different formulations of OPV. Historically, OPVs used Sabin OPV strains, for example, trivalent OPV (tOPV, containing types 1, 2, and 3), monovalent OPV (mOPV, containing type 1, 2, or 3, and identified as mOPV1, mOPV2, or mOPV3), or bivalent OPV (bOPV, containing types 1 and 3). More recently, however, the development of a novel type 2 OPV (nOPV2) strain led to its use instead of or in addition to mOPV2 in outbreak response immunization campaigns, with novel OPV types 1 and 3 rapidly being developed. In addition, while all IPV formulations remain trivalent, licensed vaccines use either wild seed strains (Salk IPV) or Sabin OPV seed strains (Sabin IPV), and delivery of IPV can occur standalone in full or fractional dosing or in combination with other antigens. All national immunization programs deliver poliovirus vaccines in their routine immunizations (RI) according to age-based national schedules. Some countries also deliver poliovirus vaccines in supplemental immunization activities (SIAs), which target individuals within a specific age range over a short period of time, either as planned preventive SIAs (pSIAs) or reactive outbreak response SIAs (oSIAs). Poliovirus modeling studies must ideally incorporate all relevant biological, epidemiological, risk, and economic data on different poliovirus types and strains to provide value to policymakers.

Since the body of literature has expanded significantly since the prior review [1], we sought to document the publications of the different modeling groups and to systematically review poliovirus transmission and economic modeling results published in English for 2020–2024.25. The prior review noted the absence of a single repository for global polio policy decisions [1], and this remains an ongoing challenge. For this update, we recognized the opportunity to review the GPEI annual reports, conclusions and recommendations of the World Health Organization Strategic Advisory Group of Experts on Immunization (SAGE) meetings, and reports of technical advisory groups to assess the impact of modeling in supporting polio policies and decisions. This review seeks to provide insights into the role and impact of modeling on national, regional, and global policies with respect to the ongoing polio endgame.

2. Materials and Methods

For each of the 102 studies that met our inclusion criteria [1–102] (Figure 1), we used the same categories and hierarchy to classify the type of modeling study as in the prior review [1]: (i) integrated modeling (i.e., including both dynamic transmission and economic modeling), (ii) dynamic transmission models, subcategorized as differential-equation-based (DEB), stochastic compartmental (SC), individual-based (IB), and/or discrete event simulation (DES), (iii) economic analyses, or (iv) other. The "other" category (i.e., polio publications not reporting poliovirus transmission or health economic modeling) applies only to the modeling groups, which we categorized as: statistical analyses (further classified as risk assessment, vaccine effectiveness, or mucosal immunity studies), reviews, discussions of policy options, or perspectives/commentaries as before [1].

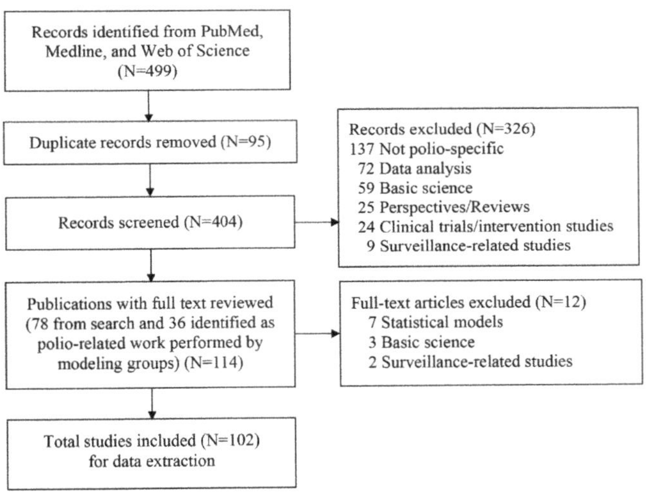

Figure 1. Literature search process.

In this review, we provide a synopsis of all poliovirus-related publications by the six modeling groups as of early 2024 and all poliovirus transmission and economic modeling studies identified in our search and published between 2020–2024.25. We also summarize trends in the numbers and types of polio-related papers published by the modeling groups and other poliovirus transmission and economic modeling papers, for which we update the summary statistics from the prior review [1]. To appropriately discuss trends, we updated the attribution of studies published 2000–2019 [1] for 2 studies led by an LSHTM researcher (Dr. Kathleen O'Reilly) with IC coauthors [111,112] from IC to LSHTM. Assuming that the GPEI data sharing agreement with LSHTM could cover other polio researchers at LSHTM, in our analysis of trends, we changed the attribution of a 2001 transmission modeling study by Dr. Paul Fine [113] from the "other" transmission modeling group in prior review [1] to LSHTM. We also added other LSHTM polio-related publications between 2000 and 2019 (i.e., statistical analyses, vaccine effectiveness and immunology studies, reviews, and perspectives [114–127]), although we note the continued exclusion of poliovirus transmission modeling papers published by these LSHTM researchers prior to 2000 [106,107]. The shift of IDM into BMGF created challenges for characterizing the contributions of IDM and BMGF modelers. We searched for and included polio publications by IDM named- staff identified in the prior review still at IDM/BMGF (i.e., Drs. Guillaume Chabot-Couture, Michael Famulare, Steve Kroiss, Hil Lyons, and Kevin McCarthy) [1]. Similar to the prior review [1], which mentioned but did not include a 2017 BMGF-led statistical analysis that characterized population immunity in the Democratic Republic of the Congo [128], this updated review excludes results from serological surveys [129,130] and a statistical approach for analyzing and presenting polio surveillance data to supplement standard performance indicators [131].

In addition to characterizing trends in the numbers and types of publications, we identified papers that covered the same themes identified in the prior review [1]. We also added themes that emerged between 2020 and 2024, including nOPV, COVID-19/pandemic modeling, secondary effects of OPV, GPEI transition and integration, and containment risks. For the subset of studies that included poliovirus transmission modeling, we identified the specific population modeled.

As noted in the prior review [1], no depository of polio policy or GPEI decisions exists, which undermines efforts to systematically review and document the decision-support provided by modeling. However, while national, regional, and global health leaders and the GPEI leaders make policy decisions that SAGE does not review, for this analysis, we reviewed the published conclusions and recommendations from SAGE biannual meetings from inception in 1999 through April 2024 [132]. We found that SAGE discussions occasionally referred to input from technical advisory groups, which led us to review all available reports from the Advisory Committee on Polio Eradication (ACPE), which met nine times during 2004–2009, and the SAGE polio working group (SPWG), which met 27 times since its creation in 2008 through April 2024. From SPWG meeting notes for the record, we extracted the model group affiliations for SPWG meeting attendance. SPWG membership included Dr. Kimberly Thompson from KRI (term, meetings 1–14, 2008–2017), Dr. Nicholas Grassly from IC (meetings 1–19, 2008–2020), Dr. Guillaume Chabot-Couture from IDM/BMGF (meetings 15–27, 2017–present), and Dr. Kathleen O'Reilly from LSHTM (meetings 20–27, 2020–present). We identified participation in SPWG meetings by representatives of the groups noting participation as a SPWG member (M) or guest (G), and we noted whether a representative of the modeling group presented its work during the meeting or if some other speaker presented work from the modeling group (e.g., another modeling group or a GPEI partner). Finally, we also reviewed the 1999–2022 GPEI Annual Reports [133–156]. From all of the available reports, we searched the references to the modeling groups, including citations of their studies, and we extracted the context and nature of the modeling mentioned.

With changes in GPEI leadership (Dr. Bruce Aylward (before 2000–2014) [157], Dr. Hamid Jafari (2015) [158], Mr. Michel Zaffran (2016–2020) [159] and Mr. Adian O'Leary (2021–present) [159]), we observed that GPEI changed its governance structure, and we separately reported how GPEI strategies and timelines evolved over time [104]. These changes included the creation of the GPEI Strategy Committee in December 2014 [157]. From experience, we know of modeling presentations made to the GPEI Strategy Committee (e.g., KRI, IC, and IDM/BMGF all presented modeling related to responding to the global situation with type 2 outbreaks in April and May 2022), but in the absence of published meeting records or minutes, we could not report on the role of modeling input in GPEI Strategy Committee decisions.

3. Results

This section begins with a brief overview of each of the 102 studies identified by the search process summarized in Figure 1 [1–102]. As before [1], we organize these by modeling group (i.e., KRI, IC, LSHTM, IDM/BMGF, SACEMA, GIT), and others. We then provide summary statistics of the included publications and characterize overall trends and themes, considering these in the context of the prior review [1]. Finally, we report the apparent impact of modeling in GPEI Annual Reports and SAGE conclusions and recommendations.

3.1. Studies That Met Inclusion Criteria Published 2020–2024.25

3.1.1. KRI

In 2020, KRI published reviews on several topics, including the prior review of modeling studies [1], potential use of vaccine patches for immunization, including IPV [2], and the performance of the United States Vaccine Injury Compensation Program (VICP): 1988–2019 [3], which highlighted VAPP risks as a key motivation for VICP establishment. KRI also published a commentary related to incentives for developing vaccine patches [4] and an economic analysis related to developing better defaults for valuing health outcomes based on health opportunity costs [5].

Prior to and during the COVID-19 pandemic, KRI published several studies related to updating the inputs of its global integrated model, including 2019 updates for iVDPV risks [160] (included in the prior review [1]). Following the release of the 2019–2023 GPEI strategic plan [161] and post-cessation strategy [162], KRI updated its integrated model inputs to use retrospective immunization and epidemiology data through the end of 2018 and prospective inputs consistent with available information about recent programmatic performance and updated plans. The third special issue of the journal *Risk Analysis* on Global Poliovirus Risk Management and Modeling, published in February 2021 [6], included many of these studies, several of which appeared online in 2020. In January 2020 (prior to the COVID-19 pandemic), the KRI update of its integrated model reported the GPEI was off-track with respect to achieving its polio eradication goals [161] and attributed this primarily to the low quality of OPV SIAs [7]. For this integrated model update [7], KRI reflected on key differences between the optimistic and ideal risk management assumptions it used prior to 2016 [163,164] and actual performance and plans after 2016 [8]. Due to its expectation of ongoing transmission of WPV1 in Pakistan and Afghanistan [7], KRI built on its prior Pakistan and Afghanistan modeling [165–168] to update its DEB model for these countries (as a single epidemiological reservoir) and identified pSIA strategies that could end WPV1 transmission within the timeline of the 2019–2023 GPEI strategic plan [9]. KRI also developed a DEB model of poliovirus transmission for northeast Nigeria to characterize the transmission of WPV1 that occurred in Borno and Yobe in 2016 [10]. Using this DEB as the basis for an SC model, KRI characterized the confidence of no circulation or undetected WPV1 transmission as a function of time for Borno and Yobe [11], which the Africa Regional Commission for the Certification of Poliomyelitis Eradication used to support its regional certification in 2020 [169]. KRI also updated its characterization of post-OPV cessation risks related to the misuse or inadvertent use of OPV after homotypic cessation, and updated its probability estimates for the need to restart OPV2 production and use in preventive immunization [12]. To support integrated analyses, KRI published updated cost estimates for poliovirus immunization and valuations of polio health outcomes [13], including consideration of health opportunity costs [5]. With global certification of WPV3 eradication in 2019 [170] and reductions of bOPV pSIAs, in late 2020, KRI published a DEB modeling study of the expected reductions of VAPP and cVDPV cases and vaccine dose requirements for a policy of globally coordinated cessation of type 3 OPV (OPV3) before type 1 OPV (OPV1) compared to ongoing bOPV use [14].

Following the May 2020 GPEI publication of an addendum to its 2019–2023 strategic plan that emphasized the use of nOPV2 for oSIAs [171], KRI applied its global model to explore the impacts of using nOPV2 compared to Sabin mOPV2 for oSIAs and reported that even with ideal characteristics, nOPV2 would not likely end all type 2 outbreaks and transmissions [15], which it also discussed in a commentary [16]. Considering pre-COVID-19 conditions, KRI updated its 2010 integrated analysis of the health and economic benefits of the GPEI [172] based on the status of the GPEI and its plans as of 2019 [17], which included consideration of the possibility of ending WPV1 transmission in Pakistan and Afghanistan [9]. KRI also applied its integrated model to consider the health and economic impacts of IPV or tOPV in RI with or without OPV use for oSIAs for different control and eradication scenarios for 2019–2029 [18].

After the emergence of COVID-19, a high-profile suggestion to use OPV to prevent COVID-19 in the United States [173,174] motivated KRI to perform a health economic analysis that estimated VAPP risks and costs with no anticipation of expected benefits for reducing COVID-19 [19] (and associated letter [175]). KRI explored the impact of disruptions caused by the COVID-19 pandemic on global polio eradication in a 2021 study [20], which included updating its assumptions related to long-range exportations. In 2021, KRI published two studies related to the hypothetical emergence of a novel poliovirus in 2020 to simulate a pandemic with poliovirus (instead of COVID-19) and demonstrated the consequences of policy decisions for control or eradication using nonpharmaceutical interventions [21] and vaccines [22]. KRI also updated its characterization of poliovirus transmission in Pakistan and Afghanistan post-COVID-19 to explore the impacts of different vaccine options for oSIAs (e.g., mOPV2, tOPV) in the context of the cocirculation of WPV1 and cVDPV2 [23]. A separate KRI study estimated the expected costs of poliovirus surveillance and immunization campaign quality monitoring for Pakistan and Afghanistan for 2019–2023 [24].

Outbreak response emerged as a theme for several KRI publications during this period. In 2021, KRI characterized the trade-offs of different OPV2 vaccines (i.e., mOPV2 or nOPV2) for oSIAs and the consequences of delaying oSIAs to wait for nOPV2 instead of using available mOPV2 [25]. This analysis emphasized the importance of responding quickly and well with available vaccine supplies (i.e., mOPV2) and anticipated that delays in waiting for nOPV2 would likely lead to over a thousand paralytic cases and greater global cVDPV2 transmission [25]. Despite this analysis, countries in the WHO African region chose to delay oSIAs to wait for nOPV2, which increased the number and spread of reported cVDPV2 cases and motivated KRI to ask, "What kind of world do we want?" in a commentary [26]. A separate commentary raised questions about the effectiveness of a nOPV2 for oSIAs and highlighted the increasingly complicated polio endgame [27].

Following up on discussions of secondary vaccine effects of OPV raised prior to the development of COVID-19 vaccines [19], KRI published a systematic review of secondary health effects of vaccines and policy insights for health economic analyses [28] and separately discussed the challenges of assessing the benefits and costs of non-polio and shared activities for polio and non-polio interventions in polio health economic analyses [29].

In 2022, following the publication of a new GPEI strategic plan for 2022–2026 [176], KRI published 2 analyses related to questions asked by GPEI partners during the development of the plan about the overall cases of polio prevented by poliovirus vaccines and GPEI [30] and the health and economic consequences of a shift to control in 2022 [31] (as an update to a 2007 KRI analysis of control vs. eradication [177]). Although KRI performed these studies in response to specific questions raised by GPEI partners, GPEI did not subsequently refer to the results of these studies.

With new milestones [104] established in the new plan [176], KRI again updated its DEB model for Pakistan and Afghanistan [32]. Assuming the application of a pSIA strategy that KRI identified as successful for ending WPV1 transmission in its model [32], KRI used this analysis as the basis for an SC model to characterize the confidence of no undetected WPV1 transmission as a function of time [33]. The Global Commission for Certification of Poliomyelitis Eradication (GCC) used these results [32,33] to support a potential shortening of the time required to certify the end of indigenous WPV1 transmission after the last reported case or positive environmental sample to less than 3 years, depending on the quality of the surveillance and immunization information [178].

In 2022, KRI removed its assumptions related to OPV restart as a policy option in its global integrated model for consistency with observed experience. This change implied the potential use of OPV vaccines available for oSIAs for the full model time horizon of prospective models, and ended KRI characterization of the probability of OPV restart as a metric to characterize OPV cessation failure [34]. One application of the KRI global model published in late 2022 showed the trade-offs of different OPV2 vaccine options and oSIA characteristics (i.e., scope, timeliness, quality) [34], which identified aggressive options that could potentially lead to a high probability of cVDPV2 transmission dying out by the end of the model time horizon and characterized the low chances of success for the *status quo* GPEI strategy and policies. A separate study applied a DEB model of a hypothetical population with cocirculation of types 1 and 2 and demonstrated the advantages of coadministration of both types (e.g., tOPV or bOPV and nOPV2) compared to sequential or alternating strategies [35]. KRI also performed a look-back analysis to learn from its prior prospective modeling of oSIAs for managing OPV2 cessation [36].

In 2023, KRI explored the complexity of modeling the increase in vaccine options (i.e., nOPVs, different IPV formulations) and the dynamics of starting and/or stopping OPV in national immunization programs after OPV cessation [37]. KRI commented on polio eradication hurdles [38] and the need for updating expectations for nOPV2 [39]. KRI also reviewed the experience with the OPV2 stockpiles and discussed the challenges of forecasting vaccine demand given uncertainty about prospective national, regional, and global policies [40]. With ongoing discussions about potential global coordination of bOPV cessation, KRI also applied its global integrated model to characterize the expected outcomes of coordinated global cessation of bOPV use in 2027 without bOPV pSIAs [41], as suggested by the 2022–2026 strategic plan [176]. In addition to exploring the expected annual paralytic cases by type over time, KRI also explored the worst-case scenarios [42]. In the context of low expectations of successful bOPV cessation, a related health economic analysis anticipated a relatively low value of antiviral drugs [43].

Finally, in 2023–2024, KRI published a DEB model of the cVDPV2 transmission and IPV oSIA for the imported cVDPV2 outbreak that occurred in 2022 in New York State [44]. KRI used this as the basis for an SC model analysis that explored confidence about no circulation as a function of time since the last positive surveillance signal [45], which helped to support the New York State and national leaders feel more confident about the end of the outbreak. KRI also explored the trade-offs of different poliovirus vaccine options for outbreak response in IPV-using countries, such as the US 2022 cVDPV2 outbreak, and considered a hypothetical cVDPV1 outbreak to show differences between poliovirus types [46], which supported the 2023 US decisions to offer IPV to adults [179] and deliberations by the Advisory Committee on Immunization Practices (ACIP) about the potential use of OPV in the US for oSIAs at its February 2024 meeting. This study also included a systematic review of modeling studies that included IPV use in outbreak response [46].

3.1.2. IC

The studies identified for IC for 2020–2024.25 showed its continued focus on statistical analyses of existing surveillance data and data collected as part of prospective trials or challenge studies and included a new focus area related to the development of a poliovirus direct detection method. With respect to transmission modeling, IC applied an SC model to characterize the spread of serotype-2 vaccine-derived-poliovirus outbreaks in Pakistan and Afghanistan to inform outbreak control strategies in the context of the COVID-19 pandemic [47], which built on a statistical analysis that quantified movement patterns and vaccination status in high-risk mobile populations [48].

Statistical analyses published by IC included an analysis of immune predictors of OPV immunogenicity among infants in South India [49]. One IC study used poliovirus genetic sequences from GenBank and demonstrated the application of phylogenetic and phylogeospatial modeling to infer geospatial transmission patterns of poliovirus transmission during the 2010 Tajikistan outbreak [50]. Another analysis characterized the variability in the sensitivity of environmental surveillance sites in Nigeria to detect poliovirus and other enteroviruses [51]. Two IC studies focused on risk factors for cVDPV2 transmission in Africa after 2016 [52,53]. The first of these highlighted the need for larger and faster OPV2 oSIAs to stop cVDPV2 transmission [52], and the second identified risk factors for VDPV2 emergence and suggested priorities for nOPV2 use [53]. IC reported the results of several vaccine effectiveness studies, including a phase 4 clinical trial on the effect of maternal immunization with multivalent vaccines containing IPV in infants [54] and the effectiveness of nOPV2 and mOPV2 against cVDPV2s in Nigeria between 2017 and 2022 [55]. IC commented on the first Africa-based nOPV2 clinical trial [56] and contributed to perspectives related to the impacts of one billion doses and WHO prequalification of nOPV2 [57] and the use of nOPV2 for oSIAs [58].

IC invested substantial effort in the research, development, and implementation of direct detection with nanopore sequencing (DDNS) for poliovirus surveillance [59–62]. This included publications that characterized rapid and sensitive direct detection and identification of poliovirus from stool and environmental surveillance samples using nanopore sequencing [59] and an analysis of the time taken to detect and respond to polio outbreaks in Africa considering the potential impact of direct molecular detection and nanopore sequencing [60]. IC also published a comparison of eleven RNA extraction methods for direct molecular detection of polioviruses from stool [61] and a prospective validation study of DDNS that reported preliminary cost estimates [62]. IC also included poliovirus surveillance in a consortium effort that it led with the goal of defining a research agenda for broad environmental wastewater surveillance of pathogens [63].

Following the detection of imported cVDPV2 transmission in the UK, IC published a commentary about the detection as a wake-up call [64] and a statistical analysis of the sustained detection by enhanced environmental surveillance in London sewage between February and July 2022 [65]. IC contributed substantially (i.e., three of eight coauthors) to a review of the use of IPV for oSIAs [66] prepared at the request of the SPWG for discussion at its 24th meeting (August 2022) and the October 2022 SAGE meeting.

3.1.3. LSHTM

Our review identified one SC modeling study that explored the effect of population partitioning on the probability of silent poliovirus transmission, which included a coauthor affiliated with both LSHTM and SACEMA [67]. The lead author of this study [67] published several poliovirus transmission modeling studies counted as "other transmission studies" in the prior review [1], in collaboration with a polio modeler from the University of Michigan (Dr. James Koopman). This study [67] represented the only publication that met the review inclusion criteria for SACEMA, although for this review, we attributed it to LSHTM.

As discussed earlier, several IC studies in the prior review included a researcher who moved to LSHTM in 2018 [1]. Not surprisingly, given prior collaboration, several LSHTM-led studies published in 2020–2024.25 included coauthors from IC [68–70]. One study included a coauthor from IDM/BMGF [71]. LSHTM reported statistical epidemiological analyses that characterized changes in the epidemiology of poliovirus serotype 2 following OPV2 cessation [68], which followed discussions held during a January 2020 meeting that included all of the groups. Other LSHTM studies explored the optimization of environmental surveillance to detect poliovirus importations into England and Wales [69] and characterized the epidemiology of cVDPV2 global outbreaks between 2016 and 2020 [70]. Another statistical analysis characterized the impact of surveillance and other factors on the detection of emergent and circulating vaccine-derived polioviruses [71]. We identified several LSHTM reviews related to the polio endgame [72], the accelerated roll-out of the nOPV2 vaccine [73], and challenges with achieving polio eradication given population immunity as of early 2024 [74]. LSHTM coauthors also commented on the challenges of informative wastewater sampling for SARS-CoV-2, considering lessons learned from polio eradication [75]. LSHTM also published a vaccine effectiveness study of an mOPV2 challenge dose given to IPV-vaccinated children [76], a mucosal immunity study for nOPV2 in healthy adults [77], and a review of polio mucosal immunity studies [78].

3.1.4. IDM/BMGF

IDM/BMGF published three poliovirus transmission modeling related studies between 2020 and 2024.25 [79–81]. Using an IB model, the first study incorporated the results from a mOPV2 clinical trial performed in Bangladesh, which suggested that household and community structure played an important role in limiting transmission [79]. In 2023, the second study described the development of a DEB model that endogenously included OPV2 reversion for the same population [80]. The third study applied a DEB model to revisit the role of time-varying viral shedding in modeling environmental surveillance using the 2013 poliovirus outbreak in Israel [81].

IDM/BMGF also published multiple statistical analyses. One study modeled the genetic sequences of type 2 polioviruses and identified positive selection and tight transmission bottlenecks that substantially influenced the early evolution of OPV2 [82]. Another study of disease surveillance investments and administrative data for Pakistan showed the limited value of the available information for improving surveillance quality [83]. Studies in 2023 developed a real-time prediction model of cVDPV2 outbreaks to aid oSIA decisions [84] and analyzed changes in population immunity for all three types of polioviruses since the 2016 shift from tOPV to bOPV for selected countries and regions [85]. The final IDM/BMGF publication applied a time series statistical model to estimate the vaccine effectiveness of nOPV2 in oSIAs in Nigeria, which also reported similar vaccine effectiveness of mOPV2, but substantially lower effectiveness for IPV than for either OPV2 [86].

3.1.5. GIT

GIT published its first two poliovirus transmission modeling studies in 2024, including a peer-reviewed conference publication [87] and a related journal article [88]. Both studies described the application of a DEB model it developed to characterize cVDPV2 transmission and the impacts of interventions that aim to control outbreaks in Nigeria, and they identified the need for more aggressive oSIAs (i.e., more rounds and broader coverage, particularly in under-vaccinated communities) [87,88].

3.1.6. Economic Analyses Published by Other Groups

The search identified two other studies published in 2020 that presented game theoretic applications to polio, which we included as other economic analyses [89,90]. The first integrated a DEB model with two age classes (i.e., [180] identified in the prior review [1]) into the game theoretic model, which led us to characterize it as an integrated model [89]. The study concluded that achieving polio eradication would require a mandatory vaccination policy [89]. The second study used survey data related to perceptions of the population benefits of OPV and statistical model inputs informed by poliovirus transmission characteristics in a model that suggested that prosocial behavior to receive bOPV in Israel contributed some to the oSIA vaccine uptake after the 2013 WPV1 outbreak [90].

The search found three other polio-related economic modeling studies. These include cost-effectiveness analyses of three poliovirus immunization schedules in Shanghai, China [91] and various immunization schedules with Sabin IPV in Hangzhou, China [92]. The final study assumed OPV could provide protection from COVID-19 due to secondary effects and suggested the need to prioritize clinical trials and other studies that could resolve the uncertainty about the effects of OPV on COVID and other non-poliovirus diseases [93].

3.1.7. Poliovirus Transmission Modeling Studies Published by Other Groups

Our review identified nine other studies that presented DEB models of poliovirus transmission for theoretical populations using different numerical simulation methods [94–102].

3.2. *Trends in Characteristics of Polio Modeling Studies*

Table 1 provides a high-level comparison between the numbers and types of studies included in this review compared to those in the prior review for 2000–2019 [1] (with the updates discussed above). Notably, the 102 studies identified for the 4.25 years covered in this review imply an increase in the annual rate of polio modeling papers published over time of approximately 2, 5, 9, 22, and 24 papers/year, respectively, for 2000–2004, 2005–2009, 2010–2014, 2015–2019, and 2020–2024.25. Among the modeling groups, KRI published the largest number of studies for 2020–2024.25 (46 publications), followed by IC (20 publications), and LSHTM (12 publications).

Table 1. Characteristics of included studies with comparison to results reported for 2000–2019 [1].

Time Period	2000–2019 [1]	2020–2024.25
Modeling group (first publication year)	Count (number excluded)	Count (number excluded) [References]
KRI (2003)	78	46 [1–46]
IC (2006)	44 [a,b] (1 [c])	20 (3 [d]) [47–66]
LSHTM (2000) *	17 [c] (1 [b])	12 [d,e,f] [67–78]
IDM/BMGF (2014/2021) *	19 (2 [a])	8 (1 [e]) [79–86]
SACEMA (2022) *	NA	0 (1 [f]) [67]
GIT (2024) *	NA	2 [87,88]
Other economic analyses (2000)	9	5 [89–93]
Other transmission modeling (2000)	23	9 [94–102]
Publication year	Count {Rate per year}	Count {Rate per year}
2000–2004	10 {2}	
2005–2009	26 {5}	
2010–2014	45 {9}	
2015–2019	109 {22}	
2020–2024.25		102 {24}
Study type	Count	Count
Integrated (DEB and economic)	12	6 [g]
DEB	42	34
SC	14	4
IB	9	1
DES, DEB	3	0
DEB, SC	2	0
DEB, IC	1	0
Economic/cost analysis only **	15	10
Risk assessment **	20	18
Vaccine effectiveness **	17	3
Mucosal immunity **	6	3
Reviews **	14	8
Discussions of policy options **	5	1
Perspectives/commentaries **	30	14

Abbreviations: BMGF, Bill and Melinda Gates Foundation; DEB, differential-equation-based model; DES, discrete-event simulation model; GIT, Georgia Institute of Technology; GPEI, Global Polio Eradication Initiative; IB, individual-based model; IC, Imperial College; IDM, Institute for Disease Modeling; KRI, Kid Risk, Inc.; LSHTM, London School of Hygiene and Tropical Medicine; SC, stochastic compartmental; SACEMA, South African Centre for Epidemiological Modelling and Analysis.

* Only KRI, IC, IDM included in the prior review as GPEI-partner-supported modeling teams covered under the GPEI Data Sharing Agreement as of 2019, although LSHTM researchers published studies noted in the prior review [1]. Other modeling groups added (including LSHTM) reflect the expansion of the GPEI Data Sharing Agreement. BMGF absorbed IDM in 2021, such that we continued to include IDM/BMGF studies published by IDM authors in the prior review [1] after 2021 as IDM/BMGF (see text).

** Categories only applicable to studies published by KRI, IC, IDM/BMGF, LSHTM, SACEMA, and GIT.

[a] Two IC studies included an IDM coauthor [1].

[b] One IC study from the prior review included an LSHTM coauthor [1].

[c] LSHTM papers published 2000–2019 are now reclassified (see Methods), including 2 papers with IC coauthors [1] now counted here [111,112], one DEB modeling study published in 2001 [113] moved from the other transmission models category [1], one statistical epidemiological study (Risk assessment) [114], four mucosal immunology studies [115–118], nine perspectives/commentaries [119–127].

[d] Three LSHTM studies included an IC coauthor [68–70].

[e] One LSHTM study included an IDM coauthor [71].

[f] One LSHTM paper included a coauthor with both an LSHTM and SACEMA affiliation [67].

[g] One game theoretic analysis is counted here as an integrated model instead of an economic or cost model due to its inclusion of a dynamic transmission model [89].

Table 2 summarizes the themes explored in the included studies by all groups with publications discussed in the prior section. We identified publications by multiple groups for several key themes from the prior review [1], as well as several new themes. Given the global situation with ongoing poliovirus transmission, particularly for cVDPV2s, we identified publications by all the groups in Table 2 on: outbreak response speed (and quality), population immunity, and novel OPV, particularly nOPV2. All groups discussed changes in population immunity in multiple publications, albeit with different definitions. As in the prior review [1], outbreak response speed and quality represented a major theme, with all groups demonstrating the need for improvements in oSIAs. With the use of nOPV2 in oSIAs starting in 2021, our review identified publications by all groups related to nOPV2, many of which included analyses related to nOPV2 use in oSIAs. With respect to OPV cessation dynamics, several groups explored the evolution of OPV, which included some prospective modeling related to potential bOPV cessation.

Table 2. Summary of themes explored and specific populations in poliovirus transmission model studies by group.

Modeling Group	KRI	IC	LSHTM	IDM /BMGF	GIT	Other
Theme						
Outbreak response speed/quality	[7,12,15,23,25,34–36,44,46]	[47,52,53,55,60,62]	[70]	[84,86]	[87,88]	[90]
Expanded age group SIAs	[34]					
Population immunity*	[7,9–12,14,15,17–23,25,30–36,41–46]	[47,52,53]	[70,74]	[82–86]	[87,88]	
OPV cessation dynamics	[14,41,42]					
Silent transmission on an IPV background/delayed detection of transmission due to IPV use	[44–46]	[52,53]	[68,70,71]	[80,85]		
Role of IPV after OPV cessation	[17,18]	[54]				[91,92]
Undetected circulation	[11,33,45]		[67,69]			
Role of IPV in oSIAs	[22,31,44,46]	[55,66]			[87,88]	
(Environmental) surveillance	[10,11,24,33,44,45]	[50,51,59–65]	[69,71,75]	[81,83]		
Vaccine stockpile	[40]					
iVDPVs	[43]					
Novel OPV (nOPV)	[13,15,16,20,22,23,25–27,34–43,46]	[55–58]	[72,73]	[86]	[87,88]	
COVID-19/pandemic modeling	[19–22]					
Secondary effects of OPV	[19,20,28,29]	[47]				[93]
GPEI transition/integration	[29]					
Containment	[12]					
Geographic area modeled for studies with poliovirus transmission models						
Global	[7,12,14,15,17,20–22,25,30,31,34,36,41–43]					
Pakistan/Afghanistan	[9,19,23,32,33]	[47]				
Nigeria	[10,11]				[87,88]	
Bangladesh				[79,80]		
Israel						
United States	[18,44–46]					
Hypothetical	[35]		[67]			[89,94–102]

Abbreviations: BMGF, Bill and Melinda Gates Foundation; GIT, Georgia Institute of Technology; GPEI, Global Polio Eradication Initiative; IC, Imperial College; IDM, Institute for Disease Modeling; IPV, inactivated poliovirus vaccine; iVDPV, immunodeficiency-associated vaccine-derived poliovirus; KRI, Kid Risk, Inc.; LSHTM, London School of Hygiene and Tropical Medicine; NA, not applicable; nOPV, novel OPV; OPV, oral poliovirus vaccine; oSIA, outbreak response SIA; SIA, supplemental immunization activity.
* Modeling groups use different definitions for population immunity [1].

Also represented in Table 2 as related to OPV cessation dynamics, we noted multiple studies by different groups on the failure of the 2016 globally coordinated cessation of OPV2 use for preventive immunization, which included retrospective statistical analyses of epidemiological data and poliovirus transmission modeling. With substantial GPEI investments in the expansion of environmental surveillance, Table 2 also shows numerous studies by different groups related to surveillance. Notably, given multiple publications by IC related to its development of DDNS, we broadened the category from environmental surveillance to surveillance.

Most of the modeling groups also published on the topic of IPV use. These publications included IPV use for oSIAs, with some studies motivated by actual experiences (e.g., the 2022 cVDPV2 outbreak in the United States). In addition, multiple groups published studies related to the role of IPV use after OPV cessation, but we did not include the studies that simply added IPV to RI consistent with the prerequisites for OPV2 cessation in Table 2. Not surprisingly, most modeling groups published studies motivated by the global experience with the COVID-19 pandemic, including many studies related to disruptions in national and GPEI immunization activities. Two groups published studies related to undetected circulation in different geographies. Only KRI published studies related to the topics of expanded age group SIAs, silent transmission on an IPV background and/or delayed detection of transmission due to IPV use, vaccine stockpile, iVDPVs, containment, secondary effects of OPV, and GPEI transition and integration.

The bottom portion of Table 2 shows the geographic scope covered by 45 studies that included poliovirus transmission modeling [7,9–12,14,15,17–23,25,30–36,41–47,67,79–81,87–89,94–102]. Not surprisingly, two groups published studies on Pakistan, Afghanistan and Nigeria, which continue to represent critical geographies for polio eradication. Populations modeled by only one group include Bangladesh, Israel, and the United States, and only KRI performed global analyses.

3.3. Modeling in GPEI Annual Reports or SAGE Conclusions and Recommendations

Table 3 provides excerpts of references to modeling and/or modeling groups and the sources for results reported that we identified in the GPEI Annual Reports. These discussions of modeling activities and/or references to studies and results published by the modeling groups provide some indication that GPEI broadly relied on modeling inputs. The rightmost two columns show the modeling group(s) referred to by name or by the journal of their publication, and the references to studies from which the GPEI Annual Reports included mention of specific results. Between 2005 and 2018, the GPEI Annual Reports referred to results from studies published by 4 modeling groups: LSHTM [121], KRI [172,177,181–183], IC [184–187], and IDM [188], and we noted multiple references to the results from older studies over time. References to the results from modeling studies occurred in 4 of 5 years for the 2005–2009, 2010–2014, and 2015–2019 time periods. In the 2020–2022 GPEI Annual Reports, only the 2022 report even alluded to the results from modeling studies by including a link to a 2022 investment case [189] that presented the results of an unpublished update of a prior study [188] and mentioned the outdated results of a 2007 publication [177]. Notably, the investment case did not mention a published 2021 updated economic analysis of the GPEI [17]. Two other relevant studies published shortly after publication of the investment case included quantification of the cases of polio prevented by polio vaccines and GPEI [30] and an update of the consequences of shifting to control in 2022 [31] (as an update for an outdated study of control vs. eradication [177]).

Table 3. Discussions of work related to polio modeling and groups in GPEI Annual Reports [133–156].

Year	Excerpt	Group	Study
2000	Refers to plans to develop a "strategy for stopping vaccination that will evaluate a number of proposed strategies, including routine immunization with the inactivated polio vaccine (IPV) or an OPV 'pulse' immunization followed by cessation"		
2001	"WHO will develop policy decision models over the next 12 months that reflect how the range of possible research outcomes would affect post-certification policy development"		
2002	A "framework has now been developed that summarizes these risks into two major categories, including (a) those due to VDPV, and (b) those due to the handling of wild poliovirus stocks"		
2003	Key decisions in 2003: 1. Cessation of oral polio vaccine (OPV) 2. No universal introduction of the inactivated polio vaccine (IPV) 3. Strategies for the Safe Cessation of OPV "Guidelines for national decision-making on OPV cessation will be completed, outlining: (a) rationale for OPV cessation; (b) risks of polio in the post-OPV era; (c) surveillance requirements; (d) post-OPV stockpile and response; and (e) implications of IPV introduction"		
2004	Concluded that "eradicating all forms of poliomyelitis paralysis will require eventually stopping use of OPV globally and that the cessation of OPV must be implemented simultaneously across the world"		

Table 3. *Cont.*

Year	Excerpt	Group	Study
2005	"A comprehensive approach must be taken to optimize the management of the risks of either the re-emergence of polio due to a cVDPV or the re-introduction of either a wild or Sabin poliovirus, following the global interruption of wild poliovirus transmission." "The ACPE, in October 2005, issued new international standards for polio outbreak response to guide countries in planning and responding to any importations of virus" and "further expansion of mOPV use in supplementary immunization activities", and "assessment was conducted on the consequences of a poliovirus release during or after OPV cessation (Fine P. E. M. and Ritchie S., Consequences of release/reintroduction of polioviruses in different geographic areas after OPV cessation. Risk Analysis, 2006)"	LSHTM, KRI	[121,181] [a,b]
2006	"Research published in Science magazine indicates monovalent OPV can boost immunity enough to stop polio in northern India." "The humanitarian and economic case for finishing eradication is sound. A new study from Harvard University demonstrates that over a 20-year period, controlling polio at high levels would cost more in human suffering and dollars than finishing eradication."	IC, KRI [a]	[177,184]
2007	"To examine the assumptions underpinning current planning for the mOPV stockpile, a Harvard University/Massachusetts Institute of Technology collaboration continues to conduct mathematical modeling of outbreak response activities for polioviruses following OPV cessation." "In close collaboration with the Imperial College of London, studies were undertaken to better estimate the efficacy of mOPV 1 and 3 in different field settings (India, Nigeria, and Pakistan)."	KRI [a], IC	[182,185]
2008	"Studies showing increased efficacy of monovalent type 1 oral polio vaccine (mOPV1) over trivalent oral polio vaccine (tOPV) in Nigeria are published in the New England Journal of Medicine, affirming the feasibility of rapidly stopping polio in that country." "In 2008, the PRC made a grant to Kid Risk Inc., formerly part of a Harvard University and Massachusetts Institute of Technology collaboration, to continue mathematical modeling of outbreak response scenarios for polioviruses following OPV cessation to further inform policy in this area."	IC, KRI	[183,186]
2009	"...An extensive program of research was accelerated in 2009 to develop the tools and policies to minimize and manage the long-term risks of polio." "To prepare for the management of long-term poliovirus risks, the GPEI is focusing research and policy development on three major areas: (1) better characterizing the primary long-term poliovirus risks (ie cVDPVs, VAPP, iVDPVs, and residual stocks of WPVs, VDPVs and Sabin viruses); (2) developing new products to manage the risks associated with OPV cessation, including the development of an international stockpile of mOPVs for cVDPV response and affordable IPV options for low-income countries that perceive the medium or long-term risks of poliovirus warrant continued routine immunization after OPV, cessation. (3) Establishing mechanisms to internationally coordinate risk management strategies, particularly the application of appropriate safeguards and bio-containment conditions for the handling and storage of residual polioviruses and potentially poliovirus-infected materials, the synchronization of the cessation of routine immunization with OPV and the adherence to internationally-agreed processes for the post-eradication use of OPV in response to new cVDPVs."		
2010	"In a rigorous evaluation of the benefits and costs of eradicating polio, a study published in Vaccine finds that the program could provide net benefits of at least US$40–50 billion by 2035, mostly in low-income countries, if transmission of wild polioviruses is interrupted within the next five years." "Jenkins et al, published in the New England Journal of Medicine in June 2010, analyzed the largest-ever recorded cVDPV outbreak detected in Nigeria."	KRI, IC	[172,187]
2011	"Mathematical modeling shows that failure to eradicate the remaining 1% puts the world at significant risk of polio resurgence, potentially leading to over 200,000 children paralyzed annually within a decade."		[177] [c]

Table 3. *Cont.*

Year	Excerpt	Group	Study
2012	"On one side of the balance, a lasting world free of polio where no child will ever know the pain of polio paralysis and US$ 50 billion in economic benefits; on the other, a resurgence of the disease resulting in 200,000 cases every year within 10 years. All countries will benefit equally from global success."		[177] [c]
2013	"Type 2 outbreak response principles were endorsed by the SAGE in November 2013. It was decided that outbreak response should utilize both monovalent OPV type 2 and IPV to rapidly boost and establish population immunity around the outbreak response zone to prevent the emergence of cVDPV. The use of mOPV2 is needed to induce intestinal immunity among those who have not been vaccinated against type-2 previously."		
2014	"In 2006, the World Health Assembly issued international outbreak response guidelines with specific measures countries should take upon detection of a polio outbreak in any polio-free area. Full implementation of these guidelines reduced the extent (in time and number of cases) of new outbreaks by 50% compared to previous outbreaks. Outbreak response is now more critical than ever, as the world is now closer than ever to being polio-free and the phased removal of oral polio vaccines (OPV) is beginning. That is why the GPEI has issued revised international outbreak response guidelines to countries, building on those from 2006."		b
2015	"A polio-free world will reap savings of more than US$ 50 billion, funds that can be used to address other pressing public health and development needs."		[172] [c]
2016	"A polio-free world will result in global savings of US$ 50 billion (mostly in developing countries)."		[172] [c]
2017	"Failure to eradicate polio would result in a drastic resurgence of the disease globally, and within the next 10 years, the world could again see 200,000 new cases every single year." "A world without polio will result in savings of more than US $50 million." ""Globally, a polio-free world will reap savings of over US$50 billion, funds that can be used to address other pressing public health needs". "Even if it has taken longer and cost more than all had anticipated, the goal of a polio-free world — so near at hand — is worth pursuing, for the benefit of all generations of children to come." "In addition to the significant humanitarian benefits associated with polio eradication, the effort is also associated with substantial economic benefits. A world free of polio will result in savings of more than US$50 billion, which can be used to address other critical public health and development needs."		[177] [c] [172] [c]
2018	"Achieving a polio-free world will generate an estimated US$14 billion in cumulative cost savings by 2050, compared to the cost countries would incur to control the virus indefinitely. In financial terms, the global effort to eradicate polio has already saved more than US$ 27 billion in health costs since 1988."		[188]
2019	"...The continued spread of existing cVDPV2 outbreaks and the emergence of new cVDPV2s pointed to the insufficient quality of outbreak response with monovalent oral polio vaccine type 2 (mOPV2). The risk that these strains spread further or that new strains emerge was magnified by an ever-increasing mucosal immunity gap to type 2 poliovirus on the continent, following the switch from trivalent oral polio vaccine (tOPV) to bivalent oral polio vaccine in 2016."		
2020	"Analysis of data for 2020 shows an increase of 0 dose cases and a decrease in 3 plus doses case both in endemic and outbreak countries. This is probably a consequence of the COVID-19 pandemic and related disruptions of immunization campaigns."		d
2021	"A statistical analysis of zero-dose children was performed in 2021 using 2016–2020 sex-disaggregated surveillance data for children aged 0–36 months. It was conducted through an intra-cluster correlation coefficient and adjusted multiple regression analysis to calculate risk at the province and district levels in endemic countries (Afghanistan and Pakistan). Age and sex were used as risk variables to calculate the risk of children being among those who do not receive any dose and to calculate if this risk was equally distributed across the countries. The results were mapped to showcase the districts in which children had a higher risk of not receiving any doses."		d

Table 3. *Cont.*

Year	Excerpt	Group	Study
2022	"The poliovirus is cornered to just a few high-risk geographies, but there is no room for complacency. Continuing to invest in polio eradication could save the world over US$ 30 billion in health care cost savings this century, compared to the cost of just controlling polio."		[e]
2023	NA		

Abbreviations: ACPE, Advisory Committee on Polio Eradication; cVDPV, circulating VDPV; GPEI, Global Polio Eradication Initiative; IC, Imperial College; IPV, inactivated poliovirus vaccine; iVDPV, immunodeficiency-associated VDPV; KRI, Kid Risk, Inc.; LSHTM, London School of Hygiene and Tropical Medicine; mOPV, monovalent OPV; NA, not available; OPV, oral poliovirus vaccine; OPV#, type # OPV (# = 1, 2, or 3); PRC, Polio Research Committee (of the GPEI); SAGE, Strategic Advisory Group of Experts on Immunization for the World Health Organization; tOPV, trivalent OPV; VAPP, vaccine-associated paralytic polio; VDPV, vaccine-derived poliovirus; WHO, World Health Organization; WPV, wild poliovirus.
[a] Kid Risk, Inc. started as the Harvard Kids Risk Project with affiliation with the Massachusetts Institute of Technology in 2004–2007.
[b] In 2005, Kid Risk, Inc. presented modeling to ACPE [190] related to improving outbreak response [181,191] that supported the 2006 outbreak response guidelines. In 2005, ACPE also heard presentations about other modeling studies published in a 2006 special issue of Risk Analysis led by KRI [192], including the cited LSHTM study [121] and another cited paper on containment [193].
[c] Results from an older study mentioned in one or more prior annual reports (see above).
[d] No source for statistical analysis was mentioned.
[e] Links to the 2022 GPEI Investment Case [189], which refers to an unpublished update of [188] and outdated results reported in [177].

Table 4 provides excerpts of discussions of polio modeling (and economic analyses) we identified in SAGE meeting conclusions and recommendations published in the *Weekly Epidemiological Record* [132]. Although every regular SAGE meeting agenda included polio eradication (annually 2000–2002 and biannually 2003–2024), Table 4 only includes meetings for which we identified discussions of polio modeling results. The third column provides references to publications specifically discussed as studies or reviews, as SAGE noted in the conclusions and recommendations. The fourth column provides references to publications we could identify in our review of available presentations to SAGE. Although we identified multiple references to modeling and/or the modeling groups, we identified only five explicit references to specific studies or reviews published by the modeling groups (i.e., KRI [172,177], IC [66,184,185]) and one acknowledgment of IC unpublished work supporting WHO. However, our review of the available presentations made to SAGE identified the inclusion of results from the modeling groups in most of its meetings. We recognized that some of the SAGE meetings included discussions of topics for which relevant modeling available at the time did not get presented (e.g., the role of older age groups in transmission, the economics of using IPV in outbreak response, trade-offs between vaccine choices for outbreak response, including in areas with cocirculation of poliovirus types 1 and 2). We identified some unpublished and not peer-reviewed (to date) modeling results presented (see notes at the bottom of Table 4), most notably predictions about the number of cVDPV2 outbreaks to expect after OPV2 cessation that did not imply any dependence on the implementation of oSIAs. We also observed multiple references to both ACPE and the SPWG. This motivated us to also review the available notes for the record from the face-to-face meetings of these groups. We know from experience that modeling groups attended and presented at some ACPE meetings, but we did not find agendas for all ACPE meetings, and we did not find specific references to the modeling publications presented in the ACPE meeting reports.

Table 4. Polio modeling discussions identified in SAGE meeting conclusions and recommendations.

Meeting Date	Excerpt	Study/Review	Presented at the Meeting
November-1999	"A delay in achieving the polio eradication target would increase the cost of the initiative by as much as US$ 100 million per year. In addition, it would be very difficult to sustain current funding levels for more than 24–36 months, a crucial point for those polio-free countries that would need to continue holding national immunization days beyond the target date to assure freedom from wild poliovirus"		
June-2002	"SAGE reaffirms the importance of the substantial programme of work now devoted to the development of polio immunization policy for the post-certification era. The immediate focus of this policy work should be in evaluating the feasibility of eventually stopping the routine use of oral polio-vaccine (OPV) worldwide" "SAGE recommends that the framework be supplemented by: [1] a peer review of the estimated burden of VAPP, cVDPV, and iVDPV; [2] a geopolitical/cultural understanding of how the 'perceived risks' that can not be answered by the scientific research agenda alone (e.g., bioterrorism, VAPP) may affect the post-certification policy in OPV-using countries; [3] an economic assessment of the various options; and [4] the completion of the research agenda to better define the risks in the post-certification era and the strengths and weaknesses of the risk management strategies"		
June-2004	"SAGE recommended that, to assist its deliberations on post-OPV immunization policy, WHO should keep it fully informed of: all related policy decisions made by the oversight groups responsible for other aspects of the OPV cessation work (i.e. the Ad-hoc Advisory Committee on Polio Eradication, the Global Commission on Certification of Polio Eradication, the Biosafety Advisory Group); the evolving understanding of the nature and magnitude of the risks of circulating polioviruses following interruption of wild poliovirus transmission and OPV cessation; and the outcomes of the continuing work to model these risks over time."		
November-2005	"SAGE also applauded the work in progress on the post-eradication strategies"		
April-2006	"SAGE noted the ratification by ACPE of the new international standards for outbreak response"		
April-2007	"An independent analysis was presented to SAGE that supported the humanitarian and economic case for investing heavily to finish eradication. The study, published in the Lancet, showed that polio "control" would cost more over a 20-year period in human and financial terms than achieving eradication."	[177]	
November-2007	"New studies in India and Nigeria showed that monovalent OPVs afford a 3-fold to 4-fold higher effectiveness per dose than trivalent OPV."	[184,185]	
November-2008	"SAGE recommends that the mathematical model(s) of post-eradication risks be evaluated by Quantitative Immunization and Vaccine Related Research Advisory Committee (QUIVER)."		
April-2009	"Areas for further study include . . . models for estimating the risk of outbreaks of vaccine-derived polio in the post-eradication era, ... SAGE underlined the need for close interaction with QUIVER, given the relevance of its work to policy-making. SAGE must be fully briefed on critical assumptions and assured of the adequacy of data and methods for models that are used to inform policy decisions." "The IPV working group presented a framework for evaluating post-eradication options for vaccination policy. SAGE was impressed with the work, but urged the working group to pay particular attention to uncertainties in mathematical modelling on the risks of emergence of vaccine-derived poliovirus."		[182]

Table 4. *Cont.*

Meeting Date	Excerpt	Study/ Review	Presented at the Meeting
April-2010	"SAGE noted that the positive current epidemiological situation, the new strategic plan, and the sound economic argument for completing eradication together form a particularly appealing product for donors, warranting substantial further investment."	[172]	
November-2010	Extended the term [for the SPWG] to "... allow the working group to benefit from considering ... further mathematical modelling of post-eradication risks..." "SAGE expanded the working group's remit by requesting it to assess whether, in view of the apparent eradication of type-2 wild poliovirus and the preponderance of circulating type-2 vaccine-derived polioviruses in recent years, trivalent OPV should be replaced with bivalent OPV for routine vaccination."		
April-2012	"SAGE also received a report from the SAGE polio working group regarding a switch from trivalent oral poliovirus vaccine (tOPV) to bivalent OPV (bOPV types 1 and 3) and related policy and technical issues, and proposed recommendations for consideration by SAGE."		[194]
April-2014	"Upon reviewing the relevant scientific evidence, SAGE endorsed updates to the existing WHO recommendations for travellers from polio-infected countries"		[195]
October-2014	"Lastly, SAGE endorsed the proposed risk-based approach for boosting immunity to type 2 poliovirus prior to OPV2 withdrawal, by ensuring that sufficient tOPV campaigns are planned and conducted to raise population immunity above the estimated threshold for transmission in areas at highest risk of cVDPV2 emergence. SAGE emphasized that planning for this risk-based approach should be done on a subnational basis."		[191,196]
April-2015	"SAGE noted the increased scope of planned tOPV SIAs that will be implemented to reduce the risk of emergence of new cVDPV2, building on the risk-based approach endorsed by SAGE in October 2014. SAGE endorsed the proposed cVDPV2 elimination strategies in Nigeria and Pakistan and the programme's risk-based approach to prevent and respond to new cVDPV2 emergence in any location."		
October-2015	"The GPEI has optimized its strategy to prevent emergence of VDPV2 through an extensive set of tOPV campaigns, more sensitive definitions of cVDPV2, immediate response to any VDPV2 detection and updated its guidelines for responding to any cVDPV outbreak."		[197] [a]
April-2016	"SAGE reviewed the Polio Working Group discussion on future polio immunization policy. The Working Group proposed to work on the following recommendations: (i) an explicit decision on whether polio vaccination should be continued after global certification of eradication; (ii) the recommended IPV schedule (number of doses, timing, formulation) after OPV withdrawal; and (iii) the criteria for when countries could stop polio vaccination (e.g. surveillance capacity, absence of immunodeficiency-related vaccine-derived poliovirus), based on vaccine and funding availability and expected vaccine price"		

Table 4. *Cont.*

Meeting Date	Excerpt	Study/ Review	Presented at the Meeting
April-2017	"SAGE also reviewed the risk of reintroduction of polioviruses after global OPV cessation. The modelling and epidemiology suggest that VDPV may emerge 0–4 years after the global cessation of OPV use."		[a,b] [198] [c]
October-2017	"SAGE acknowledged WHO's work with Imperial College, London, to grade risks in Tier 3 and 4 countries based on susceptibility, transmission, exposure, and primary immunodeficiency-associated vaccine-derived poliovirus (iVDPV) prevalence."	IC [d]	
April-2019	"SAGE proposed that the GPEI determine the criteria for requesting that OPV2- containing vaccine production be resumed. SAGE agreed that discussions on the criteria are important and should be further explored during future working group meetings"		[199] [e]
March-2020	"SAGE reviewed and agreed with the new GPEI strategy for responding to cVDPV2 outbreaks" (i.e., [160])... "SAGE recommended the strategy be more cautious about setting timelines for the introduction of nOPV2... [and] that tOPV be made available to countries for cVDPV2 outbreak response in subnational areas where there is co-circulation.... SAGE requested that GPEI further elaborate scenarios for using IPV in outbreak responses"		[68,200] [a,b]
October-2020	"SAGE recommended that IPV should not be used for outbreak response because evidence demonstrates that IPV campaigns are unlikely to reach children not reached with OPV campaigns, have limited impact on stopping transmission and have a high programmatic cost. The priority of outbreak response is to stop transmission; therefore, activities should focus on rapidly achieving high coverage with OPV."		[47]
March-2021	"SAGE acknowledged that countries are faced with complex decisions with regards to options for cVDPV2 outbreak response: should they use Sabin-based monovalent OPV type 2 (mOPV2) immediately and risk seeding new VDPV2s, or should they delay outbreak response until the country is programmatically prepared to use nOPV2? SAGE was presented with a modelling analysis of these options and agreed with the conclusion that countries facing cVDPV2 outbreaks should avoid delay and prioritize rapid, high-quality cVDPV2 outbreak response with whichever oral polio vaccine is available to them."		[25]
October-2022	"SAGE was presented with a literature review and programme experience of using IPV for poliovirus outbreak control, and the role of IPV in preventing faecal-oral and oral-oral poliovirus transmission, as requested at the April 2022 SAGE meeting."	[66]	[201,202] [f]
March-2023	"SAGE reiterated its recommendation that outbreak responses be conducted without delay. For response using oral vaccines, nOPV2 should be preferred. However, mOPV2 could be used under exceptional conditions, e.g., if supplies of nOPV2 are inadequate, if emergency use listing (EUL) readiness cannot be achieved, and tOPV in the event of co-circulation of other poliovirus serotypes" "SAGE was presented with evidence of the role of IPV in areas of persistent poliovirus transmission"		[201,203,204] [g]

Table 4. *Cont.*

Meeting Date	Excerpt	Study/ Review	Presented at the Meeting
September-2023	"Modelling analysis suggests that, if mOPV2 had been used instead of nOPV2 since March 2021, an estimated 43 new cVDPV2 emergences would have been detected by August 2023 compared with the 7 observed with nOPV2."		[h,i,j] [33] [k]
February-2024	NA		[52,68] [a]

Abbreviations: ACPE, Advisory Committee on Polio Eradication; BMGF, Bill and Melinda Gates Foundation; bOPV, bivalent OPV; cVDPV, circulating VDPV; EUL, emergency use listing; GPEI, Global Polio Eradication Initiative; IC, Imperial College; IDM, Institute for Disease Modeling; IPV, inactivated poliovirus vaccine; iVDPV, immunodeficiency-associated VDPV; KRI, Kid Risk, Inc.; LSHTM, London School of Hygiene and Tropical Medicine; mOPV, monovalent OPV; NA, not available; nOPV, novel OPV; OPV, oral poliovirus vaccine; OPV#, type # OPV (# = 1, 2, or 3); QUIVER, Quantitative Immunization and Vaccine Related Research Advisory Committee; SAGE, Strategic Advisory Group of Experts on immunization for the World Health Organization; SIA, supplemental immunization activity; SPWG, SAGE polio working group; tOPV, trivalent OPV; VAPP, vaccine-associated paralytic polio; VDPV, vaccine-derived poliovirus; VDPV#, type # VDPV (# = 1, 2, or 3); WHO, World Health Organization.

[a] Presentation included unpublished work from IDM/BMGF (cited in some instances as Global Good, Intellectual Ventures, Institute of Disease Modeling, or IDM).

[b] Unpublished work from IDM shows expected VDPV emergences each year for the first four years after global OPV cessation. Later reference in March 2020 refers to lower unpublished expected numbers than provided by IDM in 2017, with attribution of the lower numbers to the GPEI Eradication and Outbreak Management Group in a table that shows comparisons between pre-OPV2 cessation predictions and post-OPV2 cessation epidemiological experience.

[c] One presentation discussed the future immunization policy for IPV.

[d] Unpublished work by IC.

[e] One presentation discussed new guidelines for surveillance of patients with primary immunodeficiency disorders [189], although this topic did not appear in the conclusions and recommendations from the meeting.

[f] One presentation on the role of older age groups in transmission did not mention previously-published relevant modeling studies [1] or a study showing the need to target birth cohorts born since 2016 now above age 5 years of age for type 2 oSIAs [34].

[g] The evidence of the role of IPV did not include relevant studies published by KRI.

[h] The modeling mentioned in the conclusions and recommendations provided a reference to a conference abstract for modeling performed by IDM.

[i] Publications relevant to the failure of OPV2 cessation by KRI not discussed include [7,8,12,15,36].

[j] One presentation discussed outbreak responses to cocirculation that did not include relevant published modeling that did not support the recommendations made by SAGE at the meeting [35].

[k] One presentation included modeling related to the certification of WPV1 [33], although this topic did not appear in the conclusions and recommendations from the meeting.

Table 5 shows the representation of the modeling groups in the 27 face-to-face SPWG meetings and the dates of the meetings. The third through sixth columns show the roles for four of the modeling groups (i.e., KRI, IC, LSHTM, and IDM/BMGF) by indicating the meetings for which representatives from the group participated as a member (M), an invited external participant (P), or a rapporteur (R). The SPWG generally holds closed meetings, with participation limited to committee members and invited participants, although some representatives of some GPEI core partners also attended SPWG meetings. Representatives of the modeling groups, attended different numbers of total SPWG meetings to date: KRI (14), IC (22), LSHTM (12), and IDM/BMGF (24). As shown in Table 5, which uses an asterisk (*) to indicate a presentation, members frequently presented work from their groups and nearly all invited external participants presented work from their group while at the meeting. The seventh column shows the topic presented by modeling groups (and indicates the group). We identified some presentations that included work from modeling groups not attending the meeting. We included the topic of the presentation and added a note to indicate these presentations. This led to the inclusion of the topics of some presentations in the seventh column with no group indicated, as well as some notes showing presentations given by a group representative that included work from one or more other modeling groups in addition to their own work. As shown in the rightmost column in Table 5, between 2008 and 2014 the SPWG reports included references to specific studies by different modeling groups. However, since 2015, while some SPWG notes for the record mentioned presentations by modeling groups, they did not include references to specific studies (e.g., the IC review of IPV use for oSIAs [66]). In the absence of reviewing each presentation, we could not identify all of the modeling results presented to the SPWG.

Table 5. Representation of modeling at face-to-face SAGE polio workgroup meetings.

Meeting		Roles [a]				Information Extracted from the Note for the Record	
N	Date	KRI	IC	LSHTM	IDM/ BMGF	Presentation Topic (Presenting Modeling Group)	Group [Source(s)]
1	October-08	M *	M *			Modeling the risks: past and future (KRI) Modeling: The next frontiers (IC)	KRI [183]
2	June-09	M	M	P *		Cost-effectiveness of routine polio vaccination (LSHTM) Poliovirus transmission potential (LSHTM)	KRI [177,181–183,194,205–208], LSHTM [107], IC [185,186]
3	March-11	M *	M		P *	Modeling cVDPV risks/post-eradication policies (KRI) Options, risks, and prerequisites for OPV2 cessation (KRI) Modeling tools for cVDPV emergence (IDM)	
4	February-12	M *	M *		P *	Wide-spread transmission of type 2 cVDPV in Nigeria (IC) cVDPV emergence risks pre- and post-eradication (IDM) Modeling and managing VDPV risks: known and not (KRI)	NA
5	November-12	M	M				
6	June-13	M	M		P *	VDPV emergence risk for mOPV2 post-OPV2 cessation (IDM)	NA
7	October-13	M	M *		P *	Post-cessation outbreak response, OPV use, cVDPV risk (IDM)	
8	February-14	M	M *			Review of the duration of mucosal immunity to poliovirus (IC)	
9	July-14	M *	M *		P *	Modeling the risk of cVDPV emergence (KRI) Risk of VDPV emergence and spread (IC) Non-polio-AFP population immunity projections (IDM) tOPV campaigns pre-OPV2 cessation (IDM)	KRI [196,209,210] IC [b]
10	September-15	M	M *		P	Serotype 2 vaccine-derived poliovirus risk assessment (IC)	
11	January-16	M ^	M ^		P	Type 2 outbreak protocol [c] Risks of cVDPV emergence, based on modeling (IDM)	
12	August-16	M *	M *		P *	Detection of type 2 Sabin virus after the switch (IC) Needs for bOPV campaigns prior to OPV13 withdrawal (KRI) Assessment of risks and implications of bOPV use (IDM)	
13	February-17	M *	M *		P *	Roles of different vaccines in outbreaks and the endgame (KRI) Polio endgame modeling, IPV in SIAs (IDM) Impact of IPV in RI and SIA following OPV2 withdrawal (IC)	
14	September-17	M	M		P *	OPV13 cessation and SIA planning (IDM)	
15	February-18		M		M *	Risk assessment for bOPV cessation (IDM), Role of bOPV preventive SIAs pre-bOPV cessation [d]	
16	September-18		M *	R	M	Country prioritization of IPV catchup immunization (IC)	
17	February-19		M	R	M	Risks and the role of bOPV preventive SIAs pre-cessation [d]	
18	September-19		M	P *	M	VAPP analysis (LSHTM)	
19	February-20		M *	P *	M	Role of IPV for outbreak response (IC), Scenarios for initial nOPV2 use under EUL (LSHTM)	
20	September-20		P *	M *	M *	Impacts of polio eradication activity disruption (LSHTM) [e] IPV use for cVDPV and WPV outbreak response (IC) Tracing infections and micro vaccination campaigns (IDM)	
21	February-21		P *	M *	M	nOPV2 versus mOPV2 for outbreak response (IC) Transition from initial to wider nOPV2 use criteria (LSHTM)	
22	August-21			M *	M	Update on nOPV2 policy (LSHTM)	
23	March-22		P *	M *	M	Field seroprevalence and immunogenicity studies (LSHTM) nOPV2 effectiveness study (IC)	
24	August-22			M *	M	Review of data on use of IPV for outbreak response (LSHTM)	

Table 5. *Cont.*

Meeting		Roles [a]				Information Extracted from the Note for the Record	
N	Date	KRI	IC	LSHTM	IDM/ BMGF	Presentation Topic (Presenting Modeling Group)	Group [Source(s)]
25	March-23			M *	M	Update on iVDPV epidemiology (LSHTM)	
26	August-23			M *	M	Options for type 1 and 2 co-circulation outbreaks (LSHTM)	
27	February-24			M	M	bOPV cessation planning summary of modeling [f]	

Abbreviations: AFP, acute flaccid paralysis; BMGF, Bill and Melinda Gates Foundation; bOPV, bivalent OPV; cVDPV, circulating VDPV; EUL, emergency use listing; GPEI, Global Polio Eradication Initiative; IC, Imperial College; IDM, Institute for Disease Modeling; IPV, inactivated poliovirus vaccine; iVDPV, immunodeficiency-associated VDPV; KRI, Kid Risk, Inc.; LSHTM, London School of Hygiene and Tropical Medicine; mOPV, monovalent OPV; NA, not available; nOPV, novel OPV; OPV, oral poliovirus vaccine; OPV#, type # OPV (# = 1, 2, or 3); RI, routine immunization; SAGE, Strategic Advisory Group of Experts on immunization for the World Health Organization; SC, stochastic compartmental; SIA, supplemental immunization activity; SPWG, SAGE polio working group; tOPV, trivalent OPV; VAPP, vaccine-associated paralytic polio; VDPV, vaccine-derived poliovirus.
[a] M indicates attended as a SPWG member, P indicates invited external participants, R indicates rapporteur, and * indicates presented at the meeting.
[b] Also referred to an unpublished IDM analysis and an IC study ultimately published in 2016 [211].
[c] Presentation included modeling from KRI, IC, and IDM developed following a pre-meeting in-depth modeling discussion.
[d] Presentation that referred to KRI work.
[e] Presentation that referred to KRI, IC, IDM, and LSHTM work.
[f] Presentation that referred to KRI, IC, IDM/BMGF, and LSHTM work.

Overall, it appears that poliovirus transmission and economic modeling results played a much larger role in GPEI and SAGE discussions in earlier time periods than during 2020–2024.25, although we see a strong representation of consideration of the results of the modeling groups for 2000–2024.

4. Discussion

Publications by the modeling groups since 2020 have continued to show the application of different approaches and active communication of model results to policymakers. However, we observed fewer references to modeling results in GPEI Annual Reports since 2020 than during the prior 15 years, and a decrease in the impact of the results of poliovirus transmission and economic modeling on decisions. Notably, in some cases, the reduced impact of modeling occurred despite the agreement of the multiple modeling groups. For example, although multiple modeling groups recommended a rapid response to cVDPV2 outbreaks using any available OPV2 vaccine (including mOPV2) and SAGE endorsed this recommendation, some countries in the African region delayed their responses to cVDPV2 outbreaks after 2020 to wait for nOPV2 because of its perceived higher safety profile. Multiple modeling groups also published studies that highlighted the late, small, and low quality of oSIAs in some areas as a primary reason for OPV2 cessation failure.

During the past 5 years, modeling studies suggested an expected reduction in overall incremental net benefits of the global polio eradication efforts, decreased chances of a successful polio eradication endgame, expectations of increased costs of polio immunization prospectively due to the shift from OPV to IPV in RI associated with the increase in recommended IPV doses in RI, and the complexity of continued use of different formulations of OPV. However, commitment to "finishing the job" remains strong, in spite of a less favorable economic impact. Consistent with this, discussions by GPEI and SAGE trended more toward a focus on polio epidemiological studies, equity (particularly gender equity [154]), and integration of GPEI activities into national immunization programs. The increased focus on statistical analyses of polio epidemiological data reflects the reality of the increased incidence of polio cases reported since 2020 [104].

Similar to the prior review [1], we looked for areas of disagreement about recommendations from the modeling groups. We could not formally document some known differences from internal modeling group discussions because they involved unpublished results. For example, published modeling emphasized the importance of rapidly responding to cVDPV2 outbreaks using the available mOPV2 given the limited availability of nOPV2 [25,34], which unpublished modeling by one other group supported and unpublished modeling by another group did not support (it suggested that countries should wait to use nOPV2 before using mOPV2 in oSIAs). In addition, the communications to countries related to the roll out and promotion of nOPV2 in 2021 promised a better vaccine than mOPV2, which effectively disincentivized the use of mOPV2, devalued the available mOPV2 stockpile, and created challenges with respect to using any Sabin OPV in SIAs to increase and maintain population immunity.

With respect to Pakistan and Afghanistan, modeling performed by KRI, IC, and IDM did not lead to the accelerated achievement of WPV1 eradication in Pakistan and Afghanistan. We could not assess the agreement between these since some of the analyses remain unpublished, but studies by KRI and IC agreed with the need to quickly restart immunization in Pakistan and Afghanistan following disruptions caused by COVID-19 [32,47]. In addition, insights from modeling did not succeed in preventing the failure of OPV2 cessation, despite repeated warnings of its likely failure as early as 2017 in Cessation Risk Task Team meetings that occurred between June 2016 and April 2021, which included all of the modeling groups along with representatives from most GPEI core partners. Modeling support of stockpile needs prior to OPV2 cessation did not account for shifts in GPEI leadership and governance and the resulting adoption of lower prioritization of SIAs [104], decentralization of decision making, or the apparent willingness to accept increased polio cases to wait for a different vaccine (i.e., nOPV2). Notably, prior to OPV2 cessation, prospective modeling assumed aggressive oSIAs with mOPV2 would either successfully stop all type 2 poliovirus transmission or countries would restart the use of tOPV in RI [36], and thus developed estimates of demand for a time-limited OPV stockpile [40]. Instead, global efforts moved toward increased use of IPV, the development and deployment of new vaccine tools, including nOPV, and the associated extension of the polio endgame. Given the current epidemiological situation, we can anticipate that future publications of polio modeling studies may support another update of the systematic review.

Limitations of this review include our inability to evaluate whether and how national and regional decision makers interact with each other, GPEI, and other global health policy makers. Although we described some work by the modeling teams used by national and regional decision makers (e.g., New York modeling, the African Regional Certification Commission), these represent anecdotal examples, not the results of a systematic process to collect information from decision makers at all levels about their use of modeling results. Modeling results represent only one of the factors that may influence decisions.

5. Conclusions

The representatives from some modeling groups continued to serve as members on the SPWG and the modeling groups continue to increase and to publish their work at an increasing rate. By combining and updating results from prior review [1], for the full time period of 2000–2024.25 we identified 246 polio publications by the modeling groups KRI (124), IC (64), LSHTM (29), IDM/BMGF (27), and GIT (2), plus 46 publications by others (including 32 poliovirus transmission modeling papers and 14 economic analyses). With the initial target for achieving global polio eradication in 2000, the increasing number of modeling groups and rate of publications contrast notably with expectations of successful eradication and dissolution of the GPEI long before 2024. In spite of this, the GPEI core partners remain committed to delivering on the promise of polio eradication, and this suggests that opportunities and support for polio modeling will continue for the foreseeable future.

Author Contributions: Conceptualization, funding acquisition, and original draft preparation K.M.T.; Methodology, formal analysis, review and editing, and visualization, K.M.T. and K.B. All authors have read and agreed to the published version of the manuscript.

Funding: We acknowledge support for this report under Cooperative Agreement Number 5NU2RGH001915-04-00 funded by the Centers for Disease Control and Prevention. The views expressed are solely those of the authors and do not necessarily represent the official views of the Centers for Disease Control and Prevention or Department of Health and Human Services.

Acknowledgments: We thank Nicholas Grassly, Isobel Blake, Kathleen O'Reilly and Hil Lyons for comments related to our descriptions of polio publications from their respective groups.

Conflicts of Interest: The authors declare no conflicts of interest.

Abbreviations

ACPE, Advisory Committee on Polio Eradication; AFP, acute flaccid paralysis; BMGF, Bill and Melinda Gates Foundation; bOPV, bivalent OPV; cVDPV, circulating VDPV; DEB, differential equation-based; DES, discrete event simulation; EUL, emergency use listing; GIT, Georgia Institute of Technology; GPEI, Global Polio Eradication Initiative; IB, individual-based; IC, Imperial College; IDM, Institute for Disease Modeling; IPV, inactivated poliovirus vaccine; iVDPV, immunodeficiency-associated VDPV; KRI, Kid Risk, Inc.; LPV, live poliovirus; LSHTM, London School of Hygiene and Tropical Medicine; mOPV, monovalent OPV; NA, not available; nOPV, novel OPV; OPV, oral poliovirus vaccine; OPV#, type # OPV (# = 1, 2, or 3); oSIA, outbreak response SIA; PRC, GPEI polio research committee; pSIA, preventive SIA; RI, routine immunization; QUIVER, Quantitative Immunization and Vaccine Related Research Advisory Committee; SACEMA, the South African Centre for Epidemiological Modelling and Analysis; SAGE, Strategic Advisory Group of Experts on immunization for the World Health Organization; SC, stochastic compartmental; SIA, supplemental immunization activity; SPWG, SAGE polio working group; tOPV, trivalent OPV; VAPP, vaccine-associated paralytic polio; VDPV, vaccine-derived poliovirus; VICP, Vaccine Injury Compensation Program (United States); WHA, World Health Assembly; WHO, World Health Organization; WPV, wild poliovirus; WPV#, type # WPV (# = 1, 2, or 3).

References

1. Thompson, K.M.; Kalkowska, D.A. Review of poliovirus modeling performed from 2000 to 2019 to support global polio eradication. *Expert Rev. Vaccines* **2020**, *19*, 661–686. [CrossRef]
2. Badizadegan, K.; Goodson, J.L.; Rota, P.A.; Thompson, K.M. The potential role of using vaccine patches to induce immunity: Platform and pathways to innovation and commercialization. *Expert Rev. Vaccines* **2020**, *19*, 175–194. [CrossRef]
3. Thompson, K.M.; Orenstein, W.A.; Hinman, A.R. Performance of the United States Vaccine Injury Compensation Program (VICP): 1988–2019. *Vaccine* **2020**, *38*, 2136–2143. [CrossRef]
4. Thompson, K.M.; Orenstein, W.A.; Hinman, A.R. An opportunity to incentivize innovation to increase vaccine safety in the United States by improving vaccine delivery using vaccine patches. *Vaccine* **2020**, *38*, 4060–4065. [CrossRef]
5. Ochalek, J.; Claxton, K.; Lomas, J.; Thompson, K.M. Valuing health outcomes: Developing better defaults based on health opportunity costs. *Expert Rev. Pharmacoecon. Outcomes Res.* **2021**, *21*, 729–736. [CrossRef]
6. Thompson, K.M. Modeling and managing poliovirus risks: We are where we are. *Risk Anal.* **2021**, *41*, 223–228. [CrossRef]
7. Kalkowska, D.A.; Pallansch, M.A.; Wassilak, S.G.F.; Cochi, S.L.; Thompson, K.M. Global transmission of live polioviruses: Updated dynamic modeling of the polio endgame. *Risk Anal.* **2021**, *41*, 248–265. [CrossRef]
8. Thompson, K.M.; Kalkowska, D.A. Reflections on modeling poliovirus transmission and the polio eradication endgame. *Risk Anal.* **2021**, *41*, 229–247. [CrossRef]
9. Kalkowska, D.A.; Thompson, K.M. Insights from modeling preventive supplemental immunization activities as a strategy to eliminate wild poliovirus transmission in Pakistan and Afghanistan. *Risk Anal.* **2021**, *41*, 266–272. [CrossRef]
10. Kalkowska, D.A.; Franka, R.; Higgins, J.; Kovacs, S.D.; Forbi, J.C.; Wassilak, S.G.F.; Pallansch, M.A.; Thompson, K.M. Modeling poliovirus transmission in Borno and Yobe, Northeast Nigeria. *Risk Anal.* **2021**, *41*, 289–302. [CrossRef]
11. Kalkowska, D.A.; Thompson, K.M. Modeling undetected live poliovirus circulation after apparent interruption of transmission: Borno and Yobe in Northeast Nigeria. *Risk Anal.* **2021**, *41*, 303–311. [CrossRef]
12. Kalkowska, D.A.; Pallansch, M.A.; Cochi, S.L.; Kovacs, S.D.; Wassilak, S.G.F.; Thompson, K.M. Updated characterization of post-OPV cessation risks: Lessons from 2019 serotype 2 outbreaks and implications for the probability of OPV restart. *Risk Anal.* **2021**, *41*, 320–328. [CrossRef]
13. Thompson, K.M.; Kalkowska, D.A. Potential future use, costs, and value of poliovirus vaccines. *Risk Anal.* **2021**, *41*, 349–363. [CrossRef]
14. Kalkowska, D.A.; Thompson, K.M. Expected implications of globally coordinated cessation of serotype 3 oral poliovirus vaccine (OPV) before serotype 1 OPV. *Risk Anal.* **2021**, *41*, 312–319. [CrossRef]
15. Kalkowska, D.A.; Pallansch, M.A.; Wilkinson, A.; Bandyopadhyay, A.S.; Konopka-Anstadt, J.L.; Burns, C.C.; Oberste, M.S.; Wassilak, S.G.F.; Badizadegan, K.; Thompson, K.M. Updated characterization of outbreak response strategies for 2019–2029: Impacts of using a novel type 2 oral poliovirus vaccine strain. *Risk Anal.* **2021**, *41*, 329–348. [CrossRef]
16. Thompson, K.M. Poliovirus vaccine options: Another step forward. *Lancet* **2020**, *397*, 2–3. [CrossRef]

17. Thompson, K.M.; Kalkowska, D.A. An updated economic analysis of the Global Polio Eradication Initiative. *Risk Anal.* **2021**, *41*, 393–406. [CrossRef]
18. Kalkowska, D.A.; Thompson, K.M. Health and economic outcomes associated with polio vaccine policy options: 2019–2029. *Risk Anal.* **2021**, *41*, 364–375. [CrossRef]
19. Thompson, K.M.; Kalkowska, D.A.; Badizadegan, K. A health economic analysis for oral poliovirus vaccine to prevent COVID-19 in the United States. *Risk Anal.* **2021**, *41*, 376–386. [CrossRef]
20. Kalkowska, D.A.; Voorman, A.; Pallansch, M.A.; Wassilak, S.G.F.; Cochi, S.L.; Badizadegan, K.; Thompson, K.M. The impact of disruptions caused by the COVID-19 pandemic on global polio eradication. *Vaccine* **2021**, *41*, A12–A18. [CrossRef]
21. Thompson, K.M.; Kalkowska, D.A.; Badizadegan, K. Hypothetical emergence of poliovirus in 2020: Part 1. consequences of policy decisions to respond using nonpharmaceutical interventions. *Expert Rev. Vaccines* **2021**, *20*, 465–481. [CrossRef]
22. Thompson, K.M.; Kalkowska, D.A.; Badizadegan, K. Hypothetical emergence of poliovirus in 2020: Part 2. exploration of the potential role of vaccines in control and eradication. *Expert Rev. Vaccines* **2021**, *20*, 449–460. [CrossRef]
23. Kalkowska, D.A.; Pallansch, M.A.; Cochi, S.L.; Thompson, K.M. Updated Characterization of Poliovirus Transmission in Pakistan and Afghanistan and the Impacts of Different Outbreak Response Vaccine Options. *J. Infect. Dis.* **2021**, *224*, 1529–1538. [CrossRef]
24. Kalkowska, D.A.; Pallansch, M.A.; Cochi, S.L.; Thompson, K.M. Modeling Poliovirus Surveillance and Immunization Campaign Quality Monitoring Costs for Pakistan and Afghanistan for 2019–2023. *Open Forum Infect. Dis.* **2021**, *8*, ofab264. [CrossRef]
25. Kalkowska, D.A.; Pallansch, M.A.; Wassilak, S.G.F.; Cochi, S.L.; Thompson, K.M. Serotype 2 oral poliovirus vaccine (OPV2) choices and the consequences of delaying outbreak response. *Vaccine* **2023**, *41* (Suppl. 1), A136–A141. [CrossRef]
26. Thompson, K.M. Polio eradication: What kind of world do we want? *Lancet Infect. Dis.* **2022**, *22*, 161–163. [CrossRef]
27. Thompson, K.M. Effectiveness of a new vaccine for outbreak response and the increasingly complicated polio endgame. *Lancet Glob. Health* **2022**, *10*, e1697–e1698. [CrossRef]
28. Thompson, K.M.; Badizadegan, K. Health economic analyses of secondary vaccine effects: A systematic review and policy insights. *Expert Rev. Vaccines* **2022**, *21*, 297–312. [CrossRef]
29. Thompson, K.M.; Kalkowska, D.A.; Badizadegan, K. Polio health economics: Assessing the benefits and costs of polio, non-polio, and integrated activities of the Global Polio Eradication Initiative. *Gates Open Res.* **2022**, *6*, 5. [CrossRef]
30. Badizadegan, K.; Kalkowska, D.A.; Thompson, K.M. Polio by the numbers—A global perspective. *J. Infect. Dis.* **2022**, *226*, 1309–1318. [CrossRef]
31. Thompson, K.M.; Kalkowska, D.A.; Badizadegan, K. Health economic analysis of vaccine options for the polio eradication endgame: 2022-2036. *Expert Rev. Vaccines* **2022**, *21*, 1667–1674. [CrossRef] [PubMed]
32. Kalkowska, D.A.; Badizadegan, K.; Thompson, K.M. Modeling scenarios for ending poliovirus transmission in Pakistan and Afghanistan. *Risk Anal.* **2023**, *43*, 660–676. [CrossRef] [PubMed]
33. Kalkowska, D.A.; Badizadegan, K.; Thompson, K.M. Modeling undetected live type 1 wild poliovirus circulation after apparent interruption of transmission: Pakistan and Afghanistan. *Risk Anal.* **2023**, *43*, 677–685. [CrossRef] [PubMed]
34. Kalkowska, D.A.; Wassilak, S.G.F.; Pallansch, M.A.; Burns, C.C.; Wiesen, E.; Durry, E.; Badizadegan, K.; Thompson, K.M. Outbreak response strategies with type 2-containing oral poliovirus vaccines. *Vaccine* **2023**, *41* (Suppl. 1), A142–A152. [CrossRef] [PubMed]
35. Kalkowska, D.A.; Badizadegan, K.; Thompson, K.M. Outbreak management strategies for cocirculation of multiple poliovirus types. *Vaccine* **2023**, *41*, 3718–3727. [CrossRef] [PubMed]
36. Thompson, K.M.; Kalkowska, D.A.; Badizadegan, K. Looking back at prospective modeling of outbreak response strategies for managing global type 2 oral poliovirus vaccine (OPV2) cessation. *Front. Public Health* **2023**, *11*, 1098419. [CrossRef] [PubMed]
37. Kalkowska, D.; Wassilak, S.; Wiesen, E.; F Estivariz, C.; Burns, C.; Badizadegan, K.; Thompson, K. Complexity of options related to restarting oral poliovirus vaccine (OPV) in national immunization programs after OPV cessation. *Gates Open Res.* **2023**, *7*, 55. [CrossRef] [PubMed]
38. Thompson, K.M.; Lauring, A.S.; Pollard, A.J.; Andino, R.; Bandyopadhyay, A.S.; Berkley, S.; Bhutta, Z.A.; Routh, J.; Benn, C.S. Polio eradication: Addressing the hurdles on the last mile. *Cell* **2023**, *186*, 1–4. [CrossRef] [PubMed]
39. Thompson, K.M. Polio endgame complexity: Updating expectations for nOPV2. *Lancet Infect. Dis.* **2023**, *23*, 992–994. [CrossRef] [PubMed]
40. Thompson, K.M.; Kalkowska, D.A.; Badizadegan, K. Oral polio vaccine stockpile modeling: Insights from recent experience. *Expert Rev. Vaccines* **2023**, *22*, 813–825. [CrossRef]
41. Kalkowska, D.A.; Wassilak, S.G.F.; Wiesen, E.; Burns, C.C.; Pallansch, M.A.; Badizadegan, K.; Thompson, K.M. Coordinated global cessation of oral poliovirus vaccine use: Options and potential consequences. *Risk Anal.* **2023**, *44*, 366–378. [CrossRef] [PubMed]
42. Kalkowska, D.A.; Wiesen, E.; Wassilak, S.G.F.; Burns, C.C.; Pallansch, M.A.; Badizadegan, K.; Thompson, K.M. Worst-case scenarios: Modeling uncontrolled type 2 polio transmission. *Risk Anal.* **2023**, *44*, 379–389. [CrossRef] [PubMed]
43. Badizadegan, K.; Kalkowska, D.A.; Thompson, K.M. Health economic analysis of antiviral drugs in the global polio eradication endgame. *Med. Decis. Mak.* **2023**, *43*, 850–862. [CrossRef] [PubMed]
44. Thompson, K.M.; Kalkowska, D.A.; Routh, J.A.; Brenner, I.R.; Rosenberg, E.S.; Zucker, J.R.; Langdon-Embry, M.; Sugerman, D.E.; Burns, C.C.; Badizadegan, K. Modeling poliovirus transmission and responses in New York State. *J. Infect. Dis.* **2024**, *229*, 1097–1106. [CrossRef] [PubMed]

45. Kalkowska, D.A.; Badizadegan, K.; Routh, J.A.; Burns, C.C.; Rosenberg, E.S.; Brenner, I.R.; Zucker, J.R.; Langdon-Embry, M.; Thompson, K.M. Modeling undetected poliovirus circulation following the 2022 outbreak in the United States. *Expert Rev. Vaccines* **2023**, *23*, 186–195. [CrossRef] [PubMed]
46. Thompson, K.M.; Kalkowska, D.A.; Kidd, S.E.; Burns, C.C.; Badizadegan, K. Trade-offs of different poliovirus vaccine options for outbreak response in the United States and other countries that only use inactivated poliovirus vaccine (IPV) in routine immunization. *Vaccine* **2024**, *42*, 819–827. [CrossRef] [PubMed]
47. Molodecky, N.A.; Jafari, H.; Safdar, R.M.; Ahmed, J.A.; Mahamud, A.; Bandyopadhyay, A.S.; Shukla, H.; Quddus, A.; Zaffran, M.; Sutter, R.W.; et al. Modelling the spread of serotype-2 vaccine derived-poliovirus outbreak in Pakistan and Afghanistan to inform outbreak control strategies in the context of the COVID-19 pandemic. *Vaccine* **2023**, *41*, A93–A104. [CrossRef] [PubMed]
48. Molodecky, N.A.; Usman, A.; Javaid, A.; Wahdan, A.; Parker, E.P.K.; Ahmed, J.A.; Shah, N.; Agbor, J.; Mahamud, A.; Safdar, R.M. Quantifying movement patterns and vaccination status of high risk mobile populations in Pakistan and Afghanistan to inform poliovirus risk and vaccination strategy. *Vaccine* **2021**, *39*, 2124–2132. [CrossRef] [PubMed]
49. Babji, S.; Manickavasagam, P.; Chen, Y.H.; Jeyavelu, N.; Jose, N.V.; Praharaj, I.; Syed, C.; Kaliappan, S.P.; John, J.; Giri, S.; et al. Immune predictors of oral poliovirus vaccine immunogenicity among infants in South India. *NPJ Vaccines* **2020**, *5*, 27. [CrossRef] [PubMed]
50. Jorgensen, D.; Pons-Salort, M.; Shaw, A.G.; Grassly, N.C. The role of genetic sequencing and analysis in the polio eradication programme. *Virus Evol.* **2020**, *6*, veaa040. [CrossRef] [PubMed]
51. Hamisu, A.W.; Blake, I.M.; Sume, G.; Braka, F.; Jimoh, A.; Dahiru, H.; Bonos, M.; Dankoli, R.; Mamuda Bello, A.; Yusuf, K.M.; et al. Characterizing environmental surveillance sites in Nigeria and their sensitivity to detect poliovirus and other enteroviruses. *J. Infect. Dis.* **2022**, *225*, 1377–1386. [CrossRef] [PubMed]
52. Cooper, L.V.; Bandyopadhyay, A.; Gumede-Moeletsi, N.; Mach, O.; Mkanda, P.; Ndoutabé, M.; Okiror, S.O.; Ramirez-Gonzalez, A.; Touray, K.; Wanyoike, S.; et al. Risk factors for spread of vaccine-derived type 2 polioviruses in Africa following global withdrawal of trivalent oral poliovirus vaccine and impact of outbreak response with monovalent vaccine: A retrospective analysis of surveillance data. *Lancet Infect. Dis.* **2022**, *22*, 284–294. [CrossRef] [PubMed]
53. Gray, E.J.; Cooper, L.V.; Bandyopadhyay, A.S.; Blake, I.M.; Grassly, N.C. The origins and risk factors for serotype-2 vaccine-derived poliovirus (VDPV2) emergences in Africa during 2016–2019. *J. Infect. Dis.* **2023**, *228*, 80–88. [CrossRef] [PubMed]
54. Grassly, N.C.; Andrews, N.; Cooper, G.; Stephens, L.; Waight, P.; Jones, C.E.; Heath, P.T.; Calvert, A.; Southern, J.; Martin, J.; et al. Effect of maternal immunisation with multivalent vaccines containing inactivated poliovirus vaccine (IPV) on infant IPV immune response: A phase 4, multi-centre randomised trial. *Vaccine* **2023**, *41*, 1299–1302. [CrossRef] [PubMed]
55. Cooper, L.V.; Erbeto, T.B.; Danzomo, A.A.; Abdullahi, H.W.; Boateng, K.; Adamu, U.S.; Shuaib, F.; Modjirom, N.; Gray, E.J.; Bandyopadhyay, A.S.; et al. Effectiveness of poliovirus vaccines against circulating vaccine-derived type 2 poliomyelitis in Nigeria between 2017 and 2022: A case-control study. *Lancet Infect. Dis.* **2024**, *24*, 427–436. [CrossRef] [PubMed]
56. Cooper, L.V.; Blake, I.M. First Africa-based clinical trial for novel type 2 oral poliovirus vaccine. *Lancet* **2024**, *403*, 1113–1115. [CrossRef] [PubMed]
57. Bandyopadhyay, A.S.; Cooper, L.V.; Zipursky, S. One billion doses and WHO prequalification of nOPV2: Implications for the global polio situation and beyond. *PLOS Glob. Public Health* **2024**, *4*, e0002920. [CrossRef] [PubMed]
58. Kurji, F.D.; Bandyopadhyay, A.S.; Zipursky, S.; Cooper, L.V.; Gast, C.; Toher, M.; Clemens, R.; Clemens, S.A.C.; Prasad, R.; Azhari, A. Novel oral polio vaccine type 2 use for polio outbreak response: A global effort for a global health emergency. *Pathogens* **2024**, *13*, 273. [CrossRef] [PubMed]
59. Shaw, A.G.; Majumdar, M.; Troman, C.; O'Toole, A.; Benny, B.; Abraham, D.; Praharaj, I.; Kang, G.; Sharif, S.; Alam, M.M.; et al. Rapid and sensitive direct detection and identification of poliovirus from stool and environmental surveillance samples by use of nanopore sequencing. *J. Clin. Microbiol.* **2020**, *58*, 10-1128. [CrossRef] [PubMed]
60. Shaw, A.G.; Cooper, L.V.; Gumede, N.; Bandyopadhyay, A.S.; Grassly, N.C.; Blake, I.M. Time taken to detect and respond to polio outbreaks in Africa and the potential impact of direct molecular detection and nanopore sequencing. *J. Infect. Dis.* **2022**, *226*, 453–462. [CrossRef]
61. Akello, J.O.; Bujaki, E.; Shaw, A.G.; Khurshid, A.; Arshad, Y.; Troman, C.; Majumdar, M.; O'Toole, A.; Rambaut, A.; Alam, M.M.; et al. Comparison of eleven RNA extraction methods for poliovirus direct molecular detection in stool samples. *Microbiol. Spectr.* **2023**, *11*, e0425222. [CrossRef] [PubMed]
62. Shaw, A.G.; Mampuela, T.K.; Lofiko, E.L.; Pratt, C.; Troman, C.; Bujaki, E.; O'Toole, A.; Akello, J.O.; Aziza, A.A.; Lusamaki, E.K.; et al. Sensitive poliovirus detection using nested PCR and nanopore sequencing: A prospective validation study. *Nat. Microbiol.* **2023**, *8*, 1634–1640. [CrossRef] [PubMed]
63. Shaw, A.G.; Troman, C.; Akello, J.O.; O'Reilly, K.M.; Gauld, J.; Grow, S.; Grassly, N.; Steele, D.; Blazes, D.; Kumar, S.; et al. Defining a research agenda for environmental wastewater surveillance of pathogens. *Nat. Med.* **2023**, *29*, 2155–2157. [CrossRef] [PubMed]
64. Grassly, N.C. Polio's detection in London is a wake-up call. *BMJ* **2022**, *377*, o1589. [CrossRef] [PubMed]
65. Klapsa, D.; Wilton, T.; Zealand, A.; Bujaki, E.; Saxentoff, E.; Troman, C.; Shaw, A.G.; Tedcastle, A.; Majumdar, M.; Mate, R.; et al. Sustained detection of type 2 poliovirus in London sewage between February and July, 2022, by enhanced environmental surveillance. *Lancet* **2022**, *400*, 1531–1538. [CrossRef] [PubMed]
66. Bandyopadhyay, A.S.; Cavestany, R.L.; Blake, I.M.; Macklin, G.; Cooper, L.V.; Grassly, N.C.; Nery, A.L.; Mach, O. Use of inactivated poliovirus vaccine for poliovirus outbreak response. *Lancet Infect. Dis.* **2023**, *24*, e328–e342. [CrossRef] [PubMed]

67. Vallejo, C.; Pearson, C.A.B.; Koopman, J.S.; Hladish, T.J. Effect of population partitioning on the probability of silent circulation of poliovirus. *Bull. Math. Biol.* **2022**, *84*, 62. [CrossRef] [PubMed]
68. Macklin, G.R.; O'Reilly, K.M.; Grassly, N.C.; Edmunds, W.J.; Mach, O.; Santhana Gopala Krishnan, R.; Voorman, A.; Vertefeuille, J.F.; Abdelwahab, J.; Gumede, N.; et al. Evolving epidemiology of poliovirus serotype 2 following withdrawal of the serotype 2 oral poliovirus vaccine. *Science* **2020**, *368*, 401–405. [CrossRef]
69. O'Reilly, K.M.; Grassly, N.C.; Allen, D.J.; Bannister-Tyrrell, M.; Cameron, A.; Carrion Martin, A.I.; Ramsay, M.; Pebody, R.; Zambon, M. Surveillance optimisation to detect poliovirus in the pre-eradication era: A modelling study of England and Wales. *Epidemiol. Infect.* **2020**, *148*, e157. [CrossRef]
70. Macklin, G.R.; Goel, A.K.; Mach, O.; Tallis, G.; Ahmed, J.A.; O'Reilly, K.M.; Grassly, N.C.; Diop, O.M. Epidemiology of type 2 vaccine-derived poliovirus outbreaks between 2016 and 2020. *Vaccine* **2023**, *41*, A19–A24. [CrossRef]
71. Auzenbergs, M.; Fountain, H.; Macklin, G.; Lyons, H.; O'Reilly, K.M. The impact of surveillance and other factors on detection of emergent and circulating vaccine derived polioviruses. *Gates Open Res.* **2021**, *5*, 94. [CrossRef] [PubMed]
72. Bandyopadhyay, A.S.; Macklin, G.R. Final frontiers of the polio eradication endgame. *Curr. Opin. Infect. Dis.* **2020**, *33*, 404–410. [CrossRef]
73. Macklin, G.R.; Peak, C.; Eisenhawer, M.; Kurji, F.; Mach, O.; Konz, J.; Gast, C.; Bachtiar, N.S.; Bandyopadhyay, A.S.; Zipursky, S.; et al. Enabling accelerated vaccine roll-out for Public Health Emergencies of International Concern (PHEICs): Novel oral polio vaccine type 2 (nOPV2) experience. *Vaccine* **2023**, *41* (Suppl. 1), A122–A127. [CrossRef] [PubMed]
74. Fine, P.E.M. Population immunity and polio eradication. *Pathogens* **2024**, *13*, 183. [CrossRef] [PubMed]
75. O'Reilly, K.M.; Allen, D.J.; Fine, P.; Asghar, H. The challenges of informative wastewater sampling for SARS-CoV-2 must be met: Lessons from polio eradication. *Lancet Microbe* **2020**, *1*, e189–e190. [CrossRef] [PubMed]
76. Bandyopadhyay, A.S.; Gast, C.; Brickley, E.B.; Rüttimann, R.; Clemens, R.; Oberste, M.S.; Weldon, W.C.; Ackerman, M.E.; Connor, R.I.; Wieland-Alter, W.F.; et al. A randomized phase 4 study of immunogenicity and safety after monovalent oral type 2 Sabin poliovirus vaccine challenge in children vaccinated with inactivated poliovirus vaccine in Lithuania. *J. Infect. Dis.* **2021**, *223*, 119–127. [CrossRef] [PubMed]
77. Brickley, E.B.; Connor, R.I.; Wieland-Alter, W.; Weiner, J.A.; Ackerman, M.E.; Arita, M.; Gast, C.; De Coster, I.; Van Damme, P.; Bandyopadhyay, A.S.; et al. Intestinal antibody responses to 2 novel live attenuated type 2 oral poliovirus vaccines in healthy adults in Belgium. *J. Infect. Dis.* **2022**, *226*, 287–291. [CrossRef] [PubMed]
78. Connor, R.I.; Brickley, E.B.; Wieland-Alter, W.F.; Ackerman, M.E.; Weiner, J.A.; Modlin, J.F.; Bandyopadhyay, A.S.; Wright, P.F. Mucosal immunity to poliovirus. *Mucosal Immunol.* **2022**, *15*, 1–9. [CrossRef] [PubMed]
79. Famulare, M.; Wong, W.; Haque, R.; Platts-Mills, J.A.; Saha, P.; Aziz, A.B.; Ahmed, T.; Islam, M.O.; Uddin, M.J.; Bandyopadhyay, A.S.; et al. Multiscale model for forecasting Sabin 2 vaccine virus household and community transmission. *PLoS Comput. Biol.* **2021**, *17*, e1009690. [CrossRef] [PubMed]
80. Wong, W.; Gauld, J.; Famulare, M. From vaccine to pathogen: Modeling Sabin 2 vaccine virus reversion and evolutionary epidemiology in Matlab, Bangladesh. *Virus Evol.* **2023**, *9*, vead044. [CrossRef]
81. Brouwer, A.F.; Eisenberg, M.C.; Shulman, L.M.; Famulare, M.; Koopman, J.S.; Kroiss, S.J.; Hindiyeh, M.; Manor, Y.; Grotto, I.; Eisenberg, J.N.S. The role of time-varying viral shedding in modelling environmental surveillance for public health: Revisiting the 2013 poliovirus outbreak in Israel. *J. R. Soc. Interface* **2022**, *19*, 20220006. [CrossRef] [PubMed]
82. Valesano, A.L.; Taniuchi, M.; Fitzsimmons, W.J.; Islam, M.O.; Ahmed, T.; Zaman, K.; Haque, R.; Wong, W.; Famulare, M.; Lauring, A.S. The early evolution of oral poliovirus vaccine Is shaped by strong positive selection and tight transmission bottlenecks. *Cell Host Microbe* **2021**, *29*, 32–43.e34. [CrossRef] [PubMed]
83. Scott, R.P.; Cullen, A.C.; Chabot-Couture, G. Disease surveillance investments and administration: Limits to information value in Pakistan polio eradication. *Risk Anal.* **2021**, *41*, 273–288. [CrossRef] [PubMed]
84. Voorman, A.; O'Reilly, K.; Lyons, H.; Goel, A.K.; Touray, K.; Okiror, S. Real-time prediction model of cVDPV2 outbreaks to aid outbreak response vaccination strategies. *Vaccine* **2023**, *41*, A105–A112. [CrossRef] [PubMed]
85. Voorman, A.; Lyons, H.; Bennette, C.; Kovacs, S.; Makam, J.K.; F Vertefeuille, J.; Tallis, G. Analysis of population immunity to poliovirus following cessation of trivalent oral polio vaccine. *Vaccine* **2023**, *41*, A85–A92. [CrossRef] [PubMed]
86. Voorman, A.; Lyons, H.; Shuaib, F.; Adamu, U.S.; Korir, C.; Erbeto, T.; Bandyopadhyay, A.S.; Okiror, S. Impact of supplementary immunization activities using novel oral polio vaccine type 2 during a large outbreak of circulating vaccine-derived poliovirus in Nigeria. *J. Infect. Dis.* **2024**, *229*, 805–812. [CrossRef]
87. Sun, Y.; Keskinocak, P.; Steimle, L.N.; Kovacs, S.D.; Wassilak, S.G. A compartmental simulation model to improve interventions for controlling poliovirus outbreaks. In Proceedings of the 2023 Winter Simulation Conference (WSC), San Antonio, TX, USA, 10–13 December 2023; pp. 1184–1195.
88. Sun, Y.; Keskinocak, P.; Steimle, L.N.; Kovacs, S.D.; Wassilak, S.G. Modeling the spread of circulating vaccine-derived poliovirus type 2 outbreaks and interventions: A case study of Nigeria. *Vaccine X* **2024**, *18*, 100476. [CrossRef] [PubMed]
89. Cheng, E.; Gambhirrao, N.; Patel, R.; Zhowandai, A.; Rychtář, J.; Taylor, D. A game-theoretical analysis of poliomyelitis vaccination. *J. Theor. Biol.* **2020**, *499*, 110298. [CrossRef] [PubMed]
90. Wells, C.R.; Huppert, A.; Fitzpatrick, M.C.; Pandey, A.; Velan, B.; Singer, B.H.; Bauch, C.T.; Galvani, A.P. Prosocial polio vaccination in Israel. *Proc. Natl. Acad. Sci. USA* **2020**, *117*, 13138–13144. [CrossRef] [PubMed]

91. Ren, J.; Maimaiti, H.; Sun, X.; Huang, Z.; Liu, J.; Yang, J.; Li, Z.; Bai, Q.; Lu, Y. Cost-effectiveness of three poliovirus immunization schedules in Shanghai, China. *Vaccines* **2021**, *9*, 1062. [CrossRef] [PubMed]
92. Xu, Y.; Liu, Y.; Wang, J.; Che, X.; Du, J.; Zhang, X.; Gu, W.; Zhang, X.; Jiang, W. Cost-effectiveness of various immunization schedules with inactivated Sabin strain polio vaccine in Hangzhou, China. *Front. Public Health* **2022**, *10*, 990042. [CrossRef] [PubMed]
93. Chang, A.Y.; Aaby, P.; Avidan, M.S.; Benn, C.S.; Bertozzi, S.M.; Blatt, L.; Chumakov, K.; Khader, S.A.; Kottilil, S.; Nekkar, M.; et al. One vaccine to counter many diseases? Modeling the economics of oral polio vaccine against child mortality and COVID-19. *Front. Public Health* **2022**, *10*, 967920. [CrossRef] [PubMed]
94. Ahmed, N.; Macias-Diaz, J.E.; Shahid, N.; Raza, A.; Rafiq, M. A dynamically consistent computational method to solve numerically a mathematical model of polio propagation with spatial diffusion. *Comput. Methods Programs Biomed.* **2022**, *218*, 106709. [CrossRef] [PubMed]
95. Alrawajeh, F.A.; Allehiany, F.M.; Raza, A.; Abdelmohsen, S.A.M.; Cheema, T.N.; Rafiq, M.; Mohsin, M. Bio-inspired computational methods for the polio virus epidemic model. *CMC-Comput. Mater. Contin.* **2022**, *72*, 2357–2374. [CrossRef]
96. Liu, X.; Rahman, M.U.; Arfan, M.; Tchier, F.; Ahmad, S.; Inc, M.; Akinyemi, L. Fractional mathematical modeling to the spread of polio with the role of vaccination under non-singular kernal. *Fractals-Complex Geom. Patterns Scaling Nat. Soc.* **2022**, *30*, 17. [CrossRef]
97. Naveed, M.; Baleanu, D.; Raza, A.; Rafiq, M.; Soori, A.H. Treatment of polio delayed epidemic model via computer simulations. *CMC-Comput. Mater. Contin.* **2022**, *70*, 3415–3431. [CrossRef]
98. Raza, A.; Baleanu, D.; Khan, Z.U.; Mohsin, M.; Ahmed, N.; Rafiq, M.; Anwar, P. Stochastic analysis for the dynamics of a poliovirus epidemic model. *CMES-Comput. Model. Eng. Sci.* **2022**, *136*, 257–275. [CrossRef]
99. Bornaa, C.S.; Seidu, B.; Makinde, O.D. Mathematical analysis of the impact of vaccination and poor sanitation on the dynamics of poliomyelitis. *Int. J. Nonlinear Sci. Numer. Simul.* **2023**, *24*, 161–169. [CrossRef]
100. Iqbal, M.S.; Ahmed, N.; Akgül, A.; Satti, A.M.; Iqbal, Z.; Raza, A.; Rafiq, M.; Anjum, R.; Zakarya, M.; Park, C. Analysis of the fractional polio model with the Mittag-Leffler kernels. *Alex. Eng. J.* **2023**, *64*, 957–967. [CrossRef]
101. Karaagac, B.; Owolabi, K.M. Numerical analysis of polio model: A mathematical approach to epidemiological model using derivative with Mittag-Leffler Kernel. *Math. Methods Appl. Sci.* **2023**, *46*, 8175–8192. [CrossRef]
102. Wang, X.J.; Lin, G. Spreading speeds in two reaction-diffusion models for polio disease. *Commun. Nonlinear Sci. Numer. Simul.* **2023**, *118*, 18. [CrossRef]
103. World Health Assembly. *Global Eradication of Poliomyelitis by the Year 2000*; World Health Organization: Geneva, Switzerland, 1988.
104. Thompson, K.M.; Badizadegan, K. Evolution of global polio eradication strategies: Targets, vaccines, and supplemental immunization activities (SIAs). *Expert Rev. Vaccines*, 2024, *In press*.
105. World Health Organization. *Vaccines & Biologicals Annual Report 1999*; World Health Organization: Geneva, Switzerland, 2000.
106. Fine, P.E.M. Herd immunity: History, theory, practice. *Epidemiol. Rev.* **1993**, *15*, 265–302. [CrossRef] [PubMed]
107. Fine, P.E.; Carneiro, I.A. Transmissibility and persistence of oral polio vaccine viruses: Implications for the global poliomyelitis eradication initiative. *Am. J. Epidemiol.* **1999**, *150*, 1001–1021. [CrossRef]
108. Eichner, M.; Hadeler, K.P. Deterministic models for the eradication of poliomyelitis: Vaccination with the inactivated (IPV) and attenuated (OPV) polio virus vaccine. *Math. Biosci.* **1995**, *127*, 149–166. [CrossRef] [PubMed]
109. Eichner, M.; Hadeler, K.P.; Dietz, K. Stochastic models for the eradication of poliomyelitis: Minimum population size for polio virus persistence. In *Models for Infectious Human Diseases: Their Structure and Relation to Data*; Isham, V., Medley, G.F., Eds.; Cambridge University Press: New York, NY, USA, 1996; pp. 315–327.
110. Bart, K.J.; Foulds, J.; Patriarca, P. Global eradication of poliomyelitis: Benefit-cost analysis. *Bull. World Health Organ.* **1996**, *74*, 35–45. [PubMed]
111. O'Reilly, K.M.; Verity, R.; Durry, E.; Asghar, H.; Sharif, S.; Zaidi, S.Z.; Wadood, M.Z.M.; Diop, O.M.; Okayasu, H.; Safdar, R.M.; et al. Population sensitivity of acute flaccid paralysis and environmental surveillance for serotype 1 poliovirus in Pakistan: An observational study. *BMC Infect. Dis.* **2018**, *18*, 176. [CrossRef] [PubMed]
112. Macklin, G.R.; Grassly, N.C.; Sutter, R.W.; Mach, O.; Bandyopadhyay, A.S.; Edmunds, W.J.; O'Reilly, K.M. Vaccine schedules and the effect on humoral and intestinal immunity against poliovirus: A systematic review and network meta-analysis. *Lancet Infect. Dis.* **2019**, *19*, 1121–1128. [CrossRef] [PubMed]
113. Fine, P.E.; Sutter, R.W.; Orenstein, W.A. Stopping a polio outbreak in the post-eradication era. *Dev. Biol.* **2001**, *105*, 129–147; discussion 149–150.
114. Wringe, A.; Fine, P.E.; Sutter, R.W.; Kew, O.M. Estimating the extent of vaccine-derived poliovirus infection. *PLoS ONE* **2008**, *3*, e3433. [CrossRef] [PubMed]
115. Wright, P.F.; Connor, R.I.; Wieland-Alter, W.F.; Hoen, A.G.; Boesch, A.W.; Ackerman, M.E.; Oberste, M.S.; Gast, C.; Brickley, E.B.; Asturias, E.J.; et al. Vaccine-induced mucosal immunity to poliovirus: Analysis of cohorts from an open-label, randomised controlled trial in Latin American infants. *Lancet Infect. Dis.* **2016**, *16*, 1377–1384. [CrossRef] [PubMed]
116. Brickley, E.B.; Strauch, C.B.; Wieland-Alter, W.F.; Connor, R.I.; Lin, S.; Weiner, J.A.; Ackerman, M.E.; Arita, M.; Oberste, M.S.; Weldon, W.C.; et al. Intestinal immune responses to type 2 oral polio vaccine (OPV) challenge in infants previously immunized with bivalent OPV and either high-dose or standard inactivated polio vaccine. *J. Infect. Dis.* **2018**, *217*, 371–380. [CrossRef] [PubMed]

117. Brickley, E.B.; Connor, R.I.; Wieland-Alter, W.F.; Collett, M.S.; Hartford, M.; Van Der Avoort, H.; Boesch, A.W.; Weiner, J.A.; Ackerman, M.E.; McKinlay, M.A.; et al. Intestinal antibody responses to a live oral poliovirus vaccine challenge among adults previously immunized with inactivated polio vaccine in Sweden. *BMJ Glob. Health* **2019**, *4*, e001613. [CrossRef] [PubMed]
118. Brickley, E.B.; Wieland-Alter, W.; Connor, R.I.; Ackerman, M.E.; Boesch, A.W.; Arita, M.; Weldon, W.C.; O'Ryan, M.G.; Bandyopadhyay, A.S.; Wright, P.F. Intestinal immunity to poliovirus following sequential trivalent inactivated polio vaccine/bivalent oral polio vaccine and trivalent inactivated polio vaccine-only immunization schedules: Analysis of an open-label, randomized, controlled trial in Chilean infants. *Clin. Infect. Dis.* **2018**, *67*, S42–S50. [CrossRef] [PubMed]
119. Fine, P.E.M. Gaps in our knowledge about transmission of vaccine-derived polioviruses. *Bull. World Health Organ.* **2000**, *78*, 358–359. [PubMed]
120. Nathanson, N.; Fine, P.E.M. Virology. Poliomyelitis eradication—A dangerous endgame. *Science* **2002**, *296*, 269–270. [CrossRef] [PubMed]
121. Fine, P.E.; Ritchie, S. Perspective: Determinants of the severity of poliovirus outbreaks in the post eradication era. *Risk Anal.* **2006**, *26*, 1533–1540. [CrossRef] [PubMed]
122. Fine, P.E.M.; Oblapenko, G.; Sutter, R.W. Polio control after certification: Major issues outstanding. *Bull. World Health Organ.* **2004**, *82*, 47–52. [PubMed]
123. Fine, P.E. Poliomyelitis: Very small risks and very large risks. *Lancet Neurol.* **2004**, *3*, 703. [CrossRef] [PubMed]
124. Fine, P.E.; Griffiths, U.K. Global poliomyelitis eradication: Status and implications. *Lancet* **2007**, *369*, 1321–1322. [CrossRef]
125. Fine, P.E. Polio: Measuring the protection that matters most. *J. Infect. Dis.* **2009**, *200*, 673–675. [CrossRef]
126. Fine, P. Commentary: An unexpected finding that needs confirmation or rejection. *BMJ* **2000**, *321*, 1439. [PubMed]
127. Brickley, E.B.; Wright, P.F. Maximising the impact of inactivated polio vaccines. *Lancet Infect. Dis.* **2017**, *17*, 680–681. [CrossRef] [PubMed]
128. Voorman, A.; Hoff, N.A.; Doshi, R.H.; Alfonso, V.; Mukadi, P.; Muyembe-Tamfum, J.J.; Wemakoy, E.O.; Bwaka, A.; Weldon, W.; Gerber, S.; et al. Polio immunity and the impact of mass immunization campaigns in the Democratic Republic of the Congo. *Vaccine* **2017**, *35*, 5693–5699. [CrossRef] [PubMed]
129. Alfonso, V.H.; Voorman, A.; Hoff, N.A.; Weldon, W.C.; Gerber, S.; Gadoth, A.; Halbrook, M.; Goldsmith, A.; Mukadi, P.; Doshi, R.H.; et al. Poliovirus immunity among adults in the Democratic Republic of the Congo: A cross-sectional serosurvey. *BMC Infect. Dis.* **2022**, *22*, 30. [CrossRef] [PubMed]
130. Voorman, A.; Habib, M.A.; Hussain, I.; Muhammad Safdar, R.; Ahmed, J.A.; Weldon, W.C.; Ahmed, I.; Umer, M.; Partridge, J.; Soofi, S.B. Immunity and field efficacy of type 2-containing polio vaccines after cessation of trivalent oral polio vaccine: A population-based serological study in Pakistan. *Vaccine X* **2020**, *5*, 100067. [CrossRef] [PubMed]
131. VanderEnde, K.; Voorman, A.; Khan, S.; Anand, A.; Snider, C.J.; Goel, A.; Wassilak, S. New analytic approaches for analyzing and presenting polio surveillance data to supplement standard performance indicators. *Vaccine X* **2020**, *4*, 100059. [CrossRef] [PubMed]
132. World Health Organization. Strategic Advisory Group of Experts on Immunization Meetings. Available online: https://www.who.int/groups/strategic-advisory-group-of-experts-on-immunization/meetings (accessed on 28 March 2024).
133. Global Polio Eradication Initiative. Progress 1999: Every Child Counts. Available online: https://iris.who.int/bitstream/handle/10665/66964/WHO_POLIO_00.03.pdf (accessed on 13 November 2023).
134. Global Polio Eradication Initiative. Progress 2000. Available online: https://iris.who.int/bitstream/handle/10665/66763/WHO_POLIO_01.03.pdf (accessed on 13 November 2023).
135. Global Polio Eradication Initiative. Progress 2001. Available online: https://iris.who.int/bitstream/handle/10665/67417/WHO_POLIO_02.08.pd (accessed on 13 November 2023).
136. Global Polio Eradication Initiative. Progress 2002. Available online: https://iris.who.int/bitstream/handle/10665/67931/WHO_POLIO_03.02.pdf (accessed on 13 November 2023).
137. Global Polio Eradication Initiative. Progress 2003. Available online: https://iris.who.int/bitstream/handle/10665/68653/WHO_POLIO_04.02.pdf (accessed on 13 November 2023).
138. Global Polio Eradication Initiative. 2004 Annual Report. Available online: https://iris.who.int/bitstream/handle/10665/69055/WHO_POLIO_05.03.pdf (accessed on 13 November 2023).
139. Global Polio Eradication Initiative. 2005 Annual Report. Available online: https://iris.who.int/bitstream/handle/10665/70869/WHO_Polio_06.02_eng.pdf (accessed on 13 November 2023).
140. Global Polio Eradication Initiative. 2006 Annual Report. Available online: https://iris.who.int/bitstream/handle/10665/70868/WHO_Polio_07.02_eng.pdf (accessed on 13 November 2023).
141. Global Polio Eradication Initiative. 2007 Annual Report. Available online: https://iris.who.int/bitstream/handle/10665/70867/WHO_Polio_08.02_eng.pdf (accessed on 13 November 2023).
142. Global Polio Eradication Initiative. 2008 Annual Report. Available online: https://iris.who.int/bitstream/handle/10665/70866/WHO_POLIO_09.03_eng.pdf (accessed on 13 November 2023).
143. Global Polio Eradication Initiative. 2009 Annual Report. Available online: https://iris.who.int/bitstream/handle/10665/70865/WHO_Polio_10.05_eng.pdf (accessed on 13 November 2023).
144. Global Polio Eradication Initiative. 2010 Annual Report: Every Last Child. Available online: https://iris.who.int/bitstream/handle/10665/70849/WHO_POLIO_11.02_eng.pdf (accessed on 13 November 2023).

145. Global Polio Eradication Initiative. 2011 Annual Report. Available online: https://iris.who.int/bitstream/handle/10665/276243/WHO-POLIO-12.02-eng.pdf (accessed on 13 November 2023).
146. Global Polio Eradication Initiative. 2012 Annual Report. Available online: https://iris.who.int/bitstream/handle/10665/276241/WHO-POLIO-13.03-eng.pdf (accessed on 13 November 2023).
147. Global Polio Eradication Initiative. 2013 Annual Report. Available online: https://iris.who.int/bitstream/handle/10665/276239/WHO-POLIO-14.02-eng.pdf (accessed on 13 November 2023).
148. Global Polio Eradication Initiative. 2014 Annual Report: On the Threshold of a Polio Free World. Available online: https://iris.who.int/bitstream/handle/10665/276238/WHO-POLIO-15.01-eng.pdf (accessed on 13 November 2023).
149. Global Polio Eradication Initiative. 2015 Annual Report: Eradication within Reach. Available online: https://iris.who.int/bitstream/handle/10665/250145/WHO-POLIO-16.01-eng.pdf (accessed on 13 November 2023).
150. Global Polio Eradication Initiative. 2016 Annual Report: Eradication within Reach. Available online: https://iris.who.int/bitstream/handle/10665/276236/WHO-POLIO-17.03-eng.pdf (accessed on 13 November 2023).
151. Global Polio Eradication Initiative. 2017 Annual Report: Securing a Lasting World Free of All Polioviruses. Available online: https://iris.who.int/bitstream/handle/10665/276237/WHO-POLIO-18.01-eng.pdf (accessed on 13 November 2023).
152. Global Polio Eradication Initiative. 2018 Annual Report: To Achieve Lasting Success. Available online: https://polioeradication.org/wp-content/uploads/2016/07/Annual-report-2018.pdf (accessed on 13 November 2023).
153. Global Polio Eradication Initiative. 2019 Annual Report and Semi-Annual Status Updates, January–June and July–December 2019. Available online: https://iris.who.int/bitstream/handle/10665/336693/9789240013117-eng.pdf (accessed on 13 November 2023).
154. Global Polio Eradication Initiative. 2020 Annual Report and Semi-Annual Status Updates, January–June and July–December 2020. Available online: https://iris.who.int/bitstream/handle/10665/344329/9789240030763-eng.pdf (accessed on 13 November 2023).
155. Global Polio Eradication Initiative. 2021 Annual Report. Available online: https://iris.who.int/bitstream/handle/10665/364215/9789240058934-eng.pdf (accessed on 13 November 2023).
156. Global Polio Eradication Initiative. 2022 Annual Report. Available online: https://polioeradication.org/wp-content/uploads/2023/06/GPEI_2022_Expenditure_Report.pdf (accessed on 13 November 2023).
157. Polio Oversight Board. Meeting of the Polio Oversight Board, Global Polio Eradication Initiative, 12 December 2014. Available online: https://polioeradication.org/wp-content/uploads/2016/07/POB_Minutes_Mtg20141212.pdf (accessed on 10 April 2023).
158. Polio Oversight Board. Meeting of the Polio Oversight Board (Call), 13 January 2016. Available online: https://polioeradication.org/wp-content/uploads/2016/07/POB_Minutes_Mtg20160113.pdf (accessed on 10 April 2023).
159. Polio Oversight Board. Meeting of the Polio Oversight Board (POB)—Teleconference, 18 December 2020. Available online: https://polioeradication.org/wp-content/uploads/2021/02/POB-minutes-20201218.pdf (accessed on 10 April 2024).
160. Kalkowska, D.A.; Pallansch, M.A.; Thompson, K.M. Updated modelling of the prevalence of immunodeficiency-associated long-term vaccine-derived poliovirus (iVDPV) excreters. *Epidemiol. Infect.* **2019**, *147*, e295. [CrossRef] [PubMed]
161. Global Polio Eradication Initiative; World health organization. *Polio Endgame Strategy 2019–2023: Eradication, Integration, Certification and Containment*; World Health Organization: Geneva, Switzerland, 2019.
162. Global Polio Eradication Initiative. *Polio Post-Certification Strategy: A Risk Mitigation Strategy for a Polio-Free World*; World Health Organization: Geneva, Switzerland, 2018.
163. Duintjer Tebbens, R.J.; Pallansch, M.A.; Cochi, S.L.; Wassilak, S.G.F.; Thompson, K.M. An economic analysis of poliovirus risk management policy options for 2013–2052. *BMC Infect. Dis.* **2015**, *15*, 389. [CrossRef] [PubMed]
164. Duintjer Tebbens, R.J.; Pallansch, M.A.; Wassilak, S.G.; Cochi, S.L.; Thompson, K.M. Characterization of outbreak response strategies and potential vaccine stockpile needs for the polio endgame. *BMC Infect. Dis.* **2016**, *16*, 137. [CrossRef] [PubMed]
165. Duintjer Tebbens, R.J.; Pallansch, M.A.; Cochi, S.L.; Ehrhardt, D.T.; Farag, N.H.; Hadler, S.C.; Hampton, L.M.; Martinez, M.; Wassilak, S.G.F.; Thompson, K.M. Modeling poliovirus transmission in Pakistan and Afghanistan to inform vaccination strategies in undervaccinated subpopulations. *Risk Anal.* **2018**, *38*, 1701–1717. [CrossRef]
166. Kalkowska, D.A.; Duintjer Tebbens, R.J.; Thompson, K.M. Environmental surveillance system characteristics and impacts on confidence about no undetected serotype 1 wild poliovirus circulation. *Risk Anal.* **2019**, *39*, 414–425. [CrossRef] [PubMed]
167. Kalkowska, D.A.; Duintjer Tebbens, R.J.; Pallansch, M.A.; Thompson, K.M. Modeling undetected live poliovirus circulation after apparent interruption of transmission: Pakistan and Afghanistan. *Risk Anal.* **2019**, *39*, 402–413. [CrossRef] [PubMed]
168. Duintjer Tebbens, R.J.; Thompson, K.M. Evaluation of proactive and reactive strategies for polio eradication activities in Pakistan and Afghanistan. *Risk Anal.* **2019**, *39*, 389–401. [CrossRef] [PubMed]
169. African Regional Commission for the Certification of Poliomyelitis Eradication. Certifying the interruption of wild poliovirus transmission in the WHO African region on the turbulent journey to a polio-free world. *Lancet Glob. Health* **2020**, *8*, e1345–e1351. [CrossRef] [PubMed]
170. World Health Organization. Report from the Twentieth Meeting of the Global Commission for Certification of Poliomyelitis Eradication, Geneva, Switzerland, 17–18 October 2019. Available online: http://polioeradication.org/wp-content/uploads/2016/07/20th-meeting-of-the-Global-Commission-for-the-Certification-of-Eradication-of-Poliomyelitis-17-18-October-2019.pdf (accessed on 31 December 2019).

171. Global Polio Eradication Initiative; World Health Organization. *Strategy for the Response to Type 2 Circulating Vaccine-Derived Poliovirus 2020–2021: An Addendum to the Polio Endgame Strategy 2019-2023*; World Health Organization: Geneva, Switzerland, 2020.
172. Duintjer Tebbens, R.J.; Pallansch, M.A.; Cochi, S.L.; Wassilak, S.G.; Linkins, J.; Sutter, R.W.; Aylward, R.B.; Thompson, K.M. Economic analysis of the Global Polio Eradication Initiative. *Vaccine* **2010**, *29*, 334–343. [CrossRef] [PubMed]
173. Chumakov, K.; Benn, C.S.; Aaby, P.; Kottilil, S.; Gallo, R. Can existing live vaccines prevent COVID-19? *Science* **2020**, *368*, 1187–1188. [CrossRef] [PubMed]
174. Gallo, R.; Arbess, D.J. An Old Vaccine May Help against Coronavirus: A Tablet for Polio Boosts Innate Immunity, Which Fights Other Viruses. Available online: https://www.wsj.com/articles/an-old-vaccine-may-help-against-coronavirus-11593557168 (accessed on 1 July 2020).
175. Thompson, K.M.; Kalkowska, D.A.; Badizadegan, K. No role for reintroducing OPV into the United States with respect to controlling COVID-19 [Response to the letter to the Editor by Chumakov et al.]. *Risk Anal.* **2021**, *41*, 389–392. [CrossRef] [PubMed]
176. Global Polio Eradication Initiative; World Health Organization. *Polio Eradication Strategy 2022–2026: Delivering on a Promise*; World Health Organization: Geneva, Switzerland, 2021.
177. Thompson, K.M.; Duintjer Tebbens, R.J. Eradication versus control for poliomyelitis: An economic analysis. *Lancet* **2007**, *369*, 1363–1371. [CrossRef] [PubMed]
178. World Health Organization. Report from the Twenty-Second Meeting of the Global Commission for Certification of Poliomyelitis Eradication, Geneva, Switzerland, 3 June 2022. Available online: https://polioeradication.org/wp-content/uploads/2022/09/22nd-GCC-report-20220907.pdf (accessed on 12 September 2022).
179. Kidd, S.; Clark, T.; Routh, J.; Cineas, S.; Bahta, L.; Brooks, O. Use of inactivated polio vaccine among U.S. qdults: Updated recommendations of the Advisory Committee on Immunization Practices—United States, 2023. *MMWR Morb. Mortal. Wkly. Rep.* **2023**, *72*, 1327–1330. [CrossRef]
180. Bunimovich-Mendrazitsky, S.; Stone, L. Modeling polio as a disease of development. *J. Theor. Biol.* **2005**, *237*, 302–315. [CrossRef]
181. Duintjer Tebbens, R.J.; Pallansch, M.A.; Kew, O.M.; Caceres, V.M.; Sutter, R.W.; Thompson, K.M. A dynamic model of poliomyelitis outbreaks: Learning from the past to help inform the future. *Am. J. Epidemiol.* **2005**, *162*, 358–372. [CrossRef] [PubMed]
182. Thompson, K.M.; Duintjer Tebbens, R.J. The case for cooperation in managing and maintaining the end of poliomyelitis: Stockpile needs and coordinated OPV cessation. *Medscape J. Med.* **2008**, *10*, 190. [PubMed]
183. Thompson, K.M.; Tebbens, R.J.; Pallansch, M.A.; Kew, O.M.; Sutter, R.W.; Aylward, R.B.; Watkins, M.; Gary, H.E., Jr.; Alexander, J.; Jafari, H.; et al. The risks, costs, and benefits of possible future global policies for managing polioviruses. *Am. J. Public Health* **2008**, *98*, 1322–1330. [CrossRef] [PubMed]
184. Grassly, N.C.; Fraser, C.; Wenger, J.; Deshpande, J.M.; Sutter, R.W.; Heymann, D.L.; Aylward, R.B. New strategies for the elimination of polio from India. *Science* **2006**, *314*, 1150–1153. [CrossRef]
185. Grassly, N.C.; Wenger, J.; Durrani, S.; Bahl, S.; Deshpande, J.M.; Sutter, R.W.; Heymann, D.L.; Aylward, R.B. Protective efficacy of a monovalent oral type 1 poliovirus vaccine: A case-control study. *Lancet* **2007**, *369*, 1356–1362. [CrossRef] [PubMed]
186. Jenkins, H.E.; Aylward, R.B.; Gasasira, A.; Donnelly, C.A.; Abanida, E.A.; Koleosho-Adelekan, T.; Grassly, N.C. Effectiveness of immunization against paralytic poliomyelitis in Nigeria. *N. Engl. J. Med.* **2008**, *359*, 1666–1674. [CrossRef] [PubMed]
187. Jenkins, H.E.; Aylward, R.B.; Gasasira, A.; Donnelly, C.A.; Mwanza, M.; Corander, J.; Garnier, S.; Chauvin, C.; Abanida, E.; Pate, M.A.; et al. Implications of a circulating vaccine-derived poliovirus in Nigeria. *N. Engl. J. Med.* **2010**, *326*, 2360–2369. [CrossRef] [PubMed]
188. Zimmermann, M.; Hagedorn, B.; Lyons, H. Projection of costs of polio eradication compared to permanent control. *J. Infect. Dis.* **2020**, *221*, 561–565. [CrossRef] [PubMed]
189. Global Polio Eradication Initiative. *Investment Case 2022–2026*; World Health Organization: Geneva, Switzerland, 2022.
190. World Health Organization. Status of polio outbreaks in 2005. *Polio Erad. Initiat.—Polio News* **2005**, *25*, 2–3.
191. Thompson, K.M.; Duintjer Tebbens, R.J.; Pallansch, M.A. Evaluation of response scenarios to potential polio outbreaks using mathematical models. *Risk Anal.* **2006**, *26*, 1541–1556. [CrossRef] [PubMed]
192. Thompson, K.M. Poliomyelitis and the role of risk analysis in global infectious disease policy and management. *Risk Anal.* **2006**, *26*, 1419–1421. [CrossRef] [PubMed]
193. Dowdle, W.; van der Avoort, H.; de Gourville, E.; Delpeyroux, F.; Desphande, J.; Hovi, T.; Martin, J.; Pallansch, M.; Kew, O.; Wolff, C. Containment of polioviruses after eradication and OPV cessation: Characterizing risks to improve management. *Risk Anal.* **2006**, *26*, 1449–1469. [CrossRef]
194. Duintjer Tebbens, R.J.; Pallansch, M.A.; Kew, O.M.; Caceres, V.M.; Jafari, H.; Cochi, S.L.; Sutter, R.W.; Aylward, R.B.; Thompson, K.M. Risks of paralytic disease due to wild or vaccine-derived poliovirus after eradication. *Risk Anal.* **2006**, *26*, 1471–1505. [CrossRef] [PubMed]
195. Grassly, N.C.; Jafari, H.; Bahl, S.; Sethi, R.; Deshpande, J.M.; Wolff, C.; Sutter, R.W.; Aylward, R.B. Waning intestinal immunity after vaccination with oral poliovirus vaccines in India. *J. Infect. Dis.* **2012**, *205*, 1554–1561. [CrossRef] [PubMed]
196. Thompson, K.M.; Duintjer Tebbens, R.J. Modeling the dynamics of oral poliovirus vaccine cessation. *J. Infect. Dis.* **2014**, *210* (Suppl. 1), S475–S484. [CrossRef] [PubMed]

197. Pons-Salort, M.; Molodecky, N.A.; O'Reilly, K.M.; Wadood, M.Z.; Safdar, R.M.; Etsano, A.; Vaz, R.G.; Jafari, H.; Grassly, N.C.; Blake, I.M. Population immunity against serotype-2 poliomyelitis leading up to the global withdrawal of the oral poliovirus vaccine: Spatio-temporal modelling of surveillance data. *PLOS Med.* **2016**, *13*, e1002140. [CrossRef]
198. Grassly, N.C. Immunogenicity and effectiveness of routine immunization with 1 or 2 doses of inactivated poliovirus vaccine: Systematic review and meta-analysis. *J. Infect. Dis.* **2014**, *210* (Suppl. 1), S439–S446. [CrossRef] [PubMed]
199. Macklin, G.; Liao, Y.; Takane, M.; Dooling, K.; Gilmour, S.; Mach, O.; Kew, O.M.; Sutter, R.W.; iVDPV Working Group. Prolonged excretion of poliovirus among individuals with primary immunodeficiency disorder: An analysis of the World Health Organization registry. *Front. Immunol.* **2017**, *8*, 1103. [CrossRef] [PubMed]
200. Taniuchi, M.; Famulare, M.; Zaman, K.; Uddin, M.J.; Upfill-Brown, A.M.; Ahmed, T.; Saha, P.; Haque, R.; Bandyopadhyay, A.S.; Modlin, J.F.; et al. Community transmission of type 2 poliovirus after cessation of trivalent oral polio vaccine in Bangladesh: An open-label cluster-randomised trial and modelling study. *Lancet Infect. Dis.* **2017**, *17*, 1069–1079. [CrossRef]
201. Parker, E.P.; Molodecky, N.A.; Pons-Salort, M.; O'Reilly, K.M.; Grassly, N.C. Impact of inactivated poliovirus vaccine on mucosal immunity: Implications for the polio eradication endgame. *Expert Rev. Vaccines* **2015**, *14*, 1113–1123. [CrossRef] [PubMed]
202. Mangal, T.D.; Aylward, R.B.; Grassly, N.C. The potential impact of routine immunization with inactivated poliovirus vaccine on wild-type or vaccine-derived poliovirus outbreaks in a posteradication setting. *Am. J. Epidemiol.* **2013**, *178*, 1579–1587. [CrossRef] [PubMed]
203. Shirreff, G.; Wadood, M.Z.; Vaz, R.G.; Sutter, R.W.; Grassly, N.C. Estimated effect of inactivated poliovirus vaccine campaigns, Nigeria and Pakistan, January 2014–April 2016. *Emerg. Infect. Dis.* **2017**, *23*, 258–263. [CrossRef]
204. Grassly, N.C.; Wadood, M.Z.; Safdar, R.M.; Mahamud, A.S.; Sutter, R.W. Effect of inactivated poliovirus vaccine campaigns, Pakistan, 2014–2017. *Emerg. Infect. Dis.* **2018**, *24*, 2113–2115. [CrossRef] [PubMed]
205. Thompson, K.M.; Duintjer Tebbens, R.J. Retrospective cost-effectiveness analyses for polio vaccination in the United States. *Risk Anal.* **2006**, *26*, 1423–1440. [CrossRef] [PubMed]
206. Duintjer Tebbens, R.J.; Sangrujee, N.; Thompson, K.M. The costs of future polio risk management policies. *Risk Anal.* **2006**, *26*, 1507–1531. [CrossRef] [PubMed]
207. Duintjer Tebbens, R.J.; Pallansch, M.A.; Kew, O.M.; Sutter, R.W.; Bruce Aylward, R.; Watkins, M.; Gary, H.; Alexander, J.; Jafari, H.; Cochi, S.L.; et al. Uncertainty and sensitivity analyses of a decision analytic model for posteradication polio risk management. *Risk Anal.* **2008**, *28*, 855–876. [CrossRef] [PubMed]
208. Sangrujee, N.; Duintjer Tebbens, R.J.; Caceres, V.M.; Thompson, K.M. Policy decision options during the first 5 years following certification of polio eradication. *MedGenMed* **2003**, *5*, 35. [PubMed]
209. Duintjer Tebbens, R.J.; Thompson, K.M. Modeling the potential role of inactivated poliovirus vaccine to manage the risks of oral poliovirus vaccine cessation. *J. Infect. Dis.* **2014**, *210* (Suppl. 1), S485–S497. [CrossRef] [PubMed]
210. Kalkowska, D.A.; Duintjer Tebbens, R.J.; Thompson, K.M. Modeling strategies to increase population immunity and prevent poliovirus transmission in the high-risk area of northwest Nigeria. *J. Infect. Dis.* **2014**, *210* (Suppl. 1), S412–S423. [CrossRef] [PubMed]
211. Pons-Salort, M.; Burns, C.C.; Lyons, H.; Blake, I.M.; Jafari, H.; Oberste, M.S.; Kew, O.M.; Grassly, N.C. Preventing vaccine-derived poliovirus emergence during the polio endgame. *PLoS Pathog.* **2016**, *12*, e1005728. [CrossRef] [PubMed]

pathogens

MDPI

Article

Increasing Population Immunity Prior to Globally-Coordinated Cessation of Bivalent Oral Poliovirus Vaccine (bOPV)

Nima D. Badizadegan [1], Steven G. F. Wassilak [2], Concepción F. Estívariz [2], Eric Wiesen [2], Cara C. Burns [3], Omotayo Bolu [2] and Kimberly M. Thompson [1,*]

[1] Kid Risk, Inc., Orlando, FL 32819, USA
[2] Global Immunization Division, Global Health Center, Centers for Disease Control and Prevention, Atlanta, GA 30333, USA
[3] National Center for Immunization and Respiratory Diseases, Centers for Disease Control and Prevention, Atlanta, GA 30333, USA
* Correspondence: kimt@kidrisk.org; Tel.: +1-617-680-2836

Abstract: In 2022, global poliovirus modeling suggested that coordinated cessation of bivalent oral poliovirus vaccine (bOPV, containing Sabin-strain types 1 and 3) in 2027 would likely increase the risks of outbreaks and expected paralytic cases caused by circulating vaccine-derived polioviruses (cVDPVs), particularly type 1. The analysis did not include the implementation of planned, preventive supplemental immunization activities (pSIAs) with bOPV to achieve and maintain higher population immunity for types 1 and 3 prior to bOPV cessation. We reviewed prior published OPV cessation modeling studies to support bOPV cessation planning. We applied an integrated global poliovirus transmission and OPV evolution model after updating assumptions to reflect the epidemiology, immunization, and polio eradication plans through the end of 2023. We explored the effects of bOPV cessation in 2027 with and without additional bOPV pSIAs prior to 2027. Increasing population immunity for types 1 and 3 with bOPV pSIAs (i.e., intensification) could substantially reduce the expected global risks of experiencing cVDPV outbreaks and the number of expected polio cases both before and after bOPV cessation. We identified the need for substantial increases in overall bOPV coverage prior to bOPV cessation to achieve a high probability of successful bOPV cessation.

Keywords: polio; eradication; dynamic modeling; OPV cessation; immunization

1. Introduction

Well past the year 2000 target date set for poliomyelitis (polio) eradication in 1988, all three types of polioviruses (i.e., types 1, 2, and 3) continued to cause cases of paralytic polio [1], with ongoing transmission of some polioviruses reported in 2024 [2,3]. Historically, nearly all countries used oral poliovirus vaccine (OPV) in a trivalent formulation (tOPV, containing all three types) to achieve high levels of population immunity and stop the indigenous transmission of all wild polioviruses (WPVs). Countries that did not achieve and maintain sufficiently high routine immunization (RI) coverage to stop and prevent WPV transmission conducted supplemental immunization activities (SIAs) either as planned, preventive SIAs (pSIAs) or reactive, outbreak response SIAs (oSIAs) [1].

Before 2000, the potential of eradication dividends similar to smallpox eradication [4] and recognition of OPV-related risks supported discussions about ending poliovirus vaccine use after successful polio eradication, particularly OPV [1,5]. Specifically, after achieving high national immunization coverage with tOPV and eliminating indigenous WPV transmission, some high-income countries began to recognize the small but non-zero risks of OPV. First, OPV causes rare cases of vaccine-associated paralytic polio (VAPP) in vaccine recipients and their close contacts, which means a small number of expected polio cases each year as long as OPV use continues [1,5,6]. Second, low overall immunization coverage in OPV-using countries allows sustained transmission of OPV-related viruses among under-vaccinated individuals that can lead to the emergence of vaccine-derived polioviruses (VDPVs), which cause outbreaks of circulating VDPVs (cVDPV, recently also called variant polioviruses [3]) that behave identically to homotypic WPVs [6]. Last, prolonged OPV infections in some individuals with some primary immunodeficiencies can lead to very rare long-term shedding and paralytic cases due to immunodeficiency-associated VDPVs (iVDPVs) [6]. In 2008, the World Health Assembly (WHA) resolved to develop a plan "to set, if and when appropriate, a date for the eventual cessation" of OPV use in RI after the successful eradication of WPVs [7]. A 2008 health economic analysis noted that opportunities to enhance population immunity prior to OPV cessation could substantially reduce the expected burden of paralytic cases after cessation by achieving maximum population immunity, particularly in low-income countries [8].

As the Global Polio Eradication Initiative (GPEI) experienced delays in achieving polio eradication milestones, it supported the development and introduction of additional OPV formulations [1]. GPEI proposed using monovalent OPV (mOPV), and later bivalent OPV (bOPV, Sabin-strains type 1 and 3), in some SIAs in the most challenging poliovirus transmission areas to overcome relative "vaccine failure" caused by interference of type 2 in tOPV with the immune response to types 1 and 3 [1,9]. The use of Sabin-strain mOPV formulations for types 1 (mOPV1) and 3 (mOPV3) began in some SIAs in the mid-2000s, and the use of bOPV (containing types 1 and 3) started in 2009 [1]. However, any advantages of slightly increased per-dose immunogenicity for the single OPV type in mOPV (or two types in bOPV) became negligible with the administration of multiple OPV doses to the same populations in successive SIA rounds [1]. Ultimately, this strategy opened up immunity gaps for the OPV types not included in these SIAs, which allowed a resurgence of WPV3 cases (following the use of mOPV1), and vice versa and increased the risks of type 2 cVDPV (cVDPV2) emergence [10–15]. After 2009, the number of reported cVDPV2 cases increased substantially in areas using tOPV with low RI coverage and insufficient tOPV SIAs [3,16], which, along with ongoing risks of VAPP and iVDPV, led GPEI to shift to a policy of phasing OPV cessation by poliovirus type, starting with type 2 [17]. Preparations for type 2 OPV (OPV2) cessation included conducting pSIAs with tOPV to increase immunity to type 2 in populations with immunity gaps prior to April 2016. In April-May 2016, GPEI globally coordinated the cessation of all use of OPV2 for preventive immunization (i.e., RI and pSIAs), and all countries using tOPV in RI replaced it with bOPV and added at least one dose of inactivated poliovirus vaccine (IPV) into their RI schedules [17,18]. After May 2016, OPV2 became restricted to use for oSIAs with vaccine only available from a global stockpile of Sabin-strain type 2 mOPV (mOPV2) controlled by the World Health Organization (WHO) [17–21].

1.1. bOPV Cessation Planning Prior to OPV2 Cessation

At the time of OPV2 cessation, discussions among GPEI partners about the high number of cVDPV2s prior to 2015 led to the recognition of the importance of continuing to implement preventive bOPV pSIAs until bOPV cessation to ensure high population immunity for types 1 and 3. Considering the results of modeling [22,23], in October 2016, the WHO Strategic Advisory Group of Experts (SAGE) polio workgroup concluded that:

> "If the current level of routine bOPV and IPV coverage is maintained, most countries will not require additional bOPV campaigns prior to OPV cessation. However, if bOPV SIAs are not maintained and population immunity drops prior to OPV cessation, then areas with high force of infection and low RI coverage (especially in areas with under-vaccinated and/or inaccessible sub-populations), will need to conduct multiple bOPV campaigns prior to bOPV cessation to prevent cVDPVs after bOPV cessation". [24]

The workgroup further recommended maintaining the following:

"ongoing preventive SIAs in countries with low routine immunization coverage and additional bOPV campaigns prior to OPV cessation in countries (areas) where population immunity remains low". [24]

SAGE formally adopted these recommendations in 2016 [25]. GPEI strategic plans and budgets up through 2019 (with bOPV cessation anticipated to occur in 2019 [26]) included maintenance of bOPV pSIAs to sustain high levels of population immunity and mitigate the risks of outbreaks from WPV (or cVDPV) importations as well as cVDPV emergence for types 1 and 3 prior to and after OPV2 cessation [1].

1.2. bOPV Cessation PlanningFollowing OPV2 Cessation

Multiple emergences and widespread transmission of cVDPV2s after 2018 [27–29] led GPEI to shift resources budgeted for bOPV pSIAs to mOPV2 oSIAs [1,19]. GPEI also reinstated the production of tOPV for the OPV2 stockpile using existing Sabin OPV2 bulk for use in areas with co-circulation of different types of polioviruses [14,19,21,30]. Following research and development efforts initiated in 2011 that sought to genetically modify Sabin OPV strains to reduce their potential for reversion to cVDPVs, in 2019, GPEI accelerated the development of a type 2 novel OPV (nOPV2) and commissioned nOPV2 doses for the OPV2 stockpile [19,31–33]. In 2020, GPEI plans anticipated sufficient nOPV2 supply by early 2021 [34], and SAGE recommended preferential use of nOPV2 (see Section 5.4 of [35,36]), with countries in the WHO African Region opting to delay oSIAs to wait for nOPV2 instead of using Sabin-strain mOPV2. Additionally, disruptions due to the COVID-19 pandemic led to the cancellation or postponement of many oSIAs in 2020. In November 2020, nOPV2 received an emergency use listing (EUL) from WHO, and in December 2023, nOPV2 became fully licensed.

Following the GPEI shift of resources from bOPV pSIAs to OPV2 oSIAs [1], the number of cVDPV1 reported cases increased. Co-circulation of poliovirus type 1 (i.e., WPV1, cVDPV1) and 2 (i.e., cVDPV2) also emerged as an increasing challenge. During 2021–2023, GPEI reported more annual cases caused by type 1 cVDPVs (cVDPV1) than those caused by WPV1 [1–3]. In October 2020, SAGE recommended that "tOPV be made available to countries for cVDPV2 outbreak response in subnational areas where there is co-circulation or high risk of co-circulation of cVDPV2 with cVDPV1, cVDPV3 or WPV1 in order to avoid the need to conduct dual mOPV2 and bOPV campaigns" [36]. Several countries used tOPV from the OPV2 stockpile during 2021–2023 to control cVDPV2 outbreaks that occurred contemporaneously with WPV1 transmission (i.e., Afghanistan, Pakistan), cVDPV1 (i.e., Yemen) or due to high-risk of co-circulation (i.e., prior experience with a cVDPV3 outbreak in 2018 in Somalia in 2018 and ongoing concerns about risks of cVDPVs there).

Ongoing poliovirus transmission in 2024 [2,3] indicated missed milestones of the GPEI 2022–2026 strategic plan, which aimed to end all WPV1 and cVDPV transmission by the end of 2023 ([1], ([37], see page xi). Nonetheless, bOPV cessation planning discussions continue since the plan suggested that bOPV cessation could occur as early as 2027, with implementation plans developed at least two years before bOPV cessation [37]. With respect to SIAs, the plan stated: "SIAs with types 1 and 3 containing OPV (Sabin or novel) should be implemented over a period of time in the years prior to cessation and not just during the immediate pre-cessation period, to maintain persistently high population-level immunity" ([37], see page 42). This has not occurred.

Polio modeling studies continue to provide analytical support for deliberations by GPEI partners [38–42] (also see reviews of polio modeling studies published 2000–2019 [43] and 2020–2024 [44]). Recognizing that modeling studies may help with bOPV planning efforts and building on our prior studies related to bOPV cessation [22,45–49], this study aims to simulate the potential benefits of intensifying bOPV pSIAs years prior to bOPV cessation. The next section provides a review of our prior global OPV cessation modeling publications for readers unfamiliar with polio modeling. Sections 3–5 present the methods, results, and discussion of our updated modeling of bOPV cessation with and without the addition of bOPV pSIAs.

2. Global Poliovirus Transmission Modeling

2.1. Characterization of OPV Risks and Global Modeling Concepts

Prior to any decisions about OPV cessation, modeling studies identified potential variability in national preferences for vaccine options after polio eradication (i.e., IPV, OPV, or no vaccine) [8,50], the importance of global coordination of OPV cessation and creation of an OPV stockpile to support rapid oSIAs if needed [20,46,51–53], and prerequisites for OPV cessation that would help manage risks [54]. Our modeling emphasized the importance of increasing population immunity [10], which we define for the entire population relative to stopping poliovirus transmission, in contrast to other definitions of vaccine-induced immune protection from paralysis in children under a specific age (e.g., age 3 years old) [43,44]. Multiple studies identified the need to intensify tOPV pSIAs prior to OPV2 cessation to reduce the risks of emergence of cVDPV2 outbreaks after OPV cessation [14,23,55] and demonstrated the limited role of IPV in post-OPV2 cessation risk management [56]. Several studies highlighted the importance of rapidly detecting any ongoing cVDPV2 transmission after OPV2 cessation to promptly and aggressively conduct OPV2 oSIAs with high coverage to stop transmission [21,23,57]. Global modeling studies identified a small chance of failure of OPV cessation as a polio endgame strategy and the potential need to restart tOPV production and preventive use (i.e., OPV restart) if OPV cessation did not succeed [21,23].

We developed and maintained an integrated global poliovirus transmission, risk, decision, and economic model to explore the health and economic risks, costs, and benefits of polio endgame strategies (for full model description, assumptions, inputs, and equations, see [58] and its associated technical appendix). Briefly, our integrated global polio models compartmentalize the world population into subpopulations that simulate dynamic demographics, immunization activities, epidemiological histories, and characteristics relevant to poliovirus transmission, with stratifications required to characterize variability consistent with differences in actual conditions recognized through experience. For each subpopulation, which includes multiple age groups, we apply a deterministic transmission model that includes different immunity states accounting for each of the 3 different poliovirus types to simulate immunity induced by maternal antibodies, different combinations of OPV and/or IPV doses from immunization, prior infections, and waning of immunity [11]. Notably, the transmission model includes the potential for individuals with prior immunity to potentially become reinfected and participate in transmission, although only fully susceptible individuals may develop paralysis with poliovirus type-specific rates [11]. The transmission model includes a multistage infection process, and mixing occurs within model subpopulations heterogeneously by age and homogeneously in space and between subpopulations according to varied preferential mixing areas that represent larger geographical regions [11,58]. The model also includes a multistage OPV evolution process to simulate the loss of attenuating mutations and increases that occur in fitness, transmissibility, and potential for neurovirulence of OPV and OPV-related viruses in populations to mimic the emergence of cVDPVs, with infections of fully susceptible individuals with an OPV or OPV-related virus able to lead to paralysis with type- and OPV-evolution stage-specific rates [11,16]. Given the complexity of the different types and formulations of poliovirus vaccines, the model includes full consideration of their properties and appropriate adjustments for differences between populations (e.g., relatively lower or higher take rates in lower-income, temperate, or higher-income countries based on evidence from vaccine effectiveness studies) [58].

Our integrated global model introduced more complexity over time, and assumptions were modified as global conditions changed [23,28,48,49,58–63]. For all applications, the model includes a historical "burn in" period that includes retrospective deterministic inputs based on the available evidence (i.e., immunization coverage and epidemiological data) to generate appropriate initial conditions. Then, for prospective analyses, the integrated model includes numerous iterations to account for uncertain potential stochastic risk events (e.g., reintroduction from importation, containment breach, iVDPVs) and considers different potential mixing between subpopulations. Stochastic simulations yield numerous possible future realizations of the world for the different scenarios and/or policies considered, which we typically communicate in the form of expected values that average over all of the stochastic iterations and/or cumulative outcomes (e.g., cases, costs, probability of successful die-out) for the prospective model time horizon.

2.2. OPV Cessation Global Modeling Pre-OPV2 Cessation

Global modeling of the polio endgame trajectory prior to OPV2 cessation assumed that GPEI and countries would follow model- and SAGE-recommended risk management strategies to achieve the best chances of success [21,23]. These recommendations included pre-OPV2 cessation tOPV intensification, maintenance of bOPV pSIAs until bOPV cessation, sufficient and aggressive oSIAs to promptly stop outbreaks using homotypic OPV for 5 years after OPV cessation, then use IPV [23], with a separate exploration allowing homotypic OPV use for the entire model time horizon (e.g., through 2052) [21]. Additional analyses performed a larger number of stochastic iterations to identify more potential root causes for endgame failure [64] and to explore the implications of using OPV for 0 to 5 years before using IPV for oSIAs and of not conducting any oSIAs for type 2 poliovirus outbreaks after 2016 [65]. However, recognizing some chance of failure of OPV2 cessation and later bOPV cessation, the model included a threshold of 50,000 total cases (sensitivity analysis range of 1000 to 50,000) of all poliovirus types combined since OPV cessation to trigger OPV restart (i.e., tOPV use in RI and/or pSIAs) [23,29]. The pre-OPV2 cessation modeling studies assumed initial conditions as of the end of 2014 and led to an estimated 2 OPV restarts in 100 stochastic model iterations [23] and 57 OPV restarts out of 1000 stochastic iterations [64] for 2013–2052, with sensitivity analyses and different assumptions about OPV use in oSIAs leading to more expected failures and thus more OPV restarts [21,23,64,65]. Additional modeling characterized the expected increase in vulnerability of populations to restarted poliovirus transmission and outbreaks as a function of time after OPV cessation and the type of poliovirus imported [66,67].

For OPV types 1 and 3, pre-bOPV cessation modeling studies characterized (i) the expected benefit of maintaining high population immunity for types 1 and 3 with bOPV pSIAs until bOPV cessation and (ii) the expected increase in vulnerability of populations to restarted poliovirus transmission and outbreaks as a function of time after OPV cessation and type of poliovirus imported [22,45]. With the last reported case caused by WPV3 reported in 2012, studies also considered the implications of globally coordinated cessation of type 3 OPV (OPV3) prior to type 1 OPV (OPV1) [46,47].

2.3. OPV Cessation Global Modeling Post-OPV2 Cessation

After OPV2 cessation (i.e., since 2016), continued cVDPV2 transmission and delayed achievement of WPV1 eradication increased the complexity of polio endgame modeling, particularly with respect to the potential for OPV restart, bOPV cessation, increasing poliovirus vaccine options [46,68,69]. Following the release of the GPEI 2019–2023 Strategic Plan, we updated the global model to reflect the actual initial conditions as of the end of 2019 and shifted the global model time horizon to 2019–2029. At that time, we changed the OPV restart threshold to three type-specific limits of 5000 cases since homotypic OPV cessation [58]. We also updated the model inputs to include: (i) oSIAs with suboptimal performance qualities as observed since OPV2 cessation, (ii) mOPV2 use allowed for oSIAs up to 8 years after OPV2 cessation (i.e., 2024), or alternatively for the entire model time horizon, (iii) bOPV cessation in 2025 (or alternatively after the end of the model time horizon) with homotypic mOPV use for oSIAs allowed for types 1 and 3 for 5 years after bOPV cessation, and (iv) updated risk estimates for reintroduction from unexpected use of OPV after OPV cessation [28]. As efforts to develop nOPV2 accelerated, we updated the model to include bounding cases for its characteristics, and we explored the impact of using nOPV2 for oSIAs instead of mOPV2 [59]. A health economic analysis explored different options for RI vaccines assuming different scenarios for control (i.e., not pursuing bOPV cessation and either restarting tOPV or switching to 2 doses of IPV) and an eradication scenario (i.e., bOPV cessation in 2025 using modeled SIA inputs that led to successful WPV1 eradication by 2023) [70]. These studies published in 2020–2021 reported increased expected numbers of prospective stochastic model iterations with OPV restarts [28,59,70].

Following the emergence of SARS-CoV-2 and the COVID-19 pandemic, we updated the global model assumptions for long-range exportation risks and explored the impacts of disruptions in immunization and transmission due to reduced mixing during the initial stages of the pandemic, again considering mOPV2 and nOPV2 options for oSIAs [60]. This model used the same initial conditions (through the end of 2019) and a model time horizon of 2019–2023 [60]. A subsequent study focused on oSIAs with the same time horizon of 2019–2023 but started with initial conditions updated to the end of 2020 and explored the consequences of delaying oSIAs to wait for nOPV2 instead of using mOPV2 [61]. Another study using a time horizon of 2022–2026 with initial conditions updated to the end of 2021 explored the trade-offs for numerous oSIA performance characteristics (including the identification of some aggressive global strategies with more rounds, larger rounds, expanded age target age groups, improved coverage per round) and vaccine options [62]. These studies with shorter (i.e., 4-year) time horizons reported the potential for fewer expected OPV2 restarts depending on oSIA vaccine options and performance characteristics [60–62].

In 2019, GPEI did not restart the preventive use of OPV2 (i.e., in RI or pSIAs) when it commissioned new bulk production of nOPV2 for the global stockpile [71]. Following the introduction of nOPV2, GPEI shifted its outbreak response expectations to include ongoing production and exclusive use of nOPV2 for oSIAs [72] with no option for OPV restart. Consequently, since 2022, our global modeling studies have not included the possibility of OPV restarting for preventive use. Instead, we allowed OPV use for oSIAs for the entire model time horizon and focused on characterizing the probability of die-out of transmission by the end of the model time horizon [29,48,49,73]. Using a model time horizon of 2022–2026 or 2022–2035, and based on the contemporary experience of suboptimal oSIA success in stopping outbreaks, these studies reported <1% chance of dying out of type 2 transmission by the end of the model time horizon [29,48,49,59]. These studies also highlighted increased global risks of co-circulation of types 1 and 2 and the potential for substantial reductions in expected costs and cases with the use of tOPV if available or co-administered nOPV2 and bOPV in oSIAs instead of sequential oSIAs for different OPV types [29,48,49,59].

With respect to bOPV cessation, the global modeling conducted in 2022 explored the implications of projected GPEI and country plans as of the end of 2021 and assumed bOPV cessation around 1 May 2027 [48,49]. These studies reported numerous expected cVDPV1 cases both before and after bOPV cessation in the absence of bOPV pSIAs and reported a <1% chance of the die-out of type 1 transmission by the end of the model time horizon [48,49].

2.4. *Characterizing the Probability of Success (POS) for OPV Cessation*

To harmonize across the use of different metrics for OPV cessation performance in the various models described above, we broadly characterize model estimates of the probability of success (POS) for ending poliovirus transmission after OPV cessation using either (i) 1 minus the probability of OPV restart or (ii) the probability of die-out. Table 1 summarizes the evolution of published estimates with quantitative POS estimates for OPV cessation and key attributes of the studies (e.g., metric reported, model time horizon and initial conditions, poliovirus types included in the OPV restart criteria, the POS estimate(s), publication date and source) [21,23,28,48,49,59–62,64,65,70,73]. The duration of the model time horizons shortens considerably from top to bottom in Table 1, which reveals decreasing POS estimates over time while also allowing for fewer numbers of years to observe failure (i.e., increased right-censoring of the results). Pre-OPV2 cessation studies implied a high expected POS (i.e., >90% for all OPV types combined), while the expected POS for type 2 dropped to 11% for a 10-year time horizon post-OPV2 cessation [28,59,70]. Later studies with shorter (i.e., 4-year) time horizons reported potentially higher and variable type 2 POS estimates depending on oSIA vaccine options and performance characteristics [60–62], but modeling since 2022 reported expected POS results of <1% for types 1, 2, and 3, assuming GPEI continues current policies and program performance remains the same.

Table 1. Evolution of published estimates of the probability of success (POS) of OPV cessation.

Metric	Time Horizon [IC]	Type, POS [a] (Range)	Date(s) [Sources(s)]
Pre-OPV2 cessation studies (assumed OPV2 cessation would occur in 2016, bOPV cessation 2019)			
OPV restart	2013–2052 [End 2014 [b]]	All types, 98% (90–98%)	24 Sep 2015 [23] 24 Mar 2016 [21]
OPV restart	2013–2052 [End 2014 [b]]	All types, 94.3% (15–94.3%)	23 Sep 2016 [64] 1 Jun 2017 [65] (range)
Post-OPV2 cessation studies (OPV2 implemented in 2016; see text for assumptions for bOPV cessation)			
OPV restart	2019–2029 [End 2019]	Type 2, 11% (11–56%)	6 Jul 2020 [28]
OPV restart	2019–2029 [End 2019]	Type 2, 11% (33–78%)	10 Nov 2020 [59]
OPV restart	2019–2029 [c] [End 2019]	Type 2, 11% Type 1; 2; 3 [c] 80%; 56%; 100%	19 Feb 2021 [70]
OPV restart	2019–2023 [d] [End 2019]	Type 2, 67% (62–73%)	27 Apr 2021 [60]
OPV restart	2019–2023 [d] [End 2020]	Type 2, 67% (46–67%)	14 May 2021 [61]
p(die out)	2022–2026 [d] [End 2021]	Type 2, <1% (<1–95%)	17 Nov 2022 [62]
p(die out)	2022–2035 [End 2021]	Type 1; 2 <1; <1%	21 Jun 2023 [48,49] 14 Aug 2023 [73]

Abbreviations: bOPV, bivalent OPV; GPEI, Global Polio Eradication Initiative; IC, initial conditions; OPV, oral poliovirus vaccine; OPV2, type 2 OPV; p(die out), probability of die out of transmission by the end of the time horizon; POS, probability of successful OPV cessation; pSIA, preventive supplemental immunization activity; WPV1, type 1 wild poliovirus. [a] Column shows the poliovirus type(s) of POS estimates in the study and the expected POS for the modeled baseline (range of POS values for different scenarios considered, where applicable); see each study for specific details. [b] Model prospectively assumed GPEI and countries would implement all recommended OPV cessation risk management strategies. [c] For this study, baseline estimate POS of 11% for type 2, but hypothetical additional scenarios included pSIAs to achieve WPV1 eradication by 2023 and implemented bOPV cessation in 2025 with POS estimates for each type shown. [d] No consideration of bOPV cessation in this analysis since it would only potentially occur after the model time horizon.

Additional retrospective analyses identified differences between pre-OPV2 cessation model assumptions and post-OPV2 cessation experience [58,74]. A 2023 look back concluded that the authors knew then what they know now about the implementation of pre-OPV2 cessation activities and post-OPV2 cessation oSIAs; pre-OPV2 cessation modeling would not have supported expectations of a high POS for OPV2 cessation in 2016 [29]. The decline in POS estimates primarily reflects the overall failure to fully implement pre-OPV2 cessation pSIAs and model-recommended oSIA timeliness, scope, number, and quality [21]. This serves as a powerful reminder that pre-OPV cessation immunization activities, while essential for success if implemented well, do not represent the only critical factor for a successful polio endgame.

3. Materials and Methods

For this study, we started with the 2023 model of bOPV cessation without additional bOPV pSIAs (i.e., very limited use of bOPV SIAs only in some countries and no planned bOPV intensification) [48] to explore the role of bOPV pSIA intensification prior to OPV cessation. The current formulation of the global model divides the world into 72 blocks of 10 subpopulations (i.e., 720 subpopulations) of approximately 10.7 million people each, stratified by current RI vaccine use (i.e., OPV + IPV, IPV/OPV, IPV-only) and World Bank Income Level (low-income, LI; lower-middle-income, LMI; upper-middle-income, UMI; high-income, HI). The model assumed historical RI coverage consistent with

WHO/UNICEF estimates, with some transient adjustments for the disruptions associated with the COVID-19 pandemic [48]. We assume SIA performance characteristics related to coverage and repeatedly missing the same children by successive SIA rounds as in prior modeling [48]. The model detects any cases of any poliovirus type at the time of onset of paralysis, which does not account for additional delays that may exist in practice [75], and assumes that oSIAs start 45 days after detection in the model, which accounts for some delay for surveillance. All oSIAs target children < 5 years of age and include 2 oSIA rounds 30 days apart, with one recent exception noted below. The model automatically implements 2 additional rounds after any breakthrough transmission, for which we assume the oSIA occurs only in the outbreak subpopulation if its basic reproductive number (R_0) for type 1 WPV (WPV1) < 10. For other subpopulations with WPV1 $R_0 \geq 10$, oSIA rounds occur in the outbreak subpopulation and its four worst-performing neighbor subpopulations within the same block. We vary the oSIA intensity for different subpopulations, which ranges from 15% true coverage and 95% repeatedly missed probability to 80% true coverage and 50% repeatedly missed probability. We also assume the use of Sabin OPV for oSIAs prior to type-specific OPV cessation and model different OPV vaccine options after type-specific OPV cessation. When triggered in the model, oSIAs replace or delay any pSIA rounds, similar to the GPEI experience [28,48,49,58–63]. For this analysis, we assume the use of Sabin mOPV2 occurred from 2016–2021 and the use of nOPV2 from 2022 on. Similar to prior modeling, we apply bounding scenarios of (i) nOPV best, which uses type-specific nOPV for outbreak response assuming the same effectiveness as type-specific mOPV, no reversion despite transmissibility, and no VAPP, and (ii) nOPV worst, which uses type-specific nOPV for outbreak response post-type-specific OPV cessation, assumes 90% of the effectiveness of mOPV and prior assumptions for reduced reversion [59], which we further reduced here by 10%, and VAPP occurring at a rate 10% lower than the VAPP rate of mOPV in vaccine recipients [48].

Recognizing accelerated efforts to develop nOPV for types 1 and 3 (i.e., nOPV1 and nOPV3), for this analysis, we assume the availability of these vaccines for oSIAs at the time of bOPV cessation, starting 1 May 2027. Thus, we consider the implications of using nOPV2 starting at the beginning of the time horizon (in 2022) for the nOPV scenarios, with bOPV used for type 1 and/or 3 oSIAs prior to 2027 and nOPV1 and nOPV3 use after bOPV cessation. We focus on exploring the relative benefits of resuming and increasing bOPV pSIAs prior to bOPV cessation as a strategy to reduce expected cVDPV cases before and after bOPV cessation.

Since 2023 modeling [48] included implementation of some bOPV pSIAs prospectively in years 2022 and 2023 that did not occur, and it did not include some oSIAs in those years that did occur, we adjusted these baseline SIA inputs appropriately and shifted the model time horizon to 2024–2035. We also identified the very low SIA coverage in the model blocks that represent the conditions in countries such as Nigeria, the Democratic Republic of the Congo (DRC), and Yemen as barriers to success, noting that GPEI partners have invested substantial resources in these consequential geographies since 2022. This led us to assume an increase in the SIA quality in Nigeria and DRC starting in 2022 and 2023, respectively, such that for these blocks, we returned SIA quality to the pre-COVID levels (i.e., we raised the SI_L model input by one step for each). We also updated the baseline to include the use of tOPV in more SIAs than in prior modeling [48] since these SIAs actually occurred in Pakistan, Afghanistan, and Yemen, and we increased the target age range for oSIAs in Yemen to children < 10 years for consistency with reported implementation [76]. In addition, given the continuing transmission of WPV1, we postponed the assumed timing of post-eradication degradation of surveillance quality in prior global modeling [48] from 2025 to the 2035 end of the model time horizon. Maintaining the quality of surveillance significantly changed the expected numbers of polio cases after 2027 compared with prior modeling [48] because it allows for earlier outbreak detection and earlier performance of oSIAs. While we modeled these changes here, uncertainty remains about GPEI plans, finances, and potential future dissolution. Notably, GPEI already reports insufficient resources to support bOPV pSIAs due to the substantial resource needs for oSIAs [1,77]. Given these changes, we reran the baseline we used for the prior study (with no additional bOPV pSIAs [48]) for the nOPV scenarios (i.e., nOPV best and nOPV worst). We do not include an updated mOPV baseline because we assume a global shift to nOPV2 oSIA responses since 2022.

Starting with the updated baselines, we also consider the potential impact of resuming and/or increasing bOPV pSIAs in the subpopulations in the model characterized by low RI coverage and high transmission risks that correspond to countries that historically performed SIAs. We focused on increasing the number of annual bOPV pSIA rounds starting in the early part of each calendar year from 2025 through the implementation of bOPV cessation in the model on 1 May 2027. We used an iterative process to identify the specific model subpopulations that would benefit from bOPV pSIAs and sought to include enough rounds to potentially stop all ongoing cVDPV1 transmission by bOPV cessation in 2027. For 2024, we included 6–7 bOPV pSIAs in 2024 for Pakistan and Afghanistan and 2 bOPV pSIAs for high-risk areas in northern India. Figure 1 shows a histogram of the number of added bOPV pSIAs for the 720 model subpopulations for 2025 and 2026. Increasing the number of pSIAs implicitly creates more opportunity for both bOPV pSIAs and any needed type 2 oSIAs to occur. All 20 subpopulations in the model that represent populations of the endemic countries (Pakistan and Afghanistan) perform between 3 and 7 bOPV pSIAs per year, with the higher number representing implementation of SIAs in the most challenging areas. For the non-endemic countries, the note in Figure 1 provides context about the subpopulation characteristics that motivated the addition of different numbers of bOPV pSIAs.

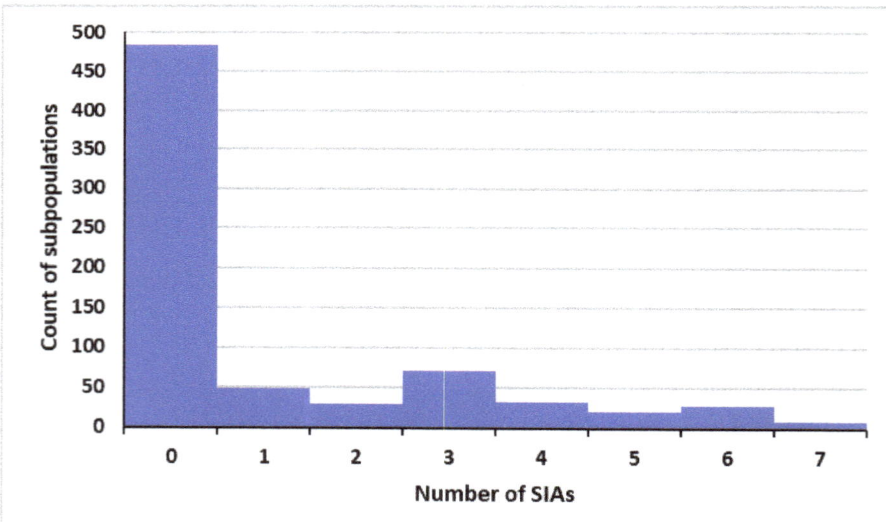

Figure 1. Histogram of bOPV pSIAs in the 720 model subpopulations with intensification *. Abbreviations: bOPV, bivalent OPV, pSIA, preventive supplemental immunization activity. * Pakistan and Afghanistan 6 pSIAs (low coverage areas 7 pSIAs), most of the Democratic Republic of the Congo, Nigeria, and Ethiopia 2–3 pSIAs (low coverage areas 4–7 pSIAs), most of India 3 pSIAs (high-risk areas, including UP and Bihar, 5–7 pSIAs), most of Somalia and South Sudan 2 pSIAs (low-coverage areas 7 pSIAs), most of Ukraine 4 pSIAs (high-risk areas 6 pSIAs), Yemen and Papua New Guinea 6 pSIAs, most of Indonesia 1 pSIA (low coverage areas 3–4 pSIAs), most of the Syrian Arab Republic 1 pSIA (low coverage areas 2–3 pSIAs), most of Bangladesh 3 pSIAs (low coverage areas 5 pSIAs), Côte d'Ivoire, Mauritania, Egypt, and Haiti 4 pSIAs, Philippines 3 pSIAs, 3–4 pSIAs in low-coverage areas

in modeled subpopulations that include countries such as: Albania, Algeria, Angola, Armenia, Azerbaijan, Benin, Bosnia and Herzegovina, Botswana, Burkina Faso, Burundi, Cambodia, Cameroon, Central African Republic, Chad, Comoros, Congo, Djibouti, Dominican Republic, El Salvador, Equatorial Guinea, Eritrea, Eswatini, Ethiopia, Gabon, Gambia, Georgia, Ghana, Guatemala, Guinea, Guinea-Bissau, Haiti, Honduras, Kazakhstan, Kyrgyzstan, Kenya, Lao People's Democratic Republic, Lesotho, Liberia, Libya, Madagascar, Malawi, Mali, Mauritius, Montenegro, Morocco, Mozambique, Myanmar, Namibia, Nicaragua, Niger, Papua New Guinea, Philippines, Republic of Moldova, Rwanda, Senegal, Serbia, Sierra Leone, Somalia, State of Palestine, Sudan, Tajikistan, The Former Yugoslavian Republic of Macedonia, Togo, Tunisia, Turkmenistan, Uganda, Ukraine, United Republic of Tanzania, Viet Nam, Zambia, and Zimbabwe. The global model includes some of these countries due to risks posed by other countries in the same block. Generally, countries with WPV1 $R_0 \geq 10$ with any levels of coverage would likely benefit from some pSIAs (e.g., the inclusion of pSIAs in India and Bangladesh), and all countries with subpopulations with coverage less than <60% would likely need 3–4 pSIAs. The model does not provide refined estimates of the number of pSIAs and may not fully account for differential decreases in coverage that occurred during COVID-19 and persist in some countries.

As in prior prospective analyses, we include stochastic risks of reintroduction of polioviruses from outbreaks into other subpopulations as well as random events (e.g., post-cessation unexpected use of OPV, excretion into the community of immunodeficiency-associated VDPVs, and/or containment breaches). We present the results of the model simulations using the expected value of 100 stochastic iterations, performed using JAVA™ programming language in the integrated development environment Eclipse™, starting with the same random number seeds and initial conditions to control the stochasticity for each scenario to focus on direct comparisons of the different scenarios.

4. Results

Figure 2 shows the expected values of the paralytic polio cases for the model time horizon for the baseline from the prior study (i.e., mOPV) [48] and for the new baselines (i.e., nOPV best and nOPV worst). The prior baseline assumed some continued bOPV pSIAs that did not actually occur and assumed mOPV2 use for oSIAs for the full-time horizon [48]. As shown in Figure 2, the baseline expected total cases for types 1 and 2 for the nOPV best and nOPV worst scenarios reflect: (i) the removal of previously modeled bOPV pSIAs for 2022 and 2023 [48], which did not actually occur, (ii) the inclusion of some tOPV and mOPV2 oSIAs that did occur, and (iii) the shift to nOPV2 for most oSIAs in 2022 and 2023. Figure 2A shows a somewhat higher overall expected burden of type 1 cases from 2024–2027, although these remain relatively low as long as bOPV use continues in RI and oSIAs. This occurs because the model includes oSIAs with bOPV for any type 1 outbreak prior to bOPV cessation, in addition to its use in RI and any pSIAs included for 2022–2027 in the polio-endemic countries of Pakistan and Afghanistan. Similar to prior modeling [48], the implementation of bOPV cessation in 2027 without additional bOPV pSIAs shows a rapid and substantial increase in expected type 1 paralytic polio cases. Figure 2B shows the expected number of annual type 2 cases. Since the introduction of nOPV2 starts in 2022, the expected cases for type 2 with oSIAs that use *mOPV*, nOPV best, or nOPV worst already differ in 2024. Figure 2B shows a much lower expected number of type 2 cases if nOPV2 exhibits unrealized properties similar to those modeled for the *nOPV2 best* bound, but the expected cases do not go to zero. The low expected number of type 3 paralytic cases shown in Figure 2C reflects the outcome of a relatively small fraction of stochastic iterations with any type 3 poliovirus transmission. Combining the expected cases for the scenarios in Figure 2D shows the dominance of the expected type 1 cases due to its relatively greater transmissibility and neurovirulence. Notably, the baseline scenario leads to increasing use of bOPV oSIAs to manage cVDPV1 outbreaks, and in some subpopulations and iterations, co-circulation of cVDPV1 and cVDPV2 outbreaks that the model manages by prioritizing oSIAs to the first outbreak type observed. The results in Figure 2 continue to reflect the model assumptions related to limited to no improvements in oSIAs and no restart of any preventive OPV use, independent of the burden of disease (i.e., no consideration of reactive policy changes).

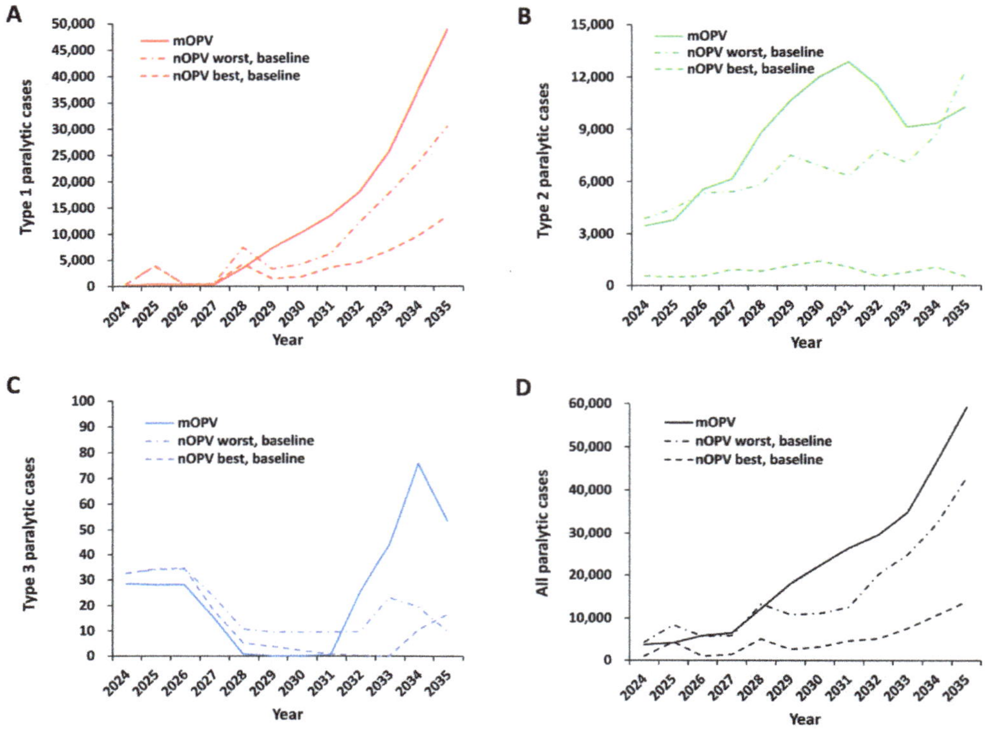

Figure 2. Expected annual polio cases for global bivalent oral poliovirus vaccine (bOPV) cessation occurring in 2027 and outbreak response for using monovalent OPV (mOPV) (assumptions and result from the prior study [48]), or using updated assumptions for novel OPV (nOPV). Outbreak response scenarios for nOPV (baseline) assume nOPV2 best or nOPV2 worst from 2022 on, and outbreak response for type 1 or 3 using Sabin-strain bOPV until 2027, and then either homotypic nOPV best or nOPV worst for types 1 and 3 (see text and prior studies [48,49] for assumed characteristics of nOPV best and nOPV worst bounds).

Figure 3 shows the expected annual cases with additional bOPV pSIAs (i.e., intensification) in some model subpopulations to intensify population immunity between 1 January 2024 and 1 May 2027, see Figure 1) compared with the baseline. In contrast with prior modeling [48] and the new baselines (Figure 2), the addition of bOPV pSIAs leads to a substantial reduction in the number of expected cases for type 1, as shown in Figure 3A for the entire time horizon. Overall, the expected number of annual cVDPV1 cases remains relatively low as long as bOPV use continues, but bOPV cessation in 2027 increases the risks of cVDPV1 outbreaks and expected cases after 2027. Due to the change in assumptions about surveillance and oSIA coverage in some high-risk geographies, the results show a less dramatic expected increase in cVDPV1 cases than prior results [48]. As expected, Figure 3B shows that adding bOPV pSIAs does not substantially change the expected annual cases for type 2, with the nOPV best and nOPV worst curves showing similar annual expected cases, although some differences occur due to some iterations with co-circulation. Adding bOPV pSIAs lowers the number of iterations with type 3 transmission and expected cases, and Figure 3C shows similar low expected annual cases compared with Figure 2C. A comparison of the total expected annual cases for the scenarios in Figure 3D shows a substantial improvement over the expected results in Figure 2D.

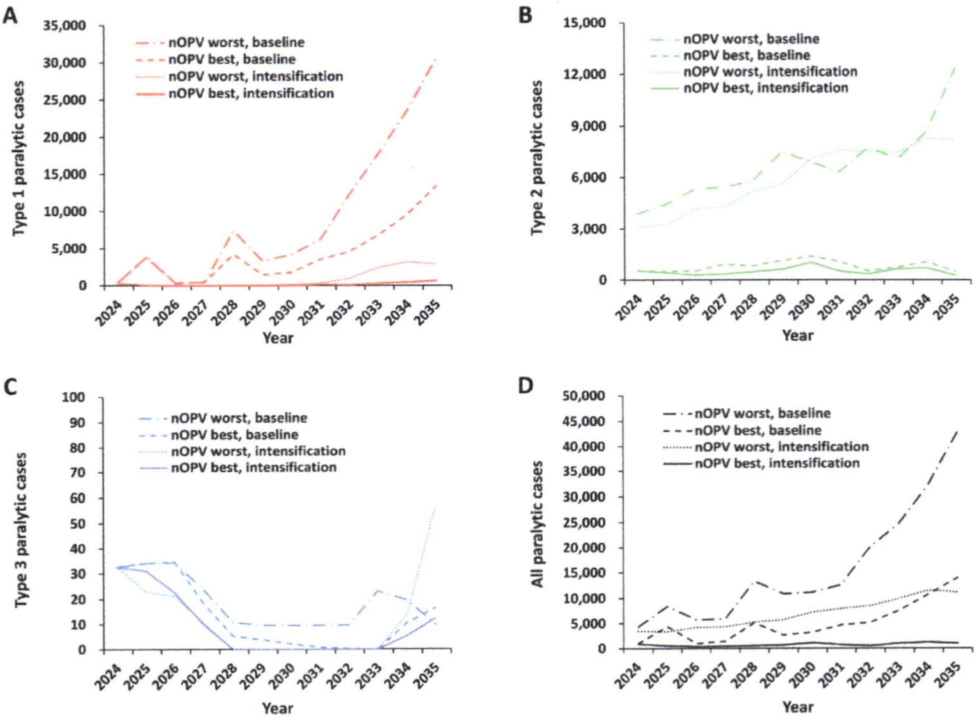

Figure 3. Expected annual polio cases for global bivalent OPV (bOPV) cessation in 2027 and outbreak response for type 2 using novel OPV (nOPV) with either nOPV2 best or nOPV2 worst from 2022 on, and outbreak response for type 1 or 3 using Sabin-strain bOPV until 2027, and then either homotypic nOPV best or nOPV worst (see text and prior studies [48,49] for assumed characteristics of nOPV best and nOPV worst bounds) after bOPV cessation without (baseline) and with additional preventive supplemental immunization activities using bOPV (i.e., intensification) added in some model subpopulations (see text and Figure 1).

Table 2 summarizes the POS estimates (and expected cases) for each type for the results of the different scenarios presented in Figures 2 and 3. The expected cases average over the variability that arises in the 100 stochastic iterations due to different risks of reintroduction. Table 2 divides the time period into pre-bOPV cessation (i.e., 2024–2027) and post-bOPV cessation (i.e., 2028–2035). The expected cases reflect estimates summed over multiple years and intended to provide context for relative comparisons for different policies, not precise estimates of future outcomes. As discussed in prior modeling, the expected annual case estimates depend on the modeled assumptions and time horizons, and they reflect substantial variability in the iterations [49]. These results suggest that intensification (i.e., increasing population immunity with additional bOPV pSIAs prior to bOPV cessation) could prevent substantial numbers of cVDPV1 cases during 2024–2027 compared with the baseline by increasing type 1 population immunity prior to the importation of cVDPV1 (or WPV1) from other countries or the development of cVDPV1 outbreaks in OPV-using countries. In addition, by adding more pSIAs in 2025 and 2026 with intensification, we reduced the competition between bOPV pSIAs and nOPV2 oSIAs in those years in some countries with co-circulation, which also led to few expected type 2 cases. The POS estimates in Table 2 show substantial improvement in the POS for both pre- and post-bOPV cessation for types 1 and 3 with bOPV pSIA intensification compared with the updated baseline with no intensification. Post-bOPV cessation, risks from the transition, iVDPVs, and containment breaches lead to some stochastic iterations, with some cases requiring outbreak response due to transmissions. The expected results in Figure 3 average over the 100 stochastic iterations, so the low numbers of expected cases for types 1 and 3 after 2028 reflect the averages of many iterations with 0 cases and some iterations with non-zero cases. Overall, as the POS increases, this reduces the expected number of cases, although for type 3, the expected annual case estimates remain below 100, and small numbers of iterations with outbreaks with intensification include a relatively higher number of cases because of their occurrence further out in time.

Table 2. Probability of success (POS) estimates (expected total cases) for different time periods by type and scenario.

Scenario and Time Period	POS (Expected Cases) for 2024–2027						POS (Expected Cases) for 2028–2035					
Type	1		2		3		1		2		3	
mOPV [a]	0	(1151)	0	(19,004)	0.68	(100)	0	(164,443)	0	(84,645)	0.41	(200)
nOPV best [a,b]	0	(932)	0	(6298)	0.81	(91)	0	(110,095)	0	(35,210)	0.41	(122)
nOPV worst [a,b]	0	(1372)	0	(26,760)	0.74	(97)	0	(143,605)	0	(93,487)	0.41	(69)
Best nOPV, baseline [b]	0	(5043)	0	(2558)	0.28	(120)	0	(45,571)	0	(7444)	0.41	(40)
Worst nOPV, baseline [b]	0	(5043)	0	(19,146)	0	(125)	0	(105,401)	0	(62,558)	0.41	(103)
Best nOPV, intensification [b,c]	0.97	(347)	0	(1661)	0.96	(96)	0.92	(1698)	0	(4797)	0.98	(18)
Worst nOPV, intensification [b,c]	0.78	(382)	0	(14,895)	0.96	(87)	0.78	(10,100)	0	(57,103)	0.98	(70)

Abbreviations: mOPV, monovalent OPV; nOPV, novel OPV; OPV, oral poliovirus vaccine; POS, probability of successful OPV cessation by the date indicated; pSIA, preventive supplemental immunization activity; VAPP, vaccine-associated paralytic polio. [a] Results for the same time periods from prior bOPV cessation modeling that included assumed degradation of surveillance quality and resultant delayed outbreak response and did not include the use of tOPV in some countries where it occurred expanded age groups targeted in Yemen or any improvements in the quality of SIAs in the consequential geographies of DRC and Nigeria [48]. [b] Similar to prior modeling [48], we apply bounding scenarios of (i) *nOPV best*, which uses type-specific nOPV for outbreak response assuming the same effectiveness as type-specific mOPV, no reversion despite transmissibility, and no VAPP [59,78], and (ii) *nOPV worst*, which uses type-specific nOPV for outbreak response post-type-specific OPV cessation, assumes 90% of the effectiveness of mOPV and prior assumptions for reduced reversion [59], which we further reduced here by 10%, and VAPP occurring at a rate 10% lower than the VAPP rate of mOPV in vaccine recipients (see text). [c] Intensification refers to the addition of bOPV pSIAs prior to bOPV cessation in 2027 to some model subpopulations (see Figure 1 and text for discussion of the impacts of the planned rounds and the expected reductions of cases for types 1 and 2 relative to the baselines).

5. Discussion

Successful control of cVDPV1 outbreaks and outbreak prevention prior to bOPV cessation should keep the expected annual cVDPV1 cases relatively low prior to bOPV cessation, depending on pSIA scope, number, and quality. In contrast, low coverage of bOPV in RI and insufficient bOPV pSIAs to end all cVDPV1 transmission prior to cessation will necessitate rapid and high-quality oSIA response to prevent outbreaks from spreading internationally after bOPV cessation. Increasing type 1 and 3 population immunity using bOPV prior to cessation in pSIAs in many countries should represent a priority for countries and GPEI. Despite these improvements, the gradual expected increase in annual type 1 cases between 2029 and 2035, Figure 3A suggested that even with the modeled intensified bOPV pSIAs, bOPV cessation still represents an option with potentially unacceptable risk for type 1 (i.e., POS < 80%, Table 2).

The ongoing expansion of poliovirus vaccine options increases the complexity of planning for the polio endgame [69]. Discussions about the potential role(s) of nOPVs for type 1 and/or 3, potential multi-valent nOPV formulations (e.g., nbOPV, ntOPV), development of polio vaccines using non-replicating vaccine strains (e.g., vaccine-like particles [VLPs]), and/or different formulations of IPV (i.e., hexavalent combination products, fractional dosing of stand-alone IPV) make global modeling of policy and national decisions for immunization schedules and financing more difficult [69]. Countries now spend and should expect to spend, substantially more money on polio immunization than in prior years, at least in the absence of changes in immunization strategy [63,70]. In the absence of a successful global interruption of cVDPV2, restarting OPV2 in RI could become preferable to countries. GPEI promoted the preferential use of nOPV2 as an innovative tool to reduce the risks of seeding new VDPV2s [79]. Experience to date shows that while nOPV2 offers some reduction in VAPP and VDPV risks, prolonged shedding allowing recombination and reversion still occurs in the context of low-quality SIAs. Additionally, nOPV2 comes with real trade-offs of lower secondary spread compared with Sabin-strain mOPV2 [59]. Due to concerns about some increased potential for virus recombination as well as clinical trial results showing lower nOPV2 immunogenicity for individual vaccine recipients of co-administered nOPV2 and bOPV compared with those given nOPV2 alone [80], in 2023, SAGE recommended against co-administering nOPV2 and bOPV [81]. Complicated by co-circulation with type 1, we expect that type 2 transmission will likely continue throughout the time horizon, given current GPEI and national plans and the continued suboptimal implementation of oSIAs. In this analysis, we did not explore options for stopping type 2.

All applications of our integrated global modeling come with limitations due to assumptions about the model framing and structure, available information, initial conditions, and uncertainties about future policies and actions [28,48,49,58–63]. These results implicitly assume unlimited vaccine supplies for purposes of directly comparing policies; however, GPEI activities for cVDPV2 outbreaks continue to face challenges due to limited nOPV2 supplies, which could lead to substantially worse outcomes. Further, this analysis does not consider the potential impacts of increasing or decreasing coverage in RI and/or SIAs that may occur prospectively and could substantially shift outcomes. In addition, the model assumes a minimum of 1 dose of IPV in RI and does not include second IPV doses in RI in blocks that represent many countries that added these in response to recent SAGE recommendations [36]. However, while IPV use in RI helps to decrease the number of paralytic cases, it does little to increase the gastrointestinal immunity that is needed to reduce poliovirus transmission in OPV-using countries with conditions conducive to relatively higher transmissibility of polioviruses. The model includes IPV in some SIAs consistent with historical use but does not include the use of IPV in SIAs for oSIAs prospectively, except in IPV-only using countries. Although SAGE recently reinstated recommendations on the use of IPV in oSIAs [81], our modeling does not show IPV delivery in SIAs as effective or cost-effective for reducing cVDPV risks above OPV alone [82]. The effects of boosting existing immunity with IPV SIAs in children with prior live-poliovirus-induced immunity likely plays a minor role in stopping outbreak transmission because these children likely play a relatively less significant role in transmission than individuals in the population with no prior live-poliovirus-induced immunity [56,82]. Future global model updates will include the addition of the second dose of IPV, updated input immunization and population data, and the characterization of nOPV2 as a licensed vaccine.

The decentralization of global health decision-making, such as the preference of the African region to delay oSIAs in 2021 pending nOPV2 availability instead of using mOPV2, implicitly demonstrates a willingness to accept more polio cases as a trade-off [61], allows expansion of outbreaks, and complicates global policy modeling, planning, and implementation. Notably, the development of global resource needs (i.e., financial, vaccines) depends on assumptions about how decision-makers will act. When the modeling assumptions differ from actual decisions, this can result in mismatches between available and needed resources [19], more extensive transmission, and more cases [29]. Uncertainty about GPEI and country plans limits the ability of global modeling efforts to predict prospective outcomes. The expected values from these analyses do not consider adaptive adjustments in strategy that could occur in the event of increasing numbers of reported cases. For example, oSIA target age groups could increase to older ages to account for increasing numbers of birth cohorts without exposure to OPV immunization with increased years since OPV cessation (as recommended by pre-OPV2 cessation modeling [21]) and/or GPEI and countries could receive additional resources that could support interventions that perform better than modeled here.

We hope that this modeling will inform the development of future national and GPEI policies related to bOPV cessation. GPEI partners and public health leaders could use these results to provide a rationale for the development of a clear multi-year plan for the necessary financial and vaccine resources required to stop all WPV and cVDPV transmission (particularly established transmission of cVDPV2) and implement bOPV cessation in a way that will prevent a repetition of the experience of OPV2 cessation.

6. Conclusions

Our modeling shows that pSIAs with bOPV could substantially reduce the expected global risks of experiencing cVDPV1 and cVDPV3 outbreaks both before and after bOPV cessation and increase the probability of success for the polio endgame for types 1 and 3 but not for type 2. The decline and absence of bOPV pSIAs since 2019 in non-endemic countries and the postponement or cancellation of the small number of bOPV pSIAs into 2024 raises the risks of cVDPV emergence. In addition, unless GPEI makes explicit plans in 2024 to resume and continue bOPV pSIAs, efforts to ensure sufficient bOPV supply could be undermined as manufacturers could prematurely reduce production ahead of expected low demand [19].

Author Contributions: Conceptualization, methodology, modeling, writing—original draft preparation, visualization, N.D.B. and K.M.T.; resources, supervision, project administration, funding acquisition, K.M.T.; data curation, writing—review and editing; All authors. All authors have read and agreed to the published version of the manuscript.

Funding: The Kid Risk: Inc. authors acknowledge support for this publication under Cooperative Agreement Number 5NU2RGH001915-03-00, funded by the Centers for Disease Control and Prevention. The views expressed are solely those of the authors and do not necessarily represent the official views of the Centers for Disease Control and Prevention or the Department of Health and Human Services.

Institutional Review Board Statement: Not applicable.

Informed Consent Statement: Not applicable.

Data Availability Statement: The original contributions presented in the study are included in the article.

Acknowledgments: We thank Dominika Kalkowska and Mark Pallansch for the helpful discussions.

Conflicts of Interest: The authors declare no conflicts of interest.

References

1. Thompson, K.M.; Badizadegan, K. Evolution of global polio eradication strategies: Targets, vaccines, and supplemental immunization activities (SIAs). *Expert. Rev. Vaccines* **2024**, *23*, 597–613. [CrossRef] [PubMed]
2. Global Polio Eradication Initiative. Wild Poliovirus List. Available online: https://polioeradication.org/wild-poliovirus-count/ (accessed on 10 September 2024).
3. Global Polio Eradication Initiative. Variant Polio (cVDPV) Cases. Available online: https://polioeradication.org/circulating-vaccine-derived-poliovirus-count/ (accessed on 10 September 2024).
4. Barrett, S. Economic considerations for the eradication endgame. *Philos. Trans. R. Soc. B Biol. Sci.* **2013**, *368*, 20120149. [CrossRef] [PubMed]
5. Fine, P.E.; Sutter, R.W.; Orenstein, W.A. Stopping a polio outbreak in the post-eradication era. *Dev. Biol.* **2001**, *105*, 129–147; discussion 149–150.
6. Duintjer Tebbens, R.J.; Pallansch, M.A.; Kew, O.M.; Caceres, V.M.; Jafari, H.; Cochi, S.L.; Sutter, R.W.; Aylward, R.B.; Thompson, K.M. Risks of paralytic disease due to wild or vaccine-derived poliovirus after eradication. *Risk Anal.* **2006**, *26*, 1471–1505. [CrossRef] [PubMed]

7. World Health Assembly. *Poliomyelitis: Mechanism for Management of Potetnial Risks to Eradication*; World Health Organization: Geneva, Switzerland, 2008.
8. Thompson, K.M.; Tebbens, R.J.; Pallansch, M.A.; Kew, O.M.; Sutter, R.W.; Aylward, R.B.; Watkins, M.; Gary, H.E., Jr.; Alexander, J.; Jafari, H.; et al. The risks, costs, and benefits of possible future global policies for managing polioviruses. *Am. J. Public Health* **2008**, *98*, 1322–1330. [CrossRef] [PubMed]
9. Frauenfelder, C. WHO is to change its polio programme in India to try to eradicate the disease. *BMJ Br. Med. J.* **2006**, *333*, 1089. [CrossRef]
10. Thompson, K.M.; Pallansch, M.A.; Duintjer Tebbens, R.J.; Wassilak, S.G.; Cochi, S.L. Modeling population immunity to support efforts to end the transmission of live polioviruses. *Risk Anal.* **2013**, *33*, 647–663. [CrossRef]
11. Duintjer Tebbens, R.J.; Pallansch, M.A.; Kalkowska, D.A.; Wassilak, S.G.; Cochi, S.L.; Thompson, K.M. Characterizing poliovirus transmission and evolution: Insights from modeling experiences with wild and vaccine-related polioviruses. *Risk Anal.* **2013**, *33*, 703–749. [CrossRef]
12. Kalkowska, D.A.; Duintjer Tebbens, R.J.; Thompson, K.M. Modeling strategies to increase population immunity and prevent poliovirus transmission in the high-risk area of northwest Nigeria. *J. Infect. Dis.* **2014**, *210* (Suppl. S1), S412–S423. [CrossRef]
13. Kalkowska, D.A.; Duintjer Tebbens, R.J.; Thompson, K.M. Modeling strategies to increase population immunity and prevent poliovirus transmission in 2 high-risk areas in northern India. *J. Infect. Dis.* **2014**, *210* (Suppl. S1), S398–S411. [CrossRef]
14. Thompson, K.M.; Duintjer Tebbens, R.J. The differential impact of oral poliovirus vaccine formulation choices on serotype-specific population immunity to poliovirus transmission. *BMC Infect. Dis.* **2015**, *15*, 376. [CrossRef]
15. Thompson, K.M.; Duintjer Tebbens, R.J. Lessons from the polio endgame: Overcoming the failure to vaccinate and the role of subpopulations in maintaining transmission. *J. Infect. Dis.* **2017**, *216*, S176–S182. [CrossRef] [PubMed]
16. Duintjer Tebbens, R.J.; Pallansch, M.A.; Kim, J.H.; Burns, C.C.; Kew, O.M.; Oberste, M.S.; Diop, O.M.; Wassilak, S.G.; Cochi, S.L.; Thompson, K.M. Oral poliovirus vaccine evolution and insights relevant to modeling the risks of circulating vaccine-derived polioviruses (cVDPVs). *Risk Anal.* **2013**, *33*, 680–702. [CrossRef] [PubMed]
17. World Health Organization. Meeting of the Strategic Advisory Group of Experts on immunization, October 2015—Conclusions and recommendations. *Wkly Epidemiol. Rec.* **2015**, *90*, 681–700.
18. Hampton, L.M.; Farrell, M.; Ramirez-Gonzalez, A.; Menning, L.; Shendale, S.; Lewis, I.; Rubin, J.; Garon, J.; Harris, J.; Hyde, T.; et al. Cessation of trivalent oral poliovirus vaccine and introduction of inactivated poliovirus vaccine—Worldwide, 2016. *MMWR* **2016**, *65*, 934–938. [CrossRef] [PubMed]
19. Thompson, K.M.; Kalkowska, D.A.; Badizadegan, K. Oral polio vaccine stockpile modeling: Insights from recent experience. *Expert. Rev. Vaccines* **2023**, *22*, 813–825. [CrossRef] [PubMed]
20. Duintjer Tebbens, R.J.; Pallansch, M.A.; Alexander, J.P.; Thompson, K.M. Optimal vaccine stockpile design for an eradicated disease: Application to polio. *Vaccine* **2010**, *28*, 4312–4327. [CrossRef] [PubMed]
21. Duintjer Tebbens, R.J.; Pallansch, M.A.; Wassilak, S.G.; Cochi, S.L.; Thompson, K.M. Characterization of outbreak response strategies and potential vaccine stockpile needs for the polio endgame. *BMC Infect. Dis.* **2016**, *16*, 137. [CrossRef]
22. Duintjer Tebbens, R.J.; Hampton, L.M.; Wassilak, S.G.F.; Pallansch, M.A.; Cochi, S.L.; Thompson, K.M. Maintenance and intensification of bivalent oral poliovirus vaccine use prior to its coordinated global cessation. *J. Vaccines Vaccin.* **2016**, *7*, 340. [CrossRef]
23. Duintjer Tebbens, R.J.; Pallansch, M.A.; Cochi, S.L.; Wassilak, S.G.; Thompson, K.M. An economic analysis of poliovirus risk management policy options for 2013–2052. *BMC Infect. Dis.* **2015**, *15*, 389. [CrossRef]
24. World Health Organization Global Polio Eradication Initiative. 12th Meeting of the SAGE Polio Working Group, Conclusions and Recommendations, Note for the Record, October 2016. Available online: https://terrance.who.int/mediacentre/data/sage/SAGE_Docs_Ppt_Oct2016/5_session_polio/Oct2016_session5_SAGE_polio-WG_2016.pdf (accessed on 30 June 2024).
25. World Health Organization. Meeting of the Strategic Advisory Group of Experts on immunization, October 2016—Conclusions and recommendations. *Wkly Epidemiol. Rec.* **2016**, *91*, 561–584.
26. Global Polio Eradication Initiative; World health organization. *Polio Eradication and Endgame Strategic Plan 2013–2018*; World Health Organization: Geneva, Switzerland, 2013.
27. Macklin, G.R.; O'Reilly, K.M.; Grassly, N.C.; Edmunds, W.J.; Mach, O.; Santhana Gopala Krishnan, R.; Voorman, A.; Vertefeuille, J.F.; Abdelwahab, J.; Gumede, N.; et al. Evolving epidemiology of poliovirus serotype 2 following withdrawal of the serotype 2 oral poliovirus vaccine. *Science* **2020**, *368*, 401–405. [CrossRef] [PubMed]
28. Kalkowska, D.A.; Pallansch, M.A.; Cochi, S.L.; Kovacs, S.D.; Wassilak, S.G.F.; Thompson, K.M. Updated characterization of post-OPV cessation risks: Lessons from 2019 serotype 2 outbreaks and implications for the probability of OPV restart. *Risk Anal.* **2021**, *41*, 320–328. [CrossRef] [PubMed]
29. Thompson, K.M.; Kalkowska, D.A.; Badizadegan, K. Looking back at prospective modeling of outbreak response strategies for managing global type 2 oral poliovirus vaccine (OPV2) cessation. *Front. Public Health* **2023**, *11*, 1098419. [CrossRef]
30. Duintjer Tebbens, R.J.; Pallansch, M.A.; Cochi, S.L.; Ehrhardt, D.T.; Farag, N.H.; Hadler, S.C.; Hampton, L.M.; Martinez, M.; Wassilak, S.G.F.; Thompson, K.M. Modeling poliovirus transmission in Pakistan and Afghanistan to inform vaccination strategies in undervaccinated subpopulations. *Risk Anal.* **2018**, *38*, 1701–1717. [CrossRef]

31. Yeh, M.T.; Bujaki, E.; Dolan, P.T.; Smith, M.; Wahid, R.; Konz, J.; Weiner, A.J.; Bandyopadhyay, A.S.; Van Damme, P.; De Coster, I.; et al. Engineering the live-attenuated polio vaccine to prevent reversion to virulence. *Cell Host Microbe* **2020**, *27*, 736–751. [CrossRef] [PubMed]
32. Konopka-Anstadt, J.L.; Campagnoli, R.; Vincent, A.; Shaw, J.; Wei, L.; Wynn, N.T.; Smithee, S.E.; Bujaki, E.; Te Yeh, M.; Laassri, M.; et al. Development of a new oral poliovirus vaccine for the eradication end game using codon deoptimization. *NPJ Vaccines* **2020**, *5*, 26. [CrossRef] [PubMed]
33. Macklin, G.R.; Peak, C.; Eisenhawer, M.; Kurji, F.; Mach, O.; Konz, J.; Gast, C.; Bachtiar, N.S.; Bandyopadhyay, A.S.; Zipursky, S.; et al. Enabling accelerated vaccine roll-out for Public Health Emergencies of International Concern (PHEICs): Novel oral polio vaccine type 2 (nOPV2) experience. *Vaccine* **2023**, *41* (Suppl. S1), A122–A127. [CrossRef] [PubMed]
34. Global Polio Eradication Initiative; World Health Organization. *Strategy for the Response to Type 2 Circulating Vaccine-Derived Poliovirus 2020–2021: An Addendum to the Polio Endgame Strategy 2019–2023*; World Health Organization: Geneva, Switzerland, 2020.
35. World Health Organization. SAGE Meeting Yellow Book: Strategic Advisory Group of Experts on Immunization 31 March–02 April 2020. Available online: https://terrance.who.int/mediacentre/data/sage/SAGE_Docs_Ppt_April2020/SAGE_Yellow_Book_March-April_2020.pdf (accessed on 30 November 2023).
36. World Health Organization. Meeting of the Strategic Advisory Group of Experts on immunization, October 2020—Conclusions and recommendations. *Wkly Epidemiol. Rec.* **2020**, *95*, 585–608.
37. Global Polio Eradication Initiative; World Health Organization. *Polio Eradication Strategy 2022–2026: Delivering on a Promise*; World Health Organization: Geneva, Switzerland, 2021.
38. Thompson, K.M.; Duintjer Tebbens, R.J.; Pallansch, M.A.; Kew, O.M.; Sutter, R.W.; Aylward, R.B.; Watkins, M.; Gary, H.; Alexander, J.P.; Venczel, L.; et al. Development and consideration of global policies for managing the future risks of poliovirus outbreaks: Insights and lessons learned through modeling. *Risk Anal.* **2006**, *26*, 1571–1580. [CrossRef] [PubMed]
39. Thompson, K.M.; Duintjer Tebbens, R.J. Using system dynamics to develop policies that matter: Global management of poliomyelitis and beyond. *Syst. Dyn. Rev.* **2008**, *24*, 433–449. [CrossRef]
40. Thompson, K.M. Modeling poliovirus risks and the legacy of polio eradication. *Risk Anal.* **2013**, *33*, 505–515. [CrossRef] [PubMed]
41. Thompson, K.M.; Duintjer Tebbens, R.J.; Pallansch, M.A.; Wassilak, S.G.F.; Cochi, S.L. Polio eradicators use integrated analytical models to make better decisions. *INFORMS J. Appl. Anal.* **2015**, *45*, 5–25. [CrossRef]
42. Duintjer Tebbens, R.J.; Thompson, K.M. Using integrated modeling to support the global eradication of vaccine-preventable diseases. *Syst. Dyn. Rev.* **2018**, *34*, 78–120. [CrossRef]
43. Thompson, K.M.; Kalkowska, D.A. Review of poliovirus modeling performed from 2000 to 2019 to support global polio eradication. *Expert Rev. Vaccines* **2020**, *19*, 661–686. [CrossRef]
44. Thompson, K.M.; Badizadegan, K. Review of poliovirus transmission and economic modeling to support global polio eradication: 2020–2024. *Pathogens* **2024**, *13*, 435. [CrossRef]
45. Duintjer Tebbens, R.J.; Hampton, L.M.; Thompson, K.M. Planning for globally coordinated cessation of bivalent oral poliovirus vaccine: Risks of non-synchronous cessation and unauthorized oral poliovirus vaccine use. *BMC Infect. Dis.* **2018**, *18*, 165. [CrossRef]
46. Thompson, K.M.; Duintjer Tebbens, R.J. Health and economic consequences of different options for timing the coordinated global cessation of the three oral poliovirus vaccine serotypes. *BMC Infect. Dis.* **2015**, *15*, 374. [CrossRef] [PubMed]
47. Kalkowska, D.A.; Thompson, K.M. Expected implications of globally coordinated cessation of serotype 3 oral poliovirus vaccine (OPV) before serotype 1 OPV. *Risk Anal.* **2021**, *41*, 312–319. [CrossRef] [PubMed]
48. Kalkowska, D.A.; Wassilak, S.G.F.; Wiesen, E.; Burns, C.C.; Pallansch, M.A.; Badizadegan, K.; Thompson, K.M. Coordinated global cessation of oral poliovirus vaccine use: Options and potential consequences. *Risk Anal.* **2024**, *44*, 366–378. [CrossRef] [PubMed]
49. Kalkowska, D.A.; Wiesen, E.; Wassilak, S.G.F.; Burns, C.C.; Pallansch, M.A.; Badizadegan, K.; Thompson, K.M. Worst-case scenarios: Modeling uncontrolled type 2 polio transmission. *Risk Anal.* **2024**, *44*, 379–389. [CrossRef] [PubMed]
50. Sangrujee, N.; Duintjer Tebbens, R.J.; Caceres, V.M.; Thompson, K.M. Policy decision options during the first 5 years following certification of polio eradication. *Med. Gen. Med.* **2003**, *5*, 35.
51. Thompson, K.M.; Duintjer Tebbens, R.J. The case for cooperation in managing and maintaining the end of poliomyelitis: Stockpile needs and coordinated OPV cessation. *Medscape J. Med.* **2008**, *10*, 190. [PubMed]
52. Thompson, K.M.; Wallace, G.S.; Tebbens, R.J.; Smith, P.J.; Barskey, A.E.; Pallansch, M.A.; Gallagher, K.M.; Alexander, J.P.; Armstrong, G.L.; Cochi, S.L.; et al. Trends in the risk of U.S. polio outbreaks and poliovirus vaccine availability for response. *Public Health Rep.* **2012**, *127*, 23–37. [CrossRef]
53. Duintjer Tebbens, R.J.; Thompson, K.M. Managing the risk of circulating vaccine-derived poliovirus during the endgame: Oral poliovirus vaccine needs. *BMC Infect. Dis.* **2015**, *15*, 390. [CrossRef]
54. Thompson, K.M.; Duintjer Tebbens, R.J. Current polio global eradication and control policy options: Perspectives from modeling and prerequisites for oral poliovirus vaccine cessation. *Expert Rev. Vaccines* **2012**, *11*, 449–459. [CrossRef]
55. Thompson, K.M.; Duintjer Tebbens, R.J. Modeling the dynamics of oral poliovirus vaccine cessation. *J. Infect. Dis.* **2014**, *210* (Suppl. S1), S475–S484. [CrossRef] [PubMed]

56. Duintjer Tebbens, R.J.; Thompson, K.M. Modeling the potential role of inactivated poliovirus vaccine to manage the risks of oral poliovirus vaccine cessation. *J. Infect. Dis.* **2014**, *210* (Suppl. S1), S485–S497. [CrossRef] [PubMed]
57. Thompson, K.M.; Duintjer Tebbens, R.J.; Pallansch, M.A. Evaluation of response scenarios to potential polio outbreaks using mathematical models. *Risk Anal.* **2006**, *26*, 1541–1556. [CrossRef] [PubMed]
58. Kalkowska, D.A.; Pallansch, M.A.; Wassilak, S.G.F.; Cochi, S.L.; Thompson, K.M. Global transmission of live polioviruses: Updated dynamic modeling of the polio endgame. *Risk Anal.* **2021**, *41*, 248–265. [CrossRef] [PubMed]
59. Kalkowska, D.A.; Pallansch, M.A.; Wilkinson, A.; Bandyopadhyay, A.S.; Konopka-Anstadt, J.L.; Burns, C.C.; Oberste, M.S.; Wassilak, S.G.F.; Badizadegan, K.; Thompson, K.M. Updated characterization of outbreak response strategies for 2019-2029: Impacts of using a novel type 2 oral poliovirus vaccine strain. *Risk Anal* **2021**, *41*, 329–348. [CrossRef] [PubMed]
60. Kalkowska, D.A.; Voorman, A.; Pallansch, M.A.; Wassilak, S.G.F.; Cochi, S.L.; Badizadegan, K.; Thompson, K.M. The impact of disruptions caused by the COVID-19 pandemic on global polio eradication. *Vaccine* **2023**, *41* (Suppl. S1), A12–A18. [CrossRef] [PubMed]
61. Kalkowska, D.A.; Pallansch, M.A.; Wassilak, S.G.F.; Cochi, S.L.; Thompson, K.M. Serotype 2 oral poliovirus vaccine (OPV2) choices and the consequences of delaying outbreak response. *Vaccine* **2023**, *41* (Suppl. S1), A136–A141. [CrossRef] [PubMed]
62. Kalkowska, D.A.; Wassilak, S.G.F.; Pallansch, M.A.; Burns, C.C.; Wiesen, E.; Durry, E.; Badizadegan, K.; Thompson, K.M. Outbreak response strategies with type 2-containing oral poliovirus vaccines. *Vaccine* **2023**, *41* (Suppl. S1), A142–A152. [CrossRef] [PubMed]
63. Thompson, K.M.; Kalkowska, D.A.; Badizadegan, K. Health economic analysis of vaccine options for the polio eradication endgame: 2022–2036. *Expert. Rev. Vaccines* **2022**, *21*, 1667–1674. [CrossRef]
64. Duintjer Tebbens, R.J.; Thompson, K.M. Uncertainty and sensitivity analysis of cost assumptions for global long-term poliovirus risk management. *J. Vaccines Vaccin.* **2016**, *7*, 1000339. [CrossRef]
65. Thompson, K.M.; Duintjer Tebbens, R.J. Lessons from globally coordinated cessation of serotype 2 oral poliovirus vaccine for the remaining serotypes. *J. Infect. Dis.* **2017**, *216*, S168–S175. [CrossRef]
66. Duintjer Tebbens, R.J.; Hampton, L.M.; Thompson, K.M. Implementation of coordinated global serotype 2 oral poliovirus vaccine cessation: Risks of inadvertent trivalent oral poliovirus vaccine use. *BMC Infect. Dis.* **2016**, *16*, 237. [CrossRef]
67. Duintjer Tebbens, R.J.; Hampton, L.M.; Thompson, K.M. Implementation of coordinated global serotype 2 oral poliovirus vaccine cessation: Risks of potential non-synchronous cessation. *BMC Infect. Dis.* **2016**, *16*, 231. [CrossRef]
68. Thompson, K.M.; Kalkowska, D.A. Logistical challenges and assumptions for modeling the failure of global cessation of oral poliovirus vaccine (OPV). *Expert. Rev. Vaccines* **2019**, *18*, 725–736. [CrossRef]
69. Kalkowska, D.; Wassilak, S.; Wiesen, E.; F Estivariz, C.; Burns, C.; Badizadegan, K.; Thompson, K. Complexity of options related to restarting oral poliovirus vaccine (OPV) in national immunization programs after OPV cessation. *Gates Open Res.* **2023**, *7*, 55. [CrossRef] [PubMed]
70. Kalkowska, D.A.; Thompson, K.M. Health and economic outcomes associated with polio vaccine policy options: 2019–2029. *Risk Anal.* **2021**, *41*, 364–375. [CrossRef] [PubMed]
71. Thompson, K.M. Modeling and managing poliovirus risks: We are where we are.... *Risk Anal.* **2021**, *41*, 223–228. [CrossRef] [PubMed]
72. Global Polio Eradication Initiative. *Global OPV Stockpile Strategy 2022–2026*; World Health Organization: Geneva, Switzerland, 2022.
73. Badizadegan, K.; Kalkowska, D.A.; Thompson, K.M. Health economic analysis of antiviral drugs in the global polio eradication endgame. *Med. Decis. Mak.* **2023**, *43*, 850–862. [CrossRef] [PubMed]
74. Thompson, K.M.; Kalkowska, D.A. Reflections on modeling poliovirus transmission and the polio eradication endgame. *Risk Anal.* **2021**, *41*, 229–247. [CrossRef] [PubMed]
75. Kalkowska, D.A.; Duintjer Tebbens, R.J.; Pallansch, M.A.; Cochi, S.L.; Wassilak, S.G.; Thompson, K.M. Modeling undetected live poliovirus circulation after apparent interruption of transmission: Implications for surveillance and vaccination. *BMC Infect. Dis.* **2015**, *15*, 66. [CrossRef]
76. Beshr, I.A.; Beshr, M.S.; Al-Qubati, H.A. Polio outbreak response, Yemen. *Bull. World Health Organ.* **2023**, *101*, 808–812. [CrossRef] [PubMed]
77. Independent Monitoring Board. Closing in on Zero: Adapting to Complexity and Risk on the Path to End Polio—Twenty-Second Report of the Independent Monitoring Board of the Global Polio Eradication Initiative. Available online: https://polioeradication.org/wp-content/uploads/2023/09/22nd-Report-of-The-Independent-Monitoring-Board-IMB.pdf (accessed on 13 November 2023).
78. Thompson, K.M.; Kalkowska, D.A.; Badizadegan, K. Hypothetical emergence of poliovirus in 2020: Part 2. exploration of the potential role of vaccines in control and eradication. *Expert. Rev. Vaccines* **2021**, *20*, 449–460. [CrossRef] [PubMed]
79. Global Polio Eradication Initiative. *Polio News—Special Edition*; World Health Organization: Geneva, Switzerland, 2020.
80. Wilkinson, A.L.; Zaman, K.; Hoque, M.; Estivariz, C.F.; Burns, C.C.; Konopka-Anstadt, J.L.; Mainou, B.A.; Kovacs, S.D.; An, Q.; Lickness, J.S.; et al. Immunogenicity of novel oral poliovirus vaccine type 2 administered concomitantly with bivalent oral poliovirus vaccine: An open-label, non-inferiority, randomised, controlled trial. *Lancet Infect. Dis.* **2023**, *23*, 1062–1071. [CrossRef]

81. World Health Organization. Meeting of the Strategic Advisory Group of Experts on immunization, September 2023: Conclusions and recommendations. *Wkly Epidemiol. Rec.* **2023**, *98*, 599–620.
82. Duintjer Tebbens, R.J.; Thompson, K.M. Costs and benefits of including inactivated in addition to oral poliovirus vaccine in outbreak response after cessation of oral poliovirus vaccine use. *MDM Policy Pract.* **2017**, *2*, 2381468317697002. [CrossRef] [PubMed]

pathogens

MDPI

Review

Antiviral Development for the Polio Endgame: Current Progress and Future Directions

Hang Xie [1,*], Eric E. Rhoden [1], Hong-Mei Liu [1], Folake Ogunsemowo [1], Bernardo A. Mainou [1], Rachel M. Burke [2] and Cara C. Burns [1]

[1] Poliovirus & Picornavirus Branch, Division of Viral Diseases, National Center for Immunization and Other Respiratory Diseases, Centers for Disease Control and Prevention, Atlanta, GA 30329, USA; imb0@cdc.gov (E.E.R.); hdl1@cdc.gov (H.-M.L.); wcm0@cdc.gov (F.O.); qlk6@cdc.gov (B.A.M.); zqd1@cdc.gov (C.C.B.)

[2] Bill & Melinda Gates Foundation, Seattle, WA 98109, USA; rachel.burke@gatesfoundation.org

* Correspondence: utk7@cdc.gov; Tel.: +1-404-718-6474

Abstract: As the world is approaching the eradication of wild poliovirus serotype 1, the last of the three wild types, the question of how to maintain a polio-free world becomes imminent. To mitigate the risk of sporadic vaccine-associated paralytic polio (VAPP) caused by oral polio vaccines (OPVs) that are routinely used in global immunization programs, the Polio Antivirals Initiative (PAI) was established in 2006. The primary goal of the PAI is to facilitate the discovery and development of antiviral drugs to stop the excretion of immunodeficiency-associated vaccine-derived poliovirus (iVDPV) in B cell-deficient individuals. This review summarizes the major progress that has been made in the development of safe and effective poliovirus antivirals and highlights the candidates that have shown promising results in vitro, in vivo, and in clinical trials.

Keywords: poliovirus; immunodeficiency-associated vaccine-derived poliovirus; picornavirus; antiviral development; small molecule-based antiviral drug; capsid-binding agent

1. Introduction

Poliomyelitis (polio) is a highly contagious and debilitating disease caused by poliovirus. Poliovirus has three serotypes; each can cause poliomyelitis in humans. Poliovirus infects human cells via the specific poliovirus receptor—CD155—and replicates primarily in the intestines [1]. It can also spread to the central nervous system, resulting in paralysis. The mode of transmission is primarily via the fecal–oral route and, less frequently, via contaminated food or water. Neonates, infants, and children under 5 years of age are the most vulnerable populations for polio [2]. In most cases, infected children have mild cold-like symptoms and can recover without medical intervention [3]. However, in rare cases (<1–2%), patients can suffer neurological damage and develop permanent paralysis or even die [3]. Since the late 1980s, the Global Polio Eradication Initiative (GPEI) has helped to distribute and administer over three billion doses of live attenuated oral polio vaccines (OPVs or Sabin vaccines) to children living in developing countries, achieving greater than a 99% reduction in global polio cases [2]. As both serotype 2 and serotype 3 wild polioviruses (WPVs) have been declared eradicated globally, and serotype 1 WPV remains in circulation in only two countries (Afghanistan and Pakistan) [4], we have never been so close to a polio-free world.

OPVs induce mucosal immunity against WPVs via limited replication in the gastrointestinal tract [5–7]. However, OPVs can also potentially cause vaccine-associated paralytic polio (VAPP), a rare adverse event when an administered OPV reverts to neurovirulence, resulting in paralysis in some recipients or unimmune persons in close contact [8–10]. The risk for VAPP has been estimated at 4.7 cases per million births globally, with incidents more frequently reported in recipients living in low-income countries who had taken more than three OPV doses and those from middle/high-income countries who were unvaccinated or who had taken only one OPV dose [11]. The persistent replication of an OPV in the gut could also lead to the reversion of virulence and allow the shedding of vaccine-derived polioviruses (VDPVs), which can spread among populations with low vaccine coverage, leading to circulating vaccine-derived polioviruses (cVDPVs) that can cause outbreaks of paralysis [12,13]. Moreover, B cell-deficient immunocompromised persons can become chronically infected, resulting in immunodeficiency-associated VDPV (iVDPV) [14–17]. Hence, these vaccine-related viruses pose great threats to a polio-free world, even after the eradication of WPVs.

In 2006, the Polio Antivirals Initiative (PAI) was established at the Task Force for Global Health as a multi-partner collaboration including the Bill & Melinda Gates Foundation, the World Health Organization (WHO), the US Centers for Disease Control and Prevention (CDC), the US National Institutes of Health (NIH), the US Food and Drug Administration (FDA), Rotary International, and the Jeffrey Modell Foundation. The PAI's primary goal is to develop safe and effective antiviral drugs to stop vaccine poliovirus shedding in immunodeficient recipients of OPVs and to mitigate the threat of prolonged poliovirus excretion to a polio-free world after the endgame (https://www.taskforce.org/polio-antivirals-initiative/ (accessed on 6 October 2024)).

This review summarizes the major efforts made in the discovery of anti-poliovirus small molecules and the progress achieved in clinical development. It also discusses the challenges encountered along the way and suggests future directions that may facilitate the discovery and development of more effective antivirals for treating infections associated with cVDPV, iVDPV, or the accidental release of other live polioviruses during or after the endgame.

2. Poliovirus Biology

Poliovirus belongs to the genus Enterovirus in the Picornaviridae family of 158 species, including many viruses (e.g., coxsackieviruses, echoviruses, hepatitis A virus, and rhinoviruses) that are known to cause significant human diseases. All picornaviruses are nonenveloped and have an icosahedral protein coat of 30 nm in diameter encapsidating a small, single-stranded positive-sense RNA genome [18].

There are three serotypes of poliovirus that are differentiated by the antigenic sites in the viral capsid protein [19]. All three serotypes are very similar in the structure of the viral capsid protein. The poliovirus capsid has 60 protomers assembled in an icosahedral structure, each containing four polypeptides (VP1, VP2, VP3, and VP4) arranged in 12 identical pentamers [20] (Figure 1a). VP4 is located on the inner side of the capsid shell in contact with the viral genome, while VP1–VP3 form star-shaped mesas covering the external surface of the shell at the five-fold axes, surrounded by deep canyons and three-bladed propellers [21]. In poliovirus, a hydrophobic pocket is formed under the canyon floor surrounding each five-fold axis of the viral capsid, which is usually occupied by one or more fatty acid-like natural ligands (pocket factors) and is accessible through a small pore [22] (Figure 1b). The interaction of the pocket factor with the hydrophobic pocket impacts virion thermal stability, and a point mutation (Phe-to-Leu) at residue 1134 of the ligand-binding site alters the temperature sensitivity of the Sabin 3 poliovirus [23]. The receptor-mediated poliovirus attachment induces a series of structural rearrangements in viral particles for subsequent uncoating and viral RNA (vRNA) transport and alters viral particle sedimentation from 160 S (mature virion) to 135 S (A particle) [24–26]. Following the translocation from the interior of the mature virion, the N-terminus of VP1 and myristoyl-VP4 become externalized in the 135 S particle to allow liposome binding and the formation of ion channels in lipid bilayers [24,25]. The 130 S particles are the intermediates in the process of receptor-mediated virus entry and are sensitive to proteases. Subsequent proteolytical removal of the first 31 amino acids of VP1 blocks the membrane association of the 135 S particles and allows vRNA release via the translocation pore in the bilayer, resulting in empty viral particles that sediment at 80 S [24–26].

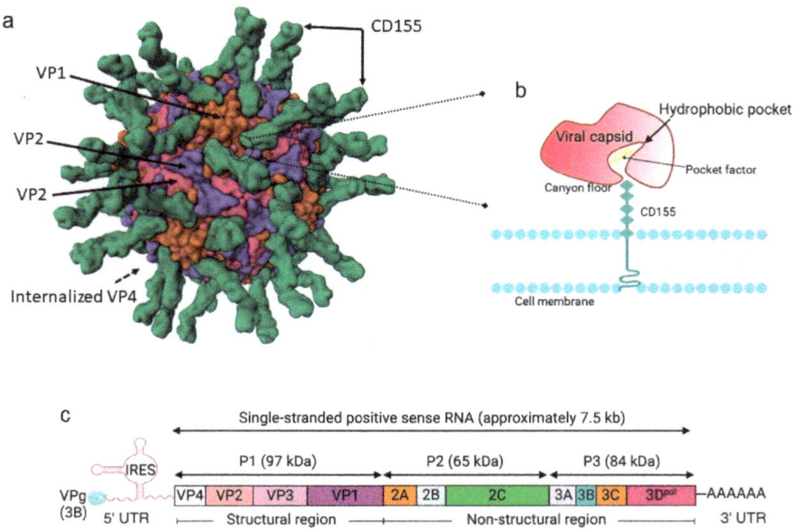

Figure 1. Poliovirus structure and viral genome and polyprotein organization. (**a**) Cryo-EM structure of poliovirus serotype 1 complexed with three domain CD155. Image from the RCSB PDB (RCSB.org) of PDB ID 1DGI [27]. (**b**) Schematic illustration of hydrophobic pocket in the viral capsid filled with pocket factor. (**c**) Organization of poliovirus genome and viral polyprotein processing (images in (**b**,**c**) were created with BioRender.com).

De novo vRNA synthesis and protein translation produce a single large polyprotein that is cleaved and processed sequentially by viral proteases (2A, 3C, and 3CD) to yield P1, P2, and P3 precursors [28–30] (Figure 1c). The P1 precursor is further cleaved by viral protease 3CD to produce VP0, VP1, and VP3, which assemble into an empty capsid. VP0 is a myristoylated immature protein that is autocatalytically processed into myristoyl-VP4 and VP2 for vRNA encapsidation [31]. The P2 precursor is cleaved to produce viral protease 2A and non-structural proteins 2B and 2C [32]. The P3 precursor is split into 3AB and 3CD, followed by a proteolytical process, resulting in membrane binding 3A, RNA priming 3B (VPg), protease 3C, and RNA-dependent polymerase 3D ($3D^{pol}$), respectively [30,32]. In addition to membrane association, viral proteins 2B, 2C, and 3A are also involved in replication complex formation, while viral protease 3C assists in capsid formation [33–35]. RNA primer VPg is covalently attached to the 5′ end of positive strand vRNA and is uridylylated by $3D^{pol}$ to form VPgpUpU for the initiation of vRNA synthesis [30,33] (Figure 1c).

3. Small Molecule-Based Antiviral Agents

3.1. Capsid-Binding Agents

Small molecule-based antiviral drug development for poliovirus has been largely focused on inhibiting virus replication by targeting the viral capsid or nonstructural proteins. Capsid-binding agents are the most extensively investigated antiviral class. These small molecules fill the hydrophobic pocket of the viral capsid by replacing the natural pocket factor. The replacement of the natural pocket factor by a small molecule increases the stability of the mature virion and prevents the capsid from undergoing conformational changes, thereby inhibiting the 135 S particle formation and blocking the viral uncoating for vRNA release [36–40].

Pleconaril (VP-63843 or Picovir) is an antiviral agent administered orally or intranasally for treating picornavirus-induced respiratory infections. It has high affinity and specificity for the hydrophobic pocket of the capsid and shows broad-spectrum antiviral activity against many common serotypes of enterovirus and rhinovirus in vitro [41]. Its predecessor, WIN 51711, was the first capsid inhibitor shown to prevent poliovirus-induced paralysis and death in mice following oral administration [42]. Pleconaril was used to treat an immunodeficient infant who acquired the poliovirus infection following an OPV administration, and it successfully eliminated Sabin 2-derived poliovirus from the cerebral spinal fluid and serum [43]. Additionally, Pleconaril combined with gamma globulin was effective in clearing prolonged poliovirus excretion in an immunocompromised child who developed VAPP after an OPV [44]. In another VAPP case, however, pleconaril in combination with immunoglobulin failed to stop virus excretion. A sequencing of virus isolates revealed the acquisition of a mutation (^{261}Met to ^{261}leu in VP1) adjacent to the binding site of pleconaril, leading to pleconaril resistance [45]. While pleconaril was shown to significantly reduce the duration of symptoms from a rhinovirus infection in two large placebo-controlled trials [46], concerns about potential drug–drug interactions (e.g., with birth control pills) have halted the further development of pleconaril to treat common colds associated with the rhinovirus infection [46]. In a randomized, double-blind, placebo-controlled trial of pleconaril for the treatment of neonatal enterovirus sepsis, an intent-to-treat analysis showed that the pleconaril-treated group had a significantly higher cumulative survival probability over 2 months (23%) than the placebo group (44%, $p = 0.02$) [47]. Hence, pleconaril was administered under compassionate use for treating children with life-threatening enterovirus infections for a few years [48,49].

Pirodavir (R77975) is another well-characterized capsid-binding agent originally developed for treating rhinovirus-induced common colds [50]. Pirodavir inhibits the replication of both serotype 2 and 3 polioviruses in vitro, but it is five- to twenty-fold less effective against serotype 1 poliovirus [51]. The pirodavir analog (R78206) binds the viral capsid in a single predominant conformation with its benzoyl ester group exposed at the open end of the pocket and exhibits stronger inhibitory effects on all three poliovirus serotypes, with half maximal effective concentration (EC_{50}) values ranging from 0.11 to 0.76 μmol/L [21,51]. However, pirodavir and its analogs are sensitive to hydrolysis of the ester bond and exhibit poor pharmacokinetics as orally administered drugs [52,53], which limits their potential as anti-poliovirus agents.

Pocapavir (V-073 or SCH 48973) and its derivatives were first developed for treating nonpolio enterovirus infections [39,53]. Many analogs in this series share common characteristics with other capsid inhibitors in that they bind in the hydrophobic pocket of the viral capsid, resulting in increased thermal stability and inhibition of the early viral replication by blocking the uncoating process [38,39]. Pocapavir exhibits antiviral activity against a spectrum of enteroviruses in vitro without direct viricidal effects [38,39]. SCH 47802, an early lead compound in this series, had a 50% inhibitory concentration (IC_{50}) of 0.04 μg/mL against serotype 2 poliovirus by a plaque reduction assay and was the only analog in the early development phase showing in vivo antiviral effects in a murine model of poliovirus-induced encephalitis [38]. Mice were protected from serotype 2 poliovirus-induced mortality when SCH 47802 was administered orally at 24 h before infection and continuously at a daily dose of 60 mg/kg for 15–21 days after infection [38]. However, other SCH 47802 derivatives in the early development phase lacked in vivo protective effects because of poor oral bioavailability, despite showing similar in vitro antiviral potency to SCH 47802 [38].

Pocapavir, a close analog of SCH 47802 with different substituting groups in the second o-chloro-p-metoxyphenol fragment, was also developed at Schering–Plough. Pocapavir has high affinity for the viral capsid, with an affinity constant of 8.85×10^{-8} M for poliovirus serotype 2, and it is potent against both serotypes 1 and 2 at IC_{50} of 0.02 μg/mL and 0.08 μg/mL in vitro, respectively [39]. ViroDefense, Inc. acquired SCH 48973 and renamed it V-073 and, later, pocapavir [54]. Unlike SCH 47802, which did not yield dose-dependent protection against poliovirus in vivo, orally administered pocapavir exerted a dose-dependent therapeutic effect in the range of 3, 10, and 20 mg/kg/day in mice infected with poliovirus serotype 2 [39]. Compared to a placebo, viral loads in the brain were 1–2 logs lower in mice receiving pocapavir orally four times at 5 mg/kg within 6–24 h post infection [39]. These results demonstrated that pocapavir has higher in vivo efficacy than SCH 47802, which is probably attributable to its better bioavailability, as SCH 47802 and other derivatives in this series are highly hydrophobic and show plateaued absorption in a range of pharmacokinetic concentrations [38].

Pocapavir has broad antiviral activity against polioviruses and inhibits 45 strains of all 3 serotypes, including WPVs, Sabin vaccine strains, cVDPVs, and iVDPVs [54]. Pocapavir shows a higher antiviral specificity for poliovirus (EC_{50} ranging 0.003–0.126 μM with mean EC_{50} value of 0.029 μM) than other nonpolio picornaviruses, such as echoviruses (EC_{50} ranging 0.009–7.08 μM with mean EC_{50} value of 0.86 μM), enteroviruses (EC_{50} ranging 0.236–14 μM with mean EC_{50} value of 3.47 μM), or coxsackieviruses (EC_{50} ranging 0.007–14 μM with mean EC_{50} value of 3.79 μM) in an in vitro cytopathic effect (CPE)-based assay [54]. Tanner et al. reported that poliovirus titers were significantly decreased in the muscles of infected Tnfr1−/− PVR+/+ transgenic mice following daily pocapavir treatment at 10 mg/kg initiated after infection, and no drug-resistant variants were selected during the treatment [55].

Pocapavir has been used to treat several cases of iVDPV in pediatric patients under expanded access (ViroDefense unpublished data). In an infant iVDPV case with the presence of neurovirulence and prolonged excretion, pocapavir was administered by mixing it with the infant formula once per day at a dose of 27 mg/kg body weight for 14 consecutive days [56]. Poliovirus shedding in stools stopped as early as Day 2, and negativity was maintained through 7 weeks posttreatment, when the last sample was tested. The infant tolerated pocapavir well during the course of treatment, without any adverse events reported [56].

In a monovalent oral poliovirus serotype 1 vaccine (mOPV1) placebo-controlled human challenge trial involving 141 healthy adults who had received a childhood inactivated poliovirus vaccine (IPV), the median clearance time was significantly shortened in pocapavir-treated subjects (10 days) compared to placebos (13 days) ($p = 0.0019$) [57]. However, a resistant virus was detected in the stools of 44% (41 out of 93) of the pocapavir recipients as well as 10% (5 out of 48) of the placebos [57]. The generation of pocapavir-resistant polioviruses in placebo-treated subjects indicates that there was significant virus transmission among subjects in the study unit.

In in vitro drug-resistance studies, pocapavir-resistant poliovirus variants emerged at the approximate frequency of $3–40 \times 10^{-5}$, with the majority of viruses bearing a point mutation in either VP1 with ^{194}Ile to ^{194}Met or ^{194}Phe (equivalent position 192 in serotype 3) or VP3 with ^{24}Ala to ^{24}Val (Tables 1 and 2) [58]. Both residues are within the hydrophobic pocket that is targeted by pocapavir. BTA798, a capsid inhibitor used for treating human rhinovirus infections, was able to inhibit the replication of pocapavir-resistant strains bearing the mutation of ^{24}Ala to ^{24}Val in VP3, but the combination of two capsid inhibitors only yielded the additive inhibition on poliovirus [59]. Although pocapavir is still available for compassionate use, the frequency of drug-resistance development in vitro and in the human challenge study suggests that pocapavir may be best used in combination with other antivirals with different mechanisms of action to treat immunodeficient poliovirus excreters.

Table 1. Susceptibility of selected poliovirus serotype 1 strains to pocapavir, imocitrelvir, or combination treatment *.

Virus	Serotype	Mutation(s)	Pocapavir		Imocitrelvir		Imocitrelvir/Pocapavir		Reference(s)
			EC_{50} (μM)	Resistance Frequency	EC_{50} (μM)	Resistance Frequency	Synergy (%) #	Resistance Frequency	
Sabin 1	Serotype 1, Vaccine strain	-	0.017–0.025	1.9×10^{-7}	0.173–0.541	Not determined	Strong (580 μM^2)	Not determined	This review & Rhoden et al. (2013) [59]
10235-DOR-WT	cVDPV1	-	0.018–0.038	3.31×10^{-5}	0.202–0.501	8.2×10^{-5}	Strong (892 μM^2)	1.9×10^{-7}	This review & Liu et al. (2012) [58]
10235-DOR-1D	cVDPV1, Pocapavir-variant	^{194}Ile to ^{194}Phe in VP1	>10	Not determined	0.316–0.612	Not determined	Weak (47 μM^2)	Not determined	This review
10235-DOR-3D	cVDPV1, Pocapavir-variant	^{24}Ala to ^{24}Val in VP3	>10	Not determined	0.287–0.657	Not determined	Weak (41 μM^2)	Not determined	
10235-DOR-4G	cVDPV1, Imocitrelvir-variant	^{165}Gly to ^{165}Ser in 3C	0.034–0.058	Not determined	8.963–9.497	Not determined	Strong (820 μM^2)	Not determined	This review
10235-DOR-6G	cVDPV1, Imocitrelvir-variant		0.027–0.061	Not determined	8.666–9.734	Not determined	Strong (834 μM^2)	Not determined	
10235-DOR-3J	cVDPV1, Imocitrelvir/Pocapavir-variant	^{24}Ala to ^{24}Val in VP3 & ^{165}Gly to ^{165}Ser in 3C	>10	Not determined	>10	Not determined	Not determined	Not determined	This review
10235-DOR-4J	cVDPV1, Imocitrelvir/Pocapavair-variant		>10	Not determined	8.873–9.107	Not determined	No (1 μM^2)	Not determined	
10235-DOR-9J	cVDPV1, Imocitrelvir/Pocapavir-variant		>10	Not determined	>10	Not determined	Not determined	Not determined	
10235-DOR-1I	cVDPV1, Imocitrelvir/Pocapavir-variant		>10	Not determined	>10	Not determined	Not determined	Not determined	

* Susceptibility of parental and drug-resistant variants was assessed by co-incubating virus with drug in a cross-titration format in HeLa or RD cells seeded onto 96-well plates. After 3 days of incubation at 37 °C, viral cytopathic effect was determined by crystal violet staining and measured by reading absorbance at 590 nm. cVDPV: circulating vaccine-derived polioviruses; EC_{50}: half maximal effective concentration. # Synergistic effects of imocitrelvir and pocapavir were determined by cross-titration based on a checkerboard dilution matrix and calculated using MacSynergy II. The synergy volume expressed in $\mu M^2\%$ is categorized as follows: strong (>100), moderate (>50–100), weak (25–50), and no (<25).

Table 2. Susceptibility of selected poliovirus serotype 2 and serotype 3 strains to pocapavir, imocitrelvir, or combination treatment *.

Virus	Serotype	Mutation(s)	Pocapavir		Imocitrelvir		Imocitrelvir/Pocapavir		Reference(s)
			EC_{50} (μM)	Resistance Frequency	EC_{50} (μM)	Resistance Frequency	Synergy (%) #	Resistance Frequency	
Sabin 2	Serotype 2, Vaccine strain	-	0.016–0.024	$<1 \times 10^{-9}$	0.305–0.340	Not determined	Strong (459 μM^2)	Not determined	This review & Rhoden et al. (2013) [59]
10230	cVDPV2	-	0.036–0.055	11.8×10^{-5}	0.314–0.502	5.4×10^{-5}	Not determined	$<1 \times 10^{-9}$	Liu et al. (2012) [58] & Rhoden et al. (2013) [59]
10230.4	cVDPV2, Pocapavir-variant	^{194}Ile to ^{194}Met in VP1	1.5	Not determined	0.292–0.344	Not determined	Not determined	Not determined	Liu et al. (2012) [58] & Rhoden et al. (2013) [59]
10230.8	cVDPV2, Pocapavir-variant	^{24}Ala to ^{24}Val in VP3	>10	Not determined	0.243–0.295	Not determined	Not determined	Not determined	Liu et al. (2012) [58] & Rhoden et al. (2013) [59]
Sabin 3	Serotype 3, Vaccine strain	-	0.020–0.048	$<1 \times 10^{-9}$	0.137–0.262	Not determined	Strong (288 μM^2)	Not determined	This review & Rhoden et al. (2013) [59]
10805	iVDPV3	-	0.024–0.034	30.8×10^{-5}	0.313–0.401	Not determined	Not determined	$<1 \times 10^{-9}$	Liu et al. (2012) [58] & Rhoden et al. (2013) [59]
10805.1	iVDPV3, Pocapavir-variant	^{194}Ile to ^{194}Phe in VP1	>10	Not determined	0.686–0.952	Not determined	Not determined	Not determined	Liu et al. (2012) [58] & Rhoden et al. (2013) [59]
10805.5	iVDPV3, Pocapavir-variant	^{24}Ala to ^{24}Val in VP3	1.1	Not determined	0.548–0.638	Not determined	Not determined	Not determined	Liu et al. (2012) [58] & Rhoden et al. (2013) [59]

* Susceptibility of parental and drug-resistant variants was assessed by co-incubating virus with drug in a cross-titration format in HeLa or RD cells seeded onto 96-well plates. After 3 days of incubation at 37 °C, viral cytopathic effect was determined by crystal violet staining and measured by reading absorbance at 590 nm. cVDPV: circulating vaccine-derived polioviruses; EC_{50}: half maximal effective concentration. # Synergistic effects of imocitrelvir and pocapavir were determined by cross-titration based on a checkerboard dilution matrix and calculated using MacSynergy II. The synergy volume expressed in μM^2% is categorized as follows: strong (>100), moderate (>50–100), weak (25–50), and no (<25).

H1PVAT is another capsid-binding agent that selectively inhibits all three poliovirus serotypes but does not affect other enteroviruses [60]. Drug-resistance results have revealed that all H1PVAT-resistant variants uniformly bear a single ^{194}Ile to ^{194}Phe mutation in VP1 [60], suggesting that H1PVAT may have a similar mechanism of action as pocapavir. Additional investigations are needed to determine whether H1PVAT has advantages over other small-molecule inhibitors to justify further advancement.

3.2. Protease 3C Inhibitors

Rupintrivir (AG7088) is an irreversible pan-3C protease inhibitor designed by Pfizer using a protein structure-based drug design strategy [61]. Rupintrivir contains peptidyl-binding elements specific for the 3C protease and an unsaturated ethyl ester Michael acceptor that can interact with the cysteine residue in the active site of the 3C protease to form an irreversible covalent bond resulting in the inactivation of the 3C protease [61]. Rupintrivir shows broad in vitro antiviral activities against human rhinoviruses, coxsackieviruses, enteroviruses, and echoviruses [62]. Rupintrivir also potently inhibits the replication of all three poliovirus serotypes, with EC_{50} values ranging between 5 and 40 nM [51]. Despite the high in vitro potency, the failure of rupintrivir to reduce the severity of natural rhinovirus infections in humans has halted its clinical development [63,64].

Imocitrelvir (V-7404) is also an irreversible protease 3C inhibitor originally developed by Pfizer for treating human rhinovirus infections [65]. This molecule, currently under development by ViroDefense, Inc., shows improved pharmacokinetic properties compared to its predecessor rupintrivir (known as Compound **1** in early studies) and has demonstrated good oral bioavailability in dogs, cynomolgus monkeys, and humans [63,66]. Compared to rupintrivir, imocitrelvir is less potent against poliovirus of all three serotypes, with EC_{50} values ranging between 0.080 and 0.674 μM [59]. However, imocitrelvir is active against all pocapavir-resistant variants, with EC_{50} values (0.218 to 0.819 μM) comparable to those (0.202–0.407 μM) for pocapavir-susceptible parent strains [59]. The available data indicate that the emergence of laboratory-derived imocitrelvir-resistant variants was at the approximate frequency of 4–8 $\times$ 10^{-5} (Tables 1 and 2), similar to that (3–40 $\times$ 10^{-5}) of laboratory-derived pocapavir-resistant variants in vitro [58]. Importantly, despite bearing a single ^{165}Gly to ^{165}Ser mutation in the 3C protease, imocitrelvir-resistant VDPV1 variants remain susceptible to pocapavir (EC_{50} value of 0.044–0.046 μM) comparable to that of the parent VDPV1 strains (EC_{50} value of 0.038 μM) (Table 1).

3.3. Imocitrelvir/Pocapavir Combination Therapy

Given that imocitrelvir-resistant variants are sensitive to pocapavir, our team tested the combination of the two drugs against poliovirus in vitro. The combination of imocitrelvir and pocapavir blocked CPE formation induced by Sabin 1, 2, and 3 [59]. Strong in vitro synergy was achieved when the combination was used to treat parental VDPV1 and imocitrelvir-resistant VDPV1 variants. Although weak synergistic effects were observed when imocitrelvir and pocapavir were used to treat pocapavir-resistant VDPV1 variants, imocitrelvir remained active against these pocapavir-resistant variants. As expected, no synergistic activity was observed on pocapavir/imocitrelvir double-resistant VDPV1 variants treated with the combination (Table 1). Pocapavir/imocitrelvir double-resistant VDPV1 variants emerged at a mean frequency of 1.9 $\times$ 10^{-7} in vitro, which is >100 times lower than that observed with VDPV1 variants resistant to either drug alone (Table 1). Laboratory-isolated double-resistant VDPV1 variants have comparable growth kinetics to their drug-sensitive parental strains in vitro but are more thermolabile (CDC unpublished data). The emergence of pocapavir/imocitrelvir double-resistant VDPV2 or VDPV3 variants is even less frequently detected in cell culture (<1 $\times$ 10^{-9}, the detection limit of the assay) (Table 2). The potent synergy and markedly reduced resistance frequency, taken together, suggest that imocitrelvir paired with pocapavir as a combination therapy could be effective for treating infections with cVDPVs or iVDPVs.

ViroDefense, Inc. has completed a Phase I double-blind, randomized, placebo-controlled clinical trial on the safety, tolerability, and pharmacokinetics of imocitrelvir alone and in combination with pocapavir orally administered in healthy adult volunteers. Imocitrelvir and its combination with pocapavir were found to be well tolerated by the subjects, with acceptable safety and pharmacokinetics profiles, after a single ascending dose or multiple ascending doses [67]. This study also provided valuable dosing data for imocitrelvir to be paired with pocapavir for the further clinical development of the combination therapy.

3.4. Protein 2C Inhibitors

Poliovirus 2C is one of the highly conserved nonstructural proteins. It has ATPase/GTPase activity and plays an important role in RNA binding, membrane binding, and viral morphology [35,68–70]. Guanidine hydrochloride (GuaHCl), a reversible 2C inhibitor, can impair poliovirus replication by blocking 2C and its precursor P2 to become membrane-bound, abolishing 2C ATPase activity and preventing the initiation of negative-stranded RNA synthesis [68–70]. Other 2C inhibitors such as 2-(a-hydroxybenzyl)-benzimidazole (HBB) and its derivative, 1-(4-fluorophenyl)-2-[(4-imino-1,4-dihydropyridin-1-yl)methyl] (MRL-1237), also reportedly inhibit poliovirus replication but are prone to drug resistance due to spontaneous mutations [71]. Most laboratory-derived MRL-1237-resistant variants are also resistant to GuaHCl [71], suggesting that these 2C inhibitors share a common mode of action. The high tendency toward drug resistance excludes 2C inhibitors from the list of potential lead antiviral candidates for further development.

3.5. Protein 3A Inhibitors

Poliovirus 3A is another highly conserved, multifunctional nonstructural protein involved in virus–host interactions, such as membrane association, host secretory pathways, RNA replication organelles, etc. [64,72,73]. Poliovirus 3A and its precursor, 3AB, can suppress host phosphatidylinositol-4 kinase III beta (PI4Kβ) and oxysterol-binding protein (OSBP) pathways to modulate the lipid microenvironment for the generation of viral RNA replication organelles [74–76].

Enviroxime, a benzimidazole derivative originally developed to treat rhinovirus-induced symptoms, inhibits the replication of all three poliovirus serotypes by targeting the 3A coding region [77]. However, single point mutations in this 3A coding region are sufficient to abolish the inhibition of enviroxime and other enviroxime-like compounds (e.g., TTP-8307, T-00127-HEV1, and GW5074) [64,77–79]. Additionally, enviroxime combined with BTA798 (capsid inhibitor) or rupintrivir (3C protease inhibitor) yielded only an additive or very weak synergistic inhibition of poliovirus [80]. In clinical studies, undesirable gastrointestinal side effects were reported in some subjects receiving an oral administration of enviroxime, and no apparent efficacy was observed in natural or experimental rhinovirus infections [64,77,81]. Because of poor pre-clinical data, the clinical development of enviroxime has been halted.

3.6. Polymerase 3D^{pol} Inhibitors

Poliovirus polymerase 3D^{pol} plays a key role in catalyzing viral RNA synthesis, which can be blocked by non-nucleoside and nucleoside analogs. Guanidine is a historic non-nucleoside inhibitor that blocks the RNA synthesis of all three poliovirus serotypes [82]. Gliotoxin, a fungal metabolite, is another non-nucleoside inhibitor that interferes with poliovirus RNA synthesis by targeting 3D^{pol} [83]. However, both guanidine and gliotoxin have toxicities that prevent them from further clinical development.

Ribavirin, a nucleoside inhibitor with a multimode mechanism of action, is a regulatory-approved drug for treating RSV and chronic HCV infections [84]. As a synthetic purine nucleoside analogue, ribavirin can act as an ambiguous purine base inhibitor that is incorporated into the poliovirus RNA genome, resulting in lethal mutagenesis and blocking the generation of progeny virus [85,86]. As ribavirin increases the number of mutations per genome, the infectivity of the resulting poliovirus RNA drops sharply [86]. However, the spontaneous RNA recombination that drives the natural evolution of the picornavirus is also suggested to contribute to ribavirin resistance [87]. Poliovirus containing ^{420}Leu in $3D^{pol}$ has higher frequencies of RNA recombination and is more resistant to ribavirin than poliovirus bearing ^{420}Ala mutation in $3D^{pol}$ [87].

3.7. New Antiviral Leads

In addition to the above antiviral drugs and candidates that have been tested or developed in the past decades, there are compounds that have recently been discovered to have antiviral activities against poliovirus. Madia et al. reported that two new oxazoline derivatives are highly potent against poliovirus of all three serotypes at submicromolar concentrations, with very low cytotoxicity [88]. These isoflavone-derived synthetic compounds likely belong to the class of capsid inhibitors by impairing virus-receptor binding or viral uncoating, but the exact mechanism(s) remain to be elucidated [88].

A novel druggable interprotomer pocket in the capsid has been discovered that is located at a conserved VP1–VP3 interprotomer interface and is conserved across multiple species of picornaviruses [89]. Preliminary structure–activity relation studies have identified several analogs targeting this pocket with broad-spectrum antiviral activities against different picornaviruses, including one against poliovirus serotype 1, with low potency [89]. Further refining of the functional groups of these early-stage inhibitors may help improve antiviral activity.

Itraconazole, an antifungal agent with anticancer activity, also has antiviral effects on enteroviruses, including poliovirus [90]. Itraconazole targets host OSBP and OSBP-related protein 4 (ORP4) and impairs the colocalization of host filipin with viral 3A to block viral replication organelle formation [90]. Although itraconazole itself does not directly inhibit PI4KIIIβ activity, mutations in the 3A protein that confer resistance to enviroxime, GW5074, or other PI4KIIIβ inhibitors also render viruses resistant to itraconazole [90].

4. Summary and Future Directions

Although extensive progress has been made in developing antiviral drugs targeting poliovirus in the past decades, none has achieved regulatory approval for therapeutic use. Poor pharmacokinetics, low oral bioavailability, toxicity, and drug resistance stand among the many issues that hinder clinical development. The standards for safety, tolerability, and oral bioavailability could be even higher for polio antiviral drug approval, considering that the potential target population is primarily children under 5 years old and immunocompromised individuals. Another significant factor is the as-yet-undefined regulatory pathway to approval for a rare condition such as iVDPV excreters.

Drug development from de novo molecule design to clinical investigation to final approval is a long, costly journey full of uncertainties even when the pathway is reasonably well defined. The entire process can easily span 10–15 years or more, from conceiving an idea to achieving the final approval. The approach of drug repurposing, which is to reinvestigate existing drugs for new applications, has gained considerable interest during the COVID-19 pandemic. In addition to reducing time and saving money, the largest benefit of repurposing licensed drugs is the ability to take an accelerated approval path for new indication(s) because licensed drugs have already passed the toxicity tests, and many have post-licensure or post-marketing surveillance data available. This approach can significantly shorten the antiviral development cycle. One such successful example is azidothymidine (AZT). Originally developed for anti-cancer treatment, AZT was discovered by the US NIH/NCI-led drug screening program to be a potent antiretroviral agent and was approved by the US FDA as a therapeutic drug for treating HIV infections in 1987 after fast-track clinical trials [91]. Remdesivir is a drug approved for treating patients with COVID-19-associated hospitalizations. Remdesivir's intracellular metabolites GS-441524 monophosphate and triphosphate are the nucleotide analogs of the viral RNA polymerase inhibitor [92]. Our team tested the potential of remdesivir and its metabolites in inhibiting poliovirus replication without success (CDC unpublished data).

In addition to repurposing licensed drugs, the pools of screened molecules can be expanded to include compounds under investigation or in databases. Previously, this strategy helped to successfully identify a synthetic agonist of peroxisome proliferator-activated receptor β/δ as a promising lead compound with broad-spectrum anti-influenza activity in vitro and in ovo after screening over 70,000 compounds in the LOPAC and Maybridge libraries [93]. Although candidate drugs selected by this approach may still need to proceed through the regular approval process, it will save considerable time in compound design and synthesis. Additionally, artificial intelligence, such as machine learning-driven frameworks, should be leveraged for more efficient drug selection and optimization. Single cell-led systems biology pipelines and other emerging technologies could also be applied to facilitate the identification of promising candidates [94].

In summary, despite the challenges and obstacles, there is progress in the development of antiviral agents that are essential in stopping the excretion of iVDPV in immune-deficient patients. At present, the most promising prospect is the combination of pocapavir and imocitrelvir (which shows synergistic antiviral activity and a very low resistance rate in vitro), which has progressed through the early stages of non-clinical and clinical development.

Author Contributions: Conceptualization, H.X. and C.C.B.; methodology, E.E.R. and H.-M.L.; investigation, E.E.R. and H.-M.L.; resources, C.C.B.; writing—original draft preparation, H.X. and F.O.; writing—review and editing, H.X., B.A.M. and R.M.B. All authors have read and agreed to the published version of the manuscript.

Funding: The Bill & Melinda Gates Foundation (BMGF) provided support for the Polio Antivirals Initiative. The completion of this review article was provided by CDC intramural support.

Conflicts of Interest: The authors declare no conflicts of interest. The opinions in this review are those of the authors and do not necessarily represent the official position of the Centers for Disease Control and Prevention. The use of trade names is for identification purposes only and does not constitute an endorsement by the Centers for Disease Control and Prevention or the US Government.

References

1. Mendelsohn, C.L.; Wimmer, E.; Racaniello, V.R. Cellular receptor for poliovirus: Molecular cloning, nucleotide sequence, and expression of a new member of the immunoglobulin superfamily. *Cell* **1989**, *56*, 855–865. [CrossRef] [PubMed]
2. WHO. Poliomyelitis: Key Facts. Available online: https://www.who.int/news-room/fact-sheets/detail/poliomyelitis (accessed on 10 August 2024).
3. ECDC. Disease Factsheet about Poliomyelitis. Available online: https://www.ecdc.europa.eu/en/poliomyelitis/facts#:~:text=All%20unimmunised%20persons%20are%20susceptible%20to%20the%20infection.,with%20sero-conversion%20rates%20of%2090%E2%80%93100%25%20among%20household%20contacts (accessed on 10 August 2024).
4. Kishore, N.; Krow-Lucal, E.; Diop, O.M.; Jorba, J.; Avagnan, T.; Grabovac, V.; Kfutwah, A.K.W.; Johnson, T.; Joshi, S.; Sangal, L.; et al. Surveillance To Track Progress Toward Polio Eradication-Worldwide, 2022–2023. *MMWR Morb. Mortal. Wkly. Rep.* **2024**, *73*, 278–285. [CrossRef] [PubMed]
5. Morimoto, N. The relationship between poliovirus multiplication, the sIgA antibody response and the serum neutralizing antibody titers after trivalent oral polio vaccination. *Kansenshogaku Zasshi* **2001**, *75*, 1030–1039. [CrossRef] [PubMed]
6. Wright, P.F.; Wieland-Alter, W.; Ilyushina, N.A.; Hoen, A.G.; Arita, M.; Boesch, A.W.; Ackerman, M.E.; van der Avoort, H.; Oberste, M.S.; Pallansch, M.A.; et al. Intestinal immunity is a determinant of clearance of poliovirus after oral vaccination. *J. Infect. Dis.* **2014**, *209*, 1628–1634. [CrossRef] [PubMed]
7. Connor, R.I.; Brickley, E.B.; Wieland-Alter, W.F.; Ackerman, M.E.; Weiner, J.A.; Modlin, J.F.; Bandyopadhyay, A.S.; Wright, P.F. Mucosal immunity to poliovirus. *Mucosal Immunol.* **2022**, *15*, 1–9. [CrossRef]
8. Polio Global Eradication Initiative Fact Sheet: Vaccine-Derived Poliovirus. Available online: https://www.who.int/docs/default-source/documents/gpei-cvdpv-factsheet-march-2017.pdf?sfvrsn=1ceef4af_2 (accessed on 10 August 2024).
9. Prevots, D.R.; Sutter, R.W.; Strebel, P.M.; Weibel, R.E.; Cochi, S.L. Completeness of reporting for paralytic poliomyelitis, United States, 1980 through 1991. Implications for estimating the risk of vaccine-associated disease. *Arch. Pediatr. Adolesc. Med.* **1994**, *148*, 479–485. [CrossRef]
10. Diop, O.M.; Burns, C.C.; Sutter, R.W.; Wassilak, S.G.; Kew, O.M.; Centers for Disease Control and Prevention (CDC). Update on Vaccine-Derived Polioviruses—Worldwide, January 2014–March 2015. *MMWR Morb. Mortal. Wkly. Rep.* **2015**, *64*, 640–646.

11. Platt, L.R.; Estivariz, C.F.; Sutter, R.W. Vaccine-associated paralytic poliomyelitis: A review of the epidemiology and estimation of the global burden. *J. Infect. Dis.* **2014**, *210* (Suppl. S1), S380–S389. [CrossRef]
12. Kew, O.; Morris-Glasgow, V.; Landaverde, M.; Burns, C.; Shaw, J.; Garib, Z.; Andre, J.; Blackman, E.; Freeman, C.J.; Jorba, J.; et al. Outbreak of poliomyelitis in Hispaniola associated with circulating type 1 vaccine-derived poliovirus. *Science* **2002**, *296*, 356–359. [CrossRef]
13. Stern, A.; Yeh, M.T.; Zinger, T.; Smith, M.; Wright, C.; Ling, G.; Nielsen, R.; Macadam, A.; Andino, R. The Evolutionary Pathway to Virulence of an RNA Virus. *Cell* **2017**, *169*, 35–46.e19. [CrossRef]
14. Mohanty, M.C.; Madkaikar, M.R.; Desai, M.; Aluri, J.; Varose, S.Y.; Taur, P.; Sharma, D.K.; Nalavade, U.P.; Rane, S.V.; Gupta, M.; et al. Natural Clearance of Prolonged VDPV Infection in a Child With Primary Immunodeficiency Disorder. *Front. Immunol.* **2019**, *10*, 1567. [CrossRef] [PubMed]
15. Macklin, G.; Diop, O.M.; Humayun, A.; Shahmahmoodi, S.; El-Sayed, Z.A.; Triki, H.; Rey, G.; Avagyan, T.; Grabovac, V.; Jorba, J.; et al. Update on Immunodeficiency-Associated Vaccine-Derived Polioviruses—Worldwide, July 2018–December 2019. *MMWR Morb. Mortal. Wkly. Rep.* **2020**, *69*, 913–917. [CrossRef] [PubMed]
16. Yao, N.; Liu, Y.; Xu, J.W.; Wang, Q.; Yin, Z.D.; Wen, N.; Yang, H.; Rodewald, L.E.; Zhang, Z.Y. Detection of a Highly Divergent Type 3 Vaccine-Derived Poliovirus in a Child with a Severe Primary Immunodeficiency Disorder—Chongqing, China, 2022. *MMWR Morb. Mortal. Wkly. Rep.* **2022**, *71*, 1148–1150. [CrossRef] [PubMed]
17. Singanayagam, A.; Klapsa, D.; Burton-Fanning, S.; Hand, J.; Wilton, T.; Stephens, L.; Mate, R.; Shillitoe, B.; Celma, C.; Slatter, M.; et al. Asymptomatic immunodeficiency-associated vaccine-derived poliovirus infections in two UK children. *Nat. Commun.* **2023**, *14*, 3413. [CrossRef] [PubMed]
18. Cifuente, J.O.; Moratorio, G. Evolutionary and Structural Overview of Human Picornavirus Capsid Antibody Evasion. *Front. Cell. Infect. Microbiol.* **2019**, *9*, 283. [CrossRef]
19. Minor, P.D.; Ferguson, M.; Evans, D.M.; Almond, J.W.; Icenogle, J.P. Antigenic structure of polioviruses of serotypes 1, 2 and 3. *J. Gen. Virol.* **1986**, *67 Pt 7*, 1283–1291. [CrossRef]
20. Hansen, J.L.; Long, A.M.; Schultz, S.C. Structure of the RNA-dependent RNA polymerase of poliovirus. *Structure* **1997**, *5*, 1109–1122. [CrossRef]
21. Grant, R.A.; Hiremath, C.N.; Filman, D.J.; Syed, R.; Andries, K.; Hogle, J.M. Structures of poliovirus complexes with anti-viral drugs: Implications for viral stability and drug design. *Curr. Biol.* **1994**, *4*, 784–797. [CrossRef]
22. Mosser, A.G.; Rueckert, R.R. WIN 51711-dependent mutants of poliovirus type 3: Evidence that virions decay after release from cells unless drug is present. *J. Virol.* **1993**, *67*, 1246–1254. [CrossRef]
23. Filman, D.J.; Syed, R.; Chow, M.; Macadam, A.J.; Minor, P.D.; Hogle, J.M. Structural factors that control conformational transitions and serotype specificity in type 3 poliovirus. *EMBO J.* **1989**, *8*, 1567–1579. [CrossRef]
24. Fricks, C.E.; Hogle, J.M. Cell-induced conformational change in poliovirus: Externalization of the amino terminus of VP1 is responsible for liposome binding. *J. Virol.* **1990**, *64*, 1934–1945. [CrossRef] [PubMed]
25. Huang, Y.; Hogle, J.M.; Chow, M. Is the 135S poliovirus particle an intermediate during cell entry? *J. Virol.* **2000**, *74*, 8757–8761. [CrossRef] [PubMed]
26. Bubeck, D.; Filman, D.J.; Cheng, N.; Steven, A.C.; Hogle, J.M.; Belnap, D.M. The structure of the poliovirus 135S cell entry intermediate at 10-angstrom resolution reveals the location of an externalized polypeptide that binds to membranes. *J. Virol.* **2005**, *79*, 7745–7755. [CrossRef] [PubMed]
27. He, Y.; Bowman, V.D.; Mueller, S.; Bator, C.M.; Bella, J.; Peng, X.; Baker, T.S.; Wimmer, E.; Kuhn, R.J.; Rossmann, M.G. Interaction of the poliovirus receptor with poliovirus. *Proc. Natl. Acad. Sci. USA* **2000**, *97*, 79–84. [CrossRef] [PubMed]
28. Kitamura, N.; Semler, B.L.; Rothberg, P.G.; Larsen, G.R.; Adler, C.J.; Dorner, A.J.; Emini, E.A.; Hanecak, R.; Lee, J.J.; van der Werf, S.; et al. Primary structure, gene organization and polypeptide expression of poliovirus RNA. *Nature* **1981**, *291*, 547–553. [CrossRef]
29. Cameron, C.E.; Oh, H.S.; Moustafa, I.M. Expanding knowledge of P3 proteins in the poliovirus lifecycle. *Future Microbiol.* **2010**, *5*, 867–881. [CrossRef]
30. Spear, A.; Ogram, S.A.; Morasco, B.J.; Smerage, L.E.; Flanegan, J.B. Viral precursor protein P3 and its processed products perform discrete and essential functions in the poliovirus RNA replication complex. *Virology* **2015**, *485*, 492–501. [CrossRef]
31. Marc, D.; Drugeon, G.; Haenni, A.L.; Girard, M.; van der Werf, S. Role of myristoylation of poliovirus capsid protein VP4 as determined by site-directed mutagenesis of its N-terminal sequence. *EMBO J.* **1989**, *8*, 2661–2668. [CrossRef]
32. Wang, S.H.; Wang, K.; Zhao, K.; Hua, S.C.; Du, J. The Structure, Function, and Mechanisms of Action of Enterovirus Non-structural Protein 2C. *Front. Microbiol.* **2020**, *11*, 615965. [CrossRef]
33. Xiang, W.; Cuconati, A.; Hope, D.; Kirkegaard, K.; Wimmer, E. Complete protein linkage map of poliovirus P3 proteins: Interaction of polymerase 3Dpol with VPg and with genetic variants of 3AB. *J. Virol.* **1998**, *72*, 6732–6741. [CrossRef]
34. Teterina, N.L.; Pinto, Y.; Weaver, J.D.; Jensen, K.S.; Ehrenfeld, E. Analysis of poliovirus protein 3A interactions with viral and cellular proteins in infected cells. *J. Virol.* **2011**, *85*, 4284–4296. [CrossRef] [PubMed]
35. Adams, P.; Kandiah, E.; Effantin, G.; Steven, A.C.; Ehrenfeld, E. Poliovirus 2C protein forms homo-oligomeric structures required for ATPase activity. *J. Biol. Chem.* **2009**, *284*, 22012–22021. [CrossRef] [PubMed]
36. McSharry, J.J.; Caliguiri, L.A.; Eggers, H.J. Inhibition of uncoating of poliovirus by arildone, a new antiviral drug. *Virology* **1979**, *97*, 307–315. [CrossRef]

37. Caliguiri, L.A.; McSharry, J.J.; Lawrence, G.W. Effect of arildone on modifications of poliovirus in vitro. *Virology* **1980**, *105*, 86–93. [CrossRef] [PubMed]
38. Cox, S.; Buontempo, P.J.; Wright-Minogue, J.; DeMartino, J.L.; Skelton, A.M.; Ferrari, E.; Schwartz, J.; Rozhon, E.J.; Linn, C.C.; Girijavallabhan, V.; et al. Antipicornavirus activity of SCH 47802 and analogs: In vitro and in vivo studies. *Antivir. Res.* **1996**, *32*, 71–79. [CrossRef] [PubMed]
39. Buontempo, P.J.; Cox, S.; Wright-Minogue, J.; DeMartino, J.L.; Skelton, A.M.; Ferrari, E.; Albin, R.; Rozhon, E.J.; Girijavallabhan, V.; Modlin, J.F.; et al. SCH 48973: A potent, broad-spectrum, antienterovirus compound. *Antimicrob. Agents Chemother.* **1997**, *41*, 1220–1225. [CrossRef]
40. Tsang, S.K.; Danthi, P.; Chow, M.; Hogle, J.M. Stabilization of poliovirus by capsid-binding antiviral drugs is due to entropic effects. *J. Mol. Biol.* **2000**, *296*, 335–340. [CrossRef]
41. Florea, N.R.; Maglio, D.; Nicolau, D.P. Pleconaril, a novel antipicornaviral agent. *Pharmacotherapy* **2003**, *23*, 339–348. [CrossRef]
42. McKinlay, M.A.; Steinberg, B.A. Oral efficacy of WIN 51711 in mice infected with human poliovirus. *Antimicrob. Agents Chemother.* **1986**, *29*, 30–32. [CrossRef]
43. Romero, J.R.; Gross, T.; Abromowitch, M.; Jung, L. Pleconaril Treatment of Vaccine-Acquired Poliovirus. *Pediatr. Res.* **1999**, *45*, 173. [CrossRef]
44. Buttinelli, G.; Donati, V.; Fiore, S.; Marturano, J.; Plebani, A.; Balestri, P.; Soresina, A.R.; Vivarelli, R.; Delpeyroux, F.; Martin, J.; et al. Nucleotide variation in Sabin type 2 poliovirus from an immunodeficient patient with poliomyelitis. *J. Gen. Virol.* **2003**, *84*, 1215–1221. [CrossRef] [PubMed]
45. MacLennan, C.; Dunn, G.; Huissoon, A.P.; Kumararatne, D.S.; Martin, J.; O'Leary, P.; Thompson, R.A.; Osman, H.; Wood, P.; Minor, P.; et al. Failure to clear persistent vaccine-derived neurovirulent poliovirus infection in an immunodeficient man. *Lancet* **2004**, *363*, 1509–1513. [CrossRef] [PubMed]
46. Hayden, F.G.; Herrington, D.T.; Coats, T.L.; Kim, K.; Cooper, E.C.; Villano, S.A.; Liu, S.; Hudson, S.; Pevear, D.C.; Collett, M.; et al. Efficacy and safety of oral pleconaril for treatment of colds due to picornaviruses in adults: Results of 2 double-blind, randomized, placebo-controlled trials. *Clin. Infect. Dis.* **2003**, *36*, 1523–1532. [CrossRef] [PubMed]
47. Abzug, M.J.; Michaels, M.G.; Wald, E.; Jacobs, R.F.; Romero, J.R.; Sanchez, P.J.; Wilson, G.; Krogstad, P.; Storch, G.A.; Lawrence, R.; et al. A Randomized, Double-Blind, Placebo-Controlled Trial of Pleconaril for the Treatment of Neonates with Enterovirus Sepsis. *J. Pediatric Infect. Dis. Soc.* **2016**, *5*, 53–62. [CrossRef]
48. Rotbart, H.A.; Webster, A.D.; Pleconaril Treatment Registry, G. Treatment of potentially life-threatening enterovirus infections with pleconaril. *Clin. Infect. Dis.* **2001**, *32*, 228–235. [CrossRef]
49. Senior, K. FDA panel rejects common cold treatment. *Lancet Infect. Dis.* **2002**, *2*, 264. [CrossRef]
50. Andries, K.; Dewindt, B.; Snoeks, J.; Willebrords, R.; van Eemeren, K.; Stokbroekx, R.; Janssen, P.A. In vitro activity of pirodavir (R 77975), a substituted phenoxy-pyridazinamine with broad-spectrum antipicornaviral activity. *Antimicrob. Agents Chemother.* **1992**, *36*, 100–107. [CrossRef]
51. De Palma, A.M.; Purstinger, G.; Wimmer, E.; Patick, A.K.; Andries, K.; Rombaut, B.; De Clercq, E.; Neyts, J. Potential use of antiviral agents in polio eradication. *Emerg. Infect. Dis.* **2008**, *14*, 545–551. [CrossRef]
52. Barnard, D.L.; Hubbard, V.D.; Smee, D.F.; Sidwell, R.W.; Watson, K.G.; Tucker, S.P.; Reece, P.A. In vitro activity of expanded-spectrum pyridazinyl oxime ethers related to pirodavir: Novel capsid-binding inhibitors with potent antipicornavirus activity. *Antimicrob. Agents Chemother.* **2004**, *48*, 1766–1772. [CrossRef]
53. Egorova, A.; Ekins, S.; Schmidtke, M.; Makarov, V. Back to the future: Advances in development of broad-spectrum capsid-binding inhibitors of enteroviruses. *Eur. J. Med. Chem.* **2019**, *178*, 606–622. [CrossRef]
54. Oberste, M.S.; Moore, D.; Anderson, B.; Pallansch, M.A.; Pevear, D.C.; Collett, M.S. In vitro antiviral activity of V-073 against polioviruses. *Antimicrob. Agents Chemother.* **2009**, *53*, 4501–4503. [CrossRef] [PubMed]
55. Tanner, E.J.; Liu, H.M.; Oberste, M.S.; Pallansch, M.; Collett, M.S.; Kirkegaard, K. Dominant drug targets suppress the emergence of antiviral resistance. *Elife* **2014**, *3*, e03830. [CrossRef] [PubMed]
56. Copelyn, J.; Hincks, J.R.; Wilmshurst, J.M.; Petersen, W.; Howard, W.; Jallow, S.; Moonsamy, S.; Seakamela, L.; Suchard, M.; Collett, M.S.; et al. Clearance of Immunodeficiency-associated Vaccine-derived Poliovirus Infection With Pocapavir. *Pediatr. Infect. Dis. J.* **2020**, *39*, 435–437. [CrossRef] [PubMed]
57. Collett, M.S.; Hincks, J.R.; Benschop, K.; Duizer, E.; van der Avoort, H.; Rhoden, E.; Liu, H.; Oberste, M.S.; McKinlay, M.A.; Hartford, M. Antiviral Activity of Pocapavir in a Randomized, Blinded, Placebo-Controlled Human Oral Poliovirus Vaccine Challenge Model. *J. Infect. Dis.* **2017**, *215*, 335–343. [CrossRef] [PubMed]
58. Liu, H.M.; Roberts, J.A.; Moore, D.; Anderson, B.; Pallansch, M.A.; Pevear, D.C.; Collett, M.S.; Oberste, M.S. Characterization of poliovirus variants selected for resistance to the antiviral compound V-073. *Antimicrob. Agents Chemother.* **2012**, *56*, 5568–5574. [CrossRef]
59. Rhoden, E.; Liu, H.M.; Wang-Chern, S.W.; Oberste, M.S. Anti-poliovirus activity of protease inhibitor AG-7404, and assessment of in vitro activity in combination with antiviral capsid inhibitor compounds. *Antivir. Res.* **2013**, *98*, 186–191. [CrossRef]
60. Tijsma, A.; Thibaut, H.J.; Spieser, S.A.; De Palma, A.; Koukni, M.; Rhoden, E.; Oberste, S.; Purstinger, G.; Volny-Luraghi, A.; Martin, J.; et al. H1PVAT is a novel and potent early-stage inhibitor of poliovirus replication that targets VP1. *Antivir. Res.* **2014**, *110*, 1–9. [CrossRef]

61. Matthews, D.A.; Dragovich, P.S.; Webber, S.E.; Fuhrman, S.A.; Patick, A.K.; Zalman, L.S.; Hendrickson, T.F.; Love, R.A.; Prins, T.J.; Marakovits, J.T.; et al. Structure-assisted design of mechanism-based irreversible inhibitors of human rhinovirus 3C protease with potent antiviral activity against multiple rhinovirus serotypes. *Proc. Natl. Acad. Sci. USA* **1999**, *96*, 11000–11007. [CrossRef]
62. Patick, A.K.; Binford, S.L.; Brothers, M.A.; Jackson, R.L.; Ford, C.E.; Diem, M.D.; Maldonado, F.; Dragovich, P.S.; Zhou, R.; Prins, T.J.; et al. In vitro antiviral activity of AG7088, a potent inhibitor of human rhinovirus 3C protease. *Antimicrob. Agents Chemother.* **1999**, *43*, 2444–2450. [CrossRef]
63. Patick, A.K.; Brothers, M.A.; Maldonado, F.; Binford, S.; Maldonado, O.; Fuhrman, S.; Petersen, A.; Smith, G.J., 3rd; Zalman, L.S.; Burns-Naas, L.A.; et al. In vitro antiviral activity and single-dose pharmacokinetics in humans of a novel, orally bioavailable inhibitor of human rhinovirus 3C protease. *Antimicrob. Agents Chemother.* **2005**, *49*, 2267–2275. [CrossRef]
64. Thibaut, H.J.; De Palma, A.M.; Neyts, J. Combating enterovirus replication: State-of-the-art on antiviral research. *Biochem. Pharmacol.* **2012**, *83*, 185–192. [CrossRef] [PubMed]
65. Dragovich, P.S.; Prins, T.J.; Zhou, R.; Brown, E.L.; Maldonado, F.C.; Fuhrman, S.A.; Zalman, L.S.; Tuntland, T.; Lee, C.A.; Patick, A.K.; et al. Structure-based design, synthesis, and biological evaluation of irreversible human rhinovirus 3C protease inhibitors. 6. Structure-activity studies of orally bioavailable, 2-pyridone-containing peptidomimetics. *J. Med. Chem.* **2002**, *45*, 1607–1623. [CrossRef] [PubMed]
66. Dragovich, P.S.; Prins, T.J.; Zhou, R.; Johnson, T.O.; Hua, Y.; Luu, H.T.; Sakata, S.K.; Brown, E.L.; Maldonado, F.C.; Tuntland, T.; et al. Structure-based design, synthesis, and biological evaluation of irreversible human rhinovirus 3C protease inhibitors. 8. Pharmacological optimization of orally bioavailable 2-pyridone-containing peptidomimetics. *J. Med. Chem.* **2003**, *46*, 4572–4585. [CrossRef]
67. Kankam, M.K.; Burns, J.M.; Collett, M.S.; Corrado, M.L.; Hincks, J.R. A Phase 1 Study of the Safety, Tolerability, and Pharmacokinetics of Single and Multiple Oral Doses of V-7404 in Healthy Adult Volunteers. *Antimicrob. Agents Chemother.* **2021**, *65*, e0102921. [CrossRef]
68. Barton, D.J.; Flanegan, J.B. Synchronous replication of poliovirus RNA: Initiation of negative-strand RNA synthesis requires the guanidine-inhibited activity of protein 2C. *J. Virol.* **1997**, *71*, 8482–8489. [CrossRef]
69. Bienz, K.; Egger, D.; Troxler, M.; Pasamontes, L. Structural organization of poliovirus RNA replication is mediated by viral proteins of the P2 genomic region. *J. Virol.* **1990**, *64*, 1156–1163. [CrossRef]
70. Pfister, T.; Wimmer, E. Characterization of the nucleoside triphosphatase activity of poliovirus protein 2C reveals a mechanism by which guanidine inhibits poliovirus replication. *J. Biol. Chem.* **1999**, *274*, 6992–7001. [CrossRef]
71. Shimizu, H.; Agoh, M.; Agoh, Y.; Yoshida, H.; Yoshii, K.; Yoneyama, T.; Hagiwara, A.; Miyamura, T. Mutations in the 2C region of poliovirus responsible for altered sensitivity to benzimidazole derivatives. *J. Virol.* **2000**, *74*, 4146–4154. [CrossRef]
72. Doedens, J.R.; Giddings, T.H., Jr.; Kirkegaard, K. Inhibition of endoplasmic reticulum-to-Golgi traffic by poliovirus protein 3A: Genetic and ultrastructural analysis. *J. Virol.* **1997**, *71*, 9054–9064. [CrossRef]
73. Dodd, D.A.; Giddings, T.H., Jr.; Kirkegaard, K. Poliovirus 3A protein limits interleukin-6 (IL-6), IL-8, and beta interferon secretion during viral infection. *J. Virol.* **2001**, *75*, 8158–8165. [CrossRef]
74. Hsu, N.Y.; Ilnytska, O.; Belov, G.; Santiana, M.; Chen, Y.H.; Takvorian, P.M.; Pau, C.; van der Schaar, H.; Kaushik-Basu, N.; Balla, T.; et al. Viral reorganization of the secretory pathway generates distinct organelles for RNA replication. *Cell* **2010**, *141*, 799–811. [CrossRef] [PubMed]
75. Arita, M. Mechanism of Poliovirus Resistance to Host Phosphatidylinositol-4 Kinase III beta Inhibitor. *ACS Infect. Dis.* **2016**, *2*, 140–148. [CrossRef] [PubMed]
76. Arita, M.; Bigay, J. Poliovirus Evolution toward Independence from the Phosphatidylinositol-4 Kinase III beta/Oxysterol-Binding Protein Family I Pathway. *ACS Infect. Dis.* **2019**, *5*, 962–973. [CrossRef] [PubMed]
77. Heinz, B.A.; Vance, L.M. The antiviral compound enviroxime targets the 3A coding region of rhinovirus and poliovirus. *J. Virol.* **1995**, *69*, 4189–4197. [CrossRef]
78. De Palma, A.M.; Thibaut, H.J.; van der Linden, L.; Lanke, K.; Heggermont, W.; Ireland, S.; Andrews, R.; Arimilli, M.; Al-Tel, T.H.; De Clercq, E.; et al. Mutations in the nonstructural protein 3A confer resistance to the novel enterovirus replication inhibitor TTP-8307. *Antimicrob. Agents Chemother.* **2009**, *53*, 1850–1857. [CrossRef]
79. Arita, M.; Kojima, H.; Nagano, T.; Okabe, T.; Wakita, T.; Shimizu, H. Phosphatidylinositol 4-kinase III beta is a target of enviroxime-like compounds for antipoliovirus activity. *J. Virol.* **2011**, *85*, 2364–2372. [CrossRef]
80. Thibaut, H.J.; Leyssen, P.; Puerstinger, G.; Muigg, A.; Neyts, J.; De Palma, A.M. Towards the design of combination therapy for the treatment of enterovirus infections. *Antivir. Res.* **2011**, *90*, 213–217. [CrossRef]
81. Phillpotts, R.J.; Wallace, J.; Tyrrell, D.A.; Tagart, V.B. Therapeutic activity of enviroxime against rhinovirus infection in volunteers. *Antimicrob. Agents Chemother.* **1983**, *23*, 671–675. [CrossRef]
82. Tershak, D.R. Inhibition of poliovirus polymerase by guanidine in vitro. *J. Virol.* **1982**, *41*, 313–318. [CrossRef]
83. Rodriguez, P.L.; Carrasco, L. Gliotoxin: Inhibitor of poliovirus RNA synthesis that blocks the viral RNA polymerase 3Dpol. *J. Virol.* **1992**, *66*, 1971–1976. [CrossRef]
84. Graci, J.D.; Cameron, C.E. Mechanisms of action of ribavirin against distinct viruses. *Rev. Med. Virol.* **2006**, *16*, 37–48. [CrossRef] [PubMed]
85. Crotty, S.; Maag, D.; Arnold, J.J.; Zhong, W.; Lau, J.Y.; Hong, Z.; Andino, R.; Cameron, C.E. The broad-spectrum antiviral ribonucleoside ribavirin is an RNA virus mutagen. *Nat. Med.* **2000**, *6*, 1375–1379. [CrossRef] [PubMed]

86. Crotty, S.; Cameron, C.E.; Andino, R. RNA virus error catastrophe: Direct molecular test by using ribavirin. *Proc. Natl. Acad. Sci. USA* **2001**, *98*, 6895–6900. [CrossRef]
87. Kempf, B.J.; Peersen, O.B.; Barton, D.J. Poliovirus Polymerase Leu420 Facilitates RNA Recombination and Ribavirin Resistance. *J. Virol.* **2016**, *90*, 8410–8421. [CrossRef]
88. Madia, V.N.; Messore, A.; Pescatori, L.; Saccoliti, F.; Tudino, V.; De Leo, A.; Scipione, L.; Fiore, L.; Rhoden, E.; Manetti, F.; et al. In Vitro Antiviral Activity of New Oxazoline Derivatives as Potent Poliovirus Inhibitors. *J. Med. Chem.* **2019**, *62*, 798–810. [CrossRef]
89. Abdelnabi, R.; Geraets, J.A.; Ma, Y.; Mirabelli, C.; Flatt, J.W.; Domanska, A.; Delang, L.; Jochmans, D.; Kumar, T.A.; Jayaprakash, V.; et al. A novel druggable interprotomer pocket in the capsid of rhino- and enteroviruses. *PLoS Biol.* **2019**, *17*, e3000281. [CrossRef]
90. Strating, J.R.; van der Linden, L.; Albulescu, L.; Bigay, J.; Arita, M.; Delang, L.; Leyssen, P.; van der Schaar, H.M.; Lanke, K.H.; Thibaut, H.J.; et al. Itraconazole inhibits enterovirus replication by targeting the oxysterol-binding protein. *Cell Rep.* **2015**, *10*, 600–615. [CrossRef]
91. Antiretroviral Drug Discovery and Development. Available online: https://www.niaid.nih.gov/diseases-conditions/antiretroviral-drug-development (accessed on 10 August 2024).
92. Warren, T.K.; Jordan, R.; Lo, M.K.; Ray, A.S.; Mackman, R.L.; Soloveva, V.; Siegel, D.; Perron, M.; Bannister, R.; Hui, H.C.; et al. Therapeutic efficacy of the small molecule GS-5734 against Ebola virus in rhesus monkeys. *Nature* **2016**, *531*, 381–385. [CrossRef]
93. Mosier, P.D.; Chiang, M.J.; Lin, Z.; Gao, Y.; Althufairi, B.; Zhou, Q.; Musayev, F.; Safo, M.K.; Xie, H.; Desai, U.R. Broad Spectrum Anti-Influenza Agents by Inhibiting Self-Association of Matrix Protein 1. *Sci. Rep.* **2016**, *6*, 32340. [CrossRef]
94. De Rosa, M.C.; Purohit, R.; Garcia-Sosa, A.T. Drug repurposing: A nexus of innovation, science, and potential. *Sci. Rep.* **2023**, *13*, 17887. [CrossRef]

pathogens

MDPI

Article

Evaluating the Effectiveness of External Molecular Proficiency Testing in the Global Polio Laboratory Network, 2021–2022

Nancy Gerloff * and Cara C. Burns

Division of Viral Diseases, Centers for Disease Control and Prevention (CDC), Atlanta, GA 30329, USA
* Correspondence: kfi4@cdc.gov

Abstract: In the Global Poliovirus Laboratory Network (GPLN), participation and successful completion in annual proficiency test (PT) panels has been a part of the WHO accreditation process for decades. The PT panel is a molecular external quality assessment (mEQA) that evaluates laboratory preparedness, technical proficiency, the accuracy of data interpretation, and result reporting. Using the Intratypic Differentiation (ITD) real-time RT-PCR kits from CDC, laboratories run screening assays and report results in accordance with the ITD algorithm to identify and type polioviruses. The mEQA panels consisted of 10 blinded, non-infectious lyophilized RNA transcripts, including programmatically relevant viruses and targets contained in the real-time PCR assays. Sample identities included wildtype, vaccine-derived (VDPV), Sabin-like polioviruses, enterovirus, and negatives, as well as categories of invalid and indeterminate. The performance of individual laboratories was assessed based on the laboratory's ability to correctly detect and characterize the serotype/genotype identities of each sample. The scoring scheme assessed the laboratory readiness following GPLN guidelines. Laboratories receiving mEQA scores of 90 or higher passed the assessment, scores of less than 90 failed and required remedial actions and re-evaluation. In 2021 and 2022, 123 and 129 GPLN laboratories were invited to request the annual PT panel, and 118 and 127 laboratories submitted results, respectively. The overall results were good, with 86% and 91.5% of laboratories passing the PT panel on their first attempt in 2021 and 2022, respectively. Most labs scored the highest score of 100, and less than one quarter scored between 90 and 95. Less than 10% of submitting laboratories failed the PT, resulting in in-depth troubleshooting to identify root causes and remediations. Most of these laboratories were issued a second PT panel for repeat testing, and almost all laboratories passed the repeat PT panel. The results of the 2021 and 2022 annual mEQA PTs showed that, despite the COVID-19 pandemic, the performance remained high in the GPLN, with most labs achieving the highest score. For these labs, the real-time PCR assay updates that were implemented during 2021–2022 were carried out with full adherence to procedures and algorithms. Even initially failing labs achieved passing scores after remediation.

Keywords: poliovirus; molecular external quality assessment; nucleic acid testing; World Health Organization; Global Polio Eradication Initiative; quality assurance program; accreditation; proficiency panel testing

1. Introduction

The Global Polio Laboratory Network (GPLN) has been the pivotal instrument for aligning poliovirus diagnostic methodologies across the global landscape of technologies. The global surveillance for acute flaccid paralysis (AFP) cases tests more than 200,000 specimens during a year [1]. The testing follows a specific algorithm using virus isolation in susceptible cell lines followed by real-time reverse transcription PCR (RT-PCR) testing and sequencing if required. Most labs perform one of the three main workstreams or a combination of them. Over the last decades, the GPLN has grown from a handful of laboratories to 144 GPLN laboratories in 2024. The accreditation process includes demonstrated proficiency in the four-tiered format for each of the tiers: (I) virus isolation for polioviruses (PV), (II) intratypic differentiation of polioviruses (real-time RT-PCR), and (III) sequencing, as well as successful completion of an on-site inspection.

In the GPLN, laboratories have participated in the annual proficiency test (PT) panel as a required component of the WHO accreditation process [2]. The molecular external quality assessment (mEQA) or molecular proficiency testing (PT) panel evaluates the ability to type poliovirus isolates in conjunction with laboratory preparedness, technical proficiency, the accuracy of data interpretation, and result reporting (Figure 1). Using the Intratypic Differentiation (ITD) primer and probes from CDC, laboratories run a suite of real-time RT-PCR screening assays and report results in accordance with the ITD algorithm to identify and type polioviruses. It is now used by GPLN laboratories in all six WHO regions.

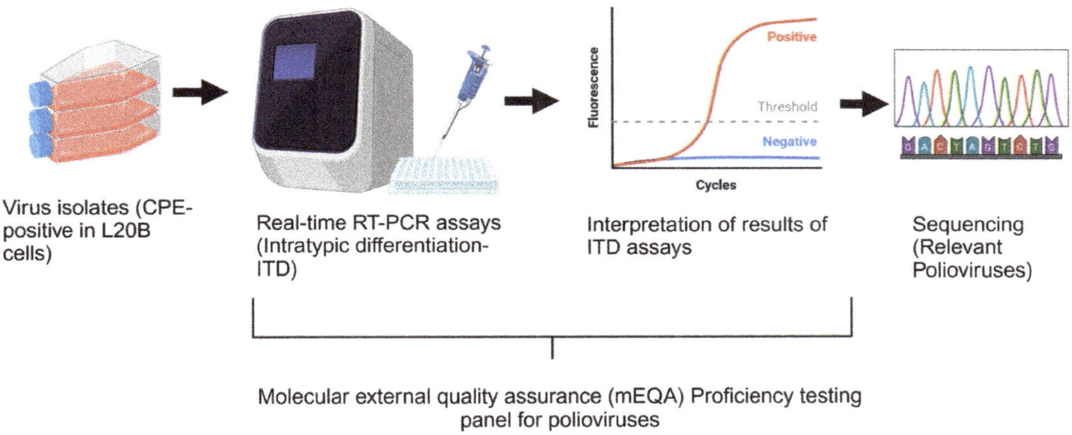

Figure 1. Scheme of annual poliovirus proficiency testing workflow for the molecular external quality assurance (mEQA) using real-time RT-PCR (ITD testing). Separate PT panels exist for virus isolation and sequencing components of poliovirus testing.

As one of the Global Specialized Laboratories, the Polio and Picornavirus Branch at the CDC in the United States has been instrumental in assay and method development, technical support, reagent provision, and the administration of the molecular proficiency testing panels. In early surveillance, laboratories performed serotyping by microneutralization using cross-adsorbed antibodies. After serotyping, ITD allowed differentiation between wild and vaccine strains [3]. Starting in 2004, the laboratory performance for methods such as probe hybridization, or ITD by ELISA, or gel-based RT-PCR, which have been replaced by a suite of real-time reverse transcription PCR (RT-PCR) assays in 2009, abbreviated as ITD [4–6]. Since 2013, the suite of real-time RT-PCR assays has undergone several iterations (version 1.0 to version 4.0) to adjust the assays for changing virus circulation patterns and vaccine usage (i.e., wildtype PV 1 genetic drift, cessation of oral polio vaccine type 2 in 2016, and the usage of novel OPV2 in 2020) [7–9]. Released in 2023, the ITD version 6.0 consists of assays with 11 targets that are tested for polioviruses [10].

Poliovirus diagnostic testing starts by inoculating acute flaccid paralysis (AFP) stool suspensions into susceptible cell lines, rhabdomyosarcoma (RD), and L20B cells (murine recombinant cells with the poliovirus receptor), followed by passaging, which is termed virus isolation. If the cytopathic effect (CPE) is observed in cells, isolates will be directly used in real-time RT-PCR without an RNA extraction step. A separate virus isolation proficiency testing panel is distributed by the Global Specialized Laboratory RIVM (The Netherlands) and aims at testing proficiency in isolation of poliovirus, cell sensitivity as well as the ability to determine CPE positivity [11]. Isolates positive in the virus isolation are tested in PCR (ITD), followed by reflex assays (VDPV assays to confirm Sabin 1 or Sabin 3). Any programmatically relevant serotypes and genotypes must be sequenced for confirmation (wildtype 1, any PV type 2, wildtype 3, and vaccine-derived polioviruses, VDPV). Oral polio vaccine strains, such as Sabin-like 1 and Sabin-like-3, do not require sequence confirmation. The ITD result is used to select appropriate sequencing primers for amplification of the complete Viral Protein 1 (VP1). The resulting Sanger sequence can be genotyped and classified as wild or vaccine-derived poliovirus [10,12].

2. Methods

2.1. Participating Laboratories and Preparation of the mEQA Panel

In 2021 and 2022, accredited and new GPLN laboratories from all six WHO regions were invited to participate in the annual proficiency testing panel. The PT panels were made available to International Reagent Resource (IRR) registrants and GPLN member labs between September 2021 and November 2021 and October 2022 and December 2022. Laboratories participating in the mEQA use the suite of ITD assays to discriminate among serotypes 1, 2, and 3, as well as distinguish wildtype viruses from vaccine-related polioviruses (Figure 1). There are two reflex real-time RT-PCR assays that are used as a screen to flag viruses that have mutated at key target sites (VDPV1 and VDPV3 assays). Use of the correct reporting scheme and correct interpretation of the assay results are crucial steps to pass the PT panel. Participating laboratories were provided with a standardized reporting sheet that collected test results and testing information, such as equipment used for testing (PCR cycler) and reagent information (lot numbers, expiration dates). In 2021–2022, the following real-time RT-PCR cyclers were validated for ITD and VDPV assays and GPLN use (AB 7500, AB 7500 Fast, QuantStudio 5 [Thermo Fisher: Applied Biosystems, Foster City, CA, USA]; CFX96 [Bio-Rad, Hercules, CA, USA]; Rotor-Gene Q [Qiagen, Germantown, PA, USA]; MxP3005X [Agilent, Santa Clara, CA, USA]).

CDC (Atlanta, GA, USA) and the IRR (Manassas, VA, USA) are the manufacturers of the PT panels. Whereas CDC designs and determines suitability in the quality assessment and quality control (QA/QC) process, IRR is responsible for aliquoting, lyophilizing, labeling, and packaging the mEQA panels for distribution in the GPLN. The mEQA panels were five versions, with each containing a randomized set of 10 blinded non-infectious RNA transcripts to test the ability to detect and type the nucleic acid of poliovirus types 1, 2, and 3 or mixtures thereof. The 10 RNAs also contained non-poliovirus transcripts made up only of Enterovirus RNA (5′ Untranslated region, 5′-UTR), Qβ bacteriophage RNA transcript, or negative template control (water). Each version was composed of multiple RNA transcripts (in total, 16 different RNA transcripts were used, for a total of 30 PT panels per version, Table 1). The mEQA addresses levels of sensitivity on different thermocyclers and assays sensitivity differences (i.e., redundant assays are positive for multiple targets for one RNA transcript). Triplicates of each of the dispensed and lyophilized RNA transcripts were tested in each of the 6 ITD assays (for ITD version 5.2 only, 5 assays were run, plus the nOPV2 Supplemental assay) and the respective VDPV assays (Sabin 1 or Sabin 3-positive transcripts only). The PT panel was evaluated on the GPLN cyclers, including AB 7500, CFX96, and Rotor Gene Q.

PT panel version numbers are omitted from the ordering catalog and box label, and the RNA transcripts are anonymized as Unknown A through Unknown J. The version of the PT panel is tracked by the CDC; version identities are not disclosed to any participating laboratory prior to testing. Labs were instructed to use either the ITD version 5.2 (or version 5.1), the Supplemental nOPV2 assay (not required for all labs), and the VPDV assay kit version 5.2 kit (or non-expired version VPDV 5.0) for testing in 2021, and 2022.

Table 1. Characteristics of the RNA transcripts used in mEQA for polio ITD and VDPV screening in the WHO GPLN, 2021–2022.

Sample ID	Composition (RNA Transcripts)	Serotype/Genotype PCR Target	Expected Result in ITD/VDPV Algorithm
1	WPV1, Sabin 1 or WPV1, Sabin 3	WPV1, Sabin 1 or WPV1, Sabin 3	NSL1 + SL1 or NSL1 + SL3
2	VDPV1 or VDPV3	VDPV1, or VDPV3	SL3 or SL1 discordant
3	Sabin 3	Sabin 3	SL3
4	Sabin 1 (low concentration), Sabin 3 (high)	Sabin 1, Sabin 3	SL1 + SL3
5	WPV1 or Sabin 1	EV 5′UTR, WPV1, or EV 5′UTR, Sabin 1	Invalid NSL1, SL1
6	WPV1, Sabin 1, Sabin 3	WPV1, Sabin 1, Sabin 3	NSL1 + SL1 + SL3
7	WPV3	WPV3	NSL3
8	Sabin 1, VPDV3	Sabin 1, VDPV3	SL1 + SL3 discordant
9	Sabin 2 or nOPV2	Sabin 2 or nOPV2	PV2
10	nOPV2, WPV1	nOPV2, WPV1	PV2 + NSL1
11	EV	EV 5′UTR	NPEV, non-polio-enterovirus
12	EV, PV	EV 5′UTR, PanPV	Indeterminate
13	Water, Qβ only	Qβ	Non-enterovirus (Qβ positive)

Note: discordant: vaccine-derived poliovirus, EV: enterovirus, invalid: PCR invalid (negative in PanPV or EV target), indeterminate: no serotype positive (PanPV and EV detected), NEV: non-enterovirus (negative), NSL: non-Sabin-like, Qβ: Qβ bacteriophage (non-poliovirus target for extraction control), PanPV: assay to detect any poliovirus, EV-5′UTR: 5′ untranslated region in enterovirus genome (including poliovirus).

2.2. Data Collection and Analysis

PT panel results were submitted using a website submission tool starting in the 2022 season. In 2021, PT panel results were evaluated after submission either through email or the GPLN management submission database, including raw data files, results following the WHO GPLN reporting scheme, and completed reporting sheets (standardized documents). Evaluation of raw data files was performed by a subject matter expert in the CDC Polio Team, and PT panel scores and comments were communicated via email or the submission tool in a standardized format. Each lab received detailed feedback about deductions, and the errors were categorized for annual tracking. Only one submission per lab was accepted for an annual score. New labs were assessed on a practice PT panel first before being invited to participate in the annual PT panel assessment and submission to the website in 2022.

3. Results

3.1. The GPLN Landscape and Overall Proficiency

The performance of individual GPLN laboratories was assessed based on the laboratory's ability to correctly detect and characterize poliovirus serotype and genotype identities deemed programmatically critical to the Global Polio Program. The scoring scheme assesses the laboratory readiness following GPLN guidelines based on relevant serotypes, interpretation, and the reporting algorithm used between 2021 and 2022 (Table 2). Laboratories receiving mEQA scores of 90 or greater passed the annual assessment; scores of less than 90 failed and required remedial actions and re-evaluation, including repetition of another PT panel.

In 2021, 123 laboratories were invited to request the annual PT panel, with five labs not participating or not submitting results by the close of the PT panel season (Figure 2). The overall results were good, with 105/123 (86%) of participants passing the PT panel on their first attempt (Table 3). About a quarter of the laboratories scored between 90 and 95 (n = 26), and all other laboratories achieved a score of 100. Thirteen failed the PT on their first attempt, resulting in in-depth troubleshooting to identify root causes for errors and remediation (Table 4). Failing laboratories were issued a second PT panel for repeat testing, eight labs passed, and one lab failed again. One laboratory was not issued a repeat PT panel because remediation was not completed until after the season was closed. Regional differences were noted but not significant, with AFR, AMR, and SEAR regions showing the best results, with all labs passing (one SEAR lab did not participate in 2021 and 2022).

Table 2. Scoring scheme for PT panel in 2021 and 2022. Abbreviations: PV2-poliovirus type 2, Qβ-bacteriophage, VDPV-vaccine-derived-poliovirus, WPV-wildtype poliovirus.

Scoring Scheme	Deduction	Comments
Major deductions for incorrect results	−15	Failure to detect/identify WPV, VDPV, PV2, or indeterminate
	−10	Failure to detect a single Sabin virus or invalid
	−5	Failure to detect a Sabin virus in a mixture
Deductions for technical issues	−10	Not recognizing failed control(s)
	−5	Failure to follow algorithm or correctly reporting results
	−5	Incorrectly interpreting curves (e.g., entering "positive" on a negative result)
	−5	Failure to correctly set up and report Qβ target in WPV1/Qβ duplex
Late reporting	−5	Per week for any results received > 7 days after panel receipt
Readiness	−15	Not ready to process panel with available reagents or personnel

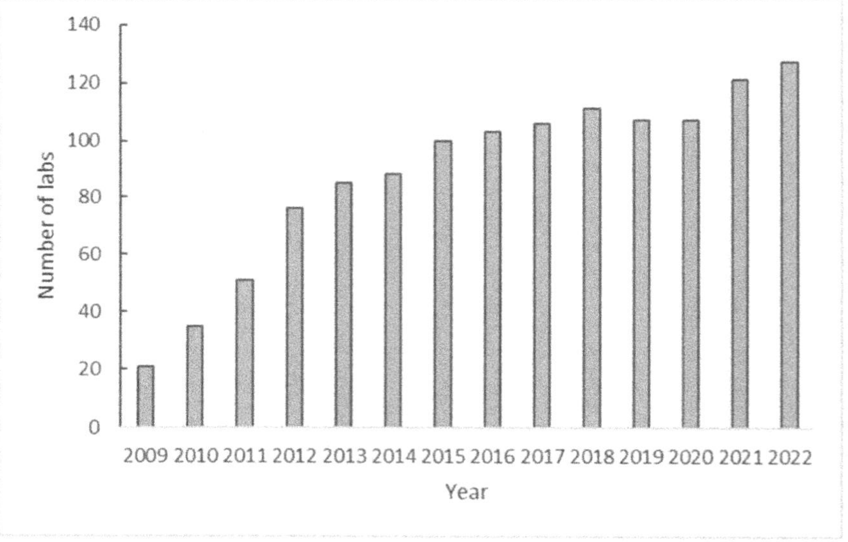

Figure 2. Number of GPLN laboratories participating in the annual mEQA PT panel between 2009 and 2022 using real-time RT-PCR (ITD testing).

In 2022, PT panels were assessed for 127 laboratories (129 labs invited) with passing scores for 118 (91.5%), and only 9 labs failed the PT panel the first time (Table 3). After the remediation, seven labs passed their second attempt. Five new labs participated for the first time in the ITD PT panel and were invited to submit their results after passing the practice panel with scores >90. Overall, most labs were highly proficient in passing the mEQA on their first attempt. There were 52 laboratories that submitted their results using the online web interface (GPLNMS), and after review of run files, the mEQA results were uploaded to the website by the CDC Polio Team, and an automated email informed the lab of the scores. Remediation was either performed by issuing a new PT panel to the lab or a virtual training using virtual PT panels (raw data files for interpretation), followed by issuance of another PT panel. In both years, only two labs were unable to repeat the panel, or communication dropped. The number of participating labs in all regions remained steady except for the EUR region, which added 14 new labs between the 2020 and 2022 seasons.

Table 3. Regional scores for mEQA PT panels in 2021 and 2022 (passing scores 90–100, failing scores < 90) and percentages of overall performances.

	Year 2021				Year 2022			
WHO Region	**Labs Invited**	**Passed**	**Failed**	**Not Participated**	**Labs Invited**	**Passed**	**Failed**	**Not Participated**
AFR	16	16	0	0	16	13	3	0
AMR	11	8	0	3	11	8	2	1
EMR	11	9	2	0	11	10	1	0
EUR	27	17	9	1	33	30	3	0
SEAR	16	15	0	1	16	15	0	1
WPR	42	40	2	0	42	42	0	0
TOTAL (%)	123 (100%)	105 (86%)	13 (11%)	5 (4%)	129 (100%)	118 (91.5%)	9 (7%)	2 (1.6%)
After remediation (%)	123	113 (91.9%)	5 (4%)	5 (4%)	129	125 (96.9%)	2 (1.6%)	2 (1.6%)

Table 4. Summary of PT panel year 2021 and 2022 by error category. Counts were reported with multiple errors per lab; Only the errors were counted if deductions were made to the overall score.

PT Panel Year		2021		2022	
Number of labs participating (total)		118		127	
Category of errors (any observation if score <100)		Number of observations	Percentage (of total labs)	Number of observations	Percentage (of total labs)
Reporting		11	9.1%	17	13.8%
Timeliness (>7 days)		2	1.7%	3	2.4%
Following algorithm		7	5.8%	8	6.5%
Technical (overall)		17	14.0%	15	12.2%
	Curve interpretation	17	14.0%	5	4.1%
	Assay set up	26	21.5%	13	10.2%
	Run method set up	9	7.4%	5	4.1%

3.2. *Variability in Laboratories*

In both years, any lab that requested the PT panel was ready to perform and report the results. Very few labs asked for a delayed delivery due to National Holiday(s) or shortages in staffing due to the conflicting diagnostic testing due to the SARS-Co-V 2 pandemic. The breakdown per error category showed that about 9% and 14% in 2021 and 2022, respectively, made reporting mistakes (incorrect poliovirus serotype or missing mixtures). For 14% and 12% of submitting labs, a combination of technical errors was observed, resulting from interpretation errors (incorrectly called a negative result positive or failed PCR controls) or due to an incorrect assay setup (such as wrong dye or no target selected), or due to an incorrect PCR run method (Table 4). Timeliness issues were observed in less than 3% of the participating labs in either year. Few labs received deductions for failure to follow the correct testing algorithm or mistakes in reporting, with little variation in 2021 and 2022 (5.8% and 6.5%). Examples included not performing the reflex assays for mixtures of Sabin-like 1 or 3-positive RNAs for any mixtures of Sabin and other poliovirus types (Table 4). Most labs were capable of reporting results correctly, but a slight increase was observed in misreporting from 9% in 2021 to 13.8% in 2022. Inversely, labs improved on assay setup in 2022 with only 13 observations instead of 26 the year prior. The most challenging RNA transcripts were samples 12 and 13, with nine labs incorrectly reporting.

Most laboratories submitted their results that were generated using AB 7500 (67%) or CFX96 cyclers (Bio-Rad, 17%), followed by Rotor Gene Q (Qiagen) and Quant Studio cyclers (Thermo Fisher Scientific). Only a few laboratories used other cyclers that had not been validated by the CDC Polio Branch, and assessments were made using either screenshots of the results (Quant Studio 12, Thermo Fisher) or specific PCR cycler software to evaluate runs (Design and Analysis version 2.6.0 software, Quant Studio 7, Thermo Fisher).

4. Discussion

The annual molecular proficiency testing for GPLN labs is part of the accreditation process in the worldwide network and has been a pillar for quality assessments and quality assurance since its inception in 1989. This study reports the results of the years 2021 and 2022 of the mEQA for poliovirus combined ITD and VDPV testing panel for the WHO GPLN laboratories in all six WHO regions. The scheme follows GPLN methods and the poliovirus testing and typing algorithm using a suite of PCR assays, followed by reflex assays for referrals. Performance within the GPLN was high, with 86% of labs scoring a passing score of 90 or greater in 2021 (in their first attempt), and this increased to 90% in 2022. Most inaccuracies were due to technical errors such as curve interpretation, assay setup or run method setup, as well as reporting errors. Several labs in the WHO European Region that have participated for the first time in the mEQA PT panel were able to pass at their first attempt, showing that the design and level of complexity can be overcome by initially assessing the lab's capability on a practice PT panel.

Remediation was initiated by regional polio laboratory coordinators and entailed a data review, repeating another PT panel, or a combination of a deeper root cause analysis performed by the laboratory, followed by virtual PT panels reviewed by the CDC Polio Team. After remediation failed for the second time, the labs were encouraged to attend training in their region to mitigate the performance issues.

Several labs used the online submission tool in GPLNMS in 2022 (n = 52), which provided a smooth experience through reporting with drop-down menus (decreasing the chance of entering an error due to incorrect terminology). The communication was streamlined through the website with automatic emails to submitters, and the PT panel grading was facilitated through concise data collection and real-time reporting. Labs uploaded all relevant PCR run files and submitted metadata, such as the lot number of PCR kits and PCR cyclers, which enabled a quicker analysis of the 2022 PT panel progress.

The PCR assays do not have any CT value cut-off, making interpretation potentially more difficult for inexperienced labs not accustomed to the assay's curves (sigmoidal curves), hence multiple errors in curve interpretation were observed, but these dropped sharply from 2021 to 2022. The PT panel composition did not vary significantly between the two years; the only difference was the randomization of each version. Due to different PCR cyclers being used in the network and the different assay sensitivities, the CT values for each of the Unknown RNA transcripts were assessed using the most common cyclers (ABI 7500 and CFX96). This is a limitation for the mEQA and previous attempts to decrease concentration for RNA transcripts failed, due to the low sensitivity of some assays that could not consistently detect the RNA target at a very low concentration (such as the least sensitive assays for WPV1, and VDPV3 targets in the ITD suite) [8,9]. Some errors that were observed in both years are largely avoidable through careful supervision by senior scientists (required since 2023). For example, the assay protocols provided inside the kit (each ITD and VDPV kit insert comes folded in the box) detail the run method and the setup of fluorescent dyes for each cycler.

Most laboratories were already IRR registrants and able to order and receive poliovirus testing reagents including PT panels. Several laboratories needed frequent email reminders and engagement by the regional coordinator before PT panels were completed in both years. Despite the RNA being non-infectious transcripts, some countries required extensive import documentation, hindering the shipment within the expected timeframe for the PT panel receipt and completion. Annual mEQA PT panels are typically released between September and November for GPLN; this can lead to issues due to national holidays. In a network of this size (n = 144 labs), it is impossible to align the release and completion for the 6 WHO regions for all PT panels (including the tiered PT panels for virus isolation or sequencing).

For future PT panels, more realistic RNA concentrations need to be assessed to prepare labs for future testing algorithms, for example, using RNA extracted from stools. One RNA transcript sample contained Qβ bacteriophage in preparation for an anticipated change in the GPLN methodology from virus isolation to RNA extraction from AFP specimens and PCR testing. In the future, Qβ will be used to monitor the RNA extraction success and assist in checking for inconsistencies due to the method's performance [13]. The Qβ target has been helpful in assessing the presence of inhibitors due to inefficient extraction. In 2023, all PT panels were reported through GPLNMS, streamlining the process of reporting results for the grading lab and the submitters. Despite the SARS-CoV-2 pandemic, the GPLN maintained its proficiency while handling an increased need for respiratory specimen testing in the National Labs during the COVID-19 pandemic.

5. Conclusions

Most laboratories participating in the GPLN maintained their proficiency in poliovirus molecular detection during the COVID-19 pandemic in 2021 and 2022. GPLN laboratories consistently performed at a high level overall, and assay updates were implemented with proper adherence to protocols and package inserts. Molecular EQA PT panel testing provides WHO and the Global Polio Laboratory Network with valuable data to understand testing capabilities as well as identify training and technical support needs.

Author Contributions: Conceptualization, N.G. and C.C.B.; methodology, N.G.; formal analysis, N.G.; investigation, N.G.; data curation, N.G.; writing—original draft preparation, N.G.; writing—review and editing, C.C.B.; visualization, N.G.; supervision, C.C.B. All authors have read and agreed to the published version of the manuscript.

Funding: This research received no external funding.

Institutional Review Board Statement: Not applicable.

Informed Consent Statement: Not applicable.

Data Availability Statement: The datasets presented in this article are not readily available because the data are part of the restricted system supporting the accreditation of the Global Polio Network Laboratories, individual laboratory data will not be disclosed due to GPEI and WHO limitations. Requests to access the datasets should be directed to www.polioeradication.org.

Acknowledgments: The authors would like to thank the WHO regional coordinators and the WHO headquarters for the support in the PT panel administration providing guidance and provision of the website tool for submission, especially the Global Polio Laboratory Coordinator Ousmane M. Diop, and Technical Coordinator Shahzad Shaukat. The authors also thank the Polio Molecular Diagnostic Development team for the quality assessment of RNA transcripts, grading, and laboratory support activities, especially Hong Sun, Stacey Jeffries Miles, Brandon Short, Paula L. Marcet. We thank Chelsea Harrington, and Everardo M. Vega for support of previous mEQA seasons.

Conflicts of Interest: The authors declare no conflicts of interest.

Disclaimer: The findings and conclusions in this report are those of the author(s) and do not necessarily represent the official position of the Centers for Disease Control and Prevention. The use of trade names is for identification only and does not imply endorsement by the CDC or the US government.

References

1. Lickness, J.S.; Gardner, T.; Diop, O.M.; Chavan, S.; Jorba, J.; Ahmed, J.; Gumede, N.; Johnson, T.; Butt, O.; Asghar, H.; et al. Surveillance to Track Progress Toward Polio Eradication—Worldwide, 2018–2019. *MMWR Morb. Mortal. Wkly. Rep.* **2020**, *69*, 623–629. [CrossRef] [PubMed]
2. Zaidi, S.S.Z.; Asghar, H.; Sharif, S.; Alam, M.M. Poliovirus Laboratory Based Surveillance: An Overview. In *Poliovirus: Methods and Protocols*; Martín, J., Ed.; Springer: New York, NY, USA, 2016; pp. 11–18. [CrossRef]

3. Hull, B.P.; Dowdle, W.R. Poliovirus Surveillance: Building the Global Polio Laboratory Network. *J. Infect. Dis.* **1997**, *175*, S113–S116. [CrossRef] [PubMed]
4. Kilpatrick, D.R.; Nottay, B.; Yang, C.F.; Yang, S.J.; Da Silva, E.; Penaranda, S.; Pallansch, M.; Kew, O. Serotype-specific identification of polioviruses by PCR using primers containing mixed-base or deoxyinosine residues at positions of codon degeneracy. *J. Clin. Microbiol.* **1998**, *36*, 352–357. [CrossRef] [PubMed]
5. Kilpatrick, D.R.; Nottay, B.; Yang, C.F.; Yang, S.J.; Mulders, M.N.; Holloway, B.P.; Pallansch, M.A.; Kew, O.M. Group-specific identification of polioviruses by PCR using primers containing mixed-base or deoxyinosine residue at positions of codon degeneracy. *J. Clin. Microbiol.* **1996**, *34*, 2990–2996. [CrossRef] [PubMed]
6. Kilpatrick, D.R.; Yang, C.F.; Ching, K.; Vincent, A.; Iber, J.; Campagnoli, R.; Mandelbaum, M.; De, L.; Yang, S.J.; Nix, A.; et al. Rapid group-, serotype-, and vaccine strain-specific identification of poliovirus isolates by real-time reverse transcription-PCR using degenerate primers and probes containing deoxyinosine residues. *J. Clin. Microbiol.* **2009**, *47*, 1939–1941. [CrossRef] [PubMed]
7. GPEI. Updates on ITD Molecular Testing. 2016. Available online: https://polioeradication.org/wp-content/uploads/2024/05/GP2-Updates-on-ITD-molecular-testing.pdf (accessed on 4 October 2024).
8. Gerloff, N.; Sun, H.; Mandelbaum, M.; Maher, C.; Nix, W.A.; Zaidi, S.; Shaukat, S.; Seakamela, L.; Nalavade, U.P.; Sharma, D.K.; et al. Diagnostic Assay Development for Poliovirus Eradication. *J. Clin. Microbiol.* **2018**, *56*, e01624-17. [CrossRef] [PubMed]
9. Sun, H.; Harrington, C.; Gerloff, N.; Mandelbaum, M.; Jeffries-Miles, S.; Apostol, L.N.G.; Valencia, M.A.D.; Shaukat, S.; Angez, M.; Sharma, D.K.; et al. Validation of a redesigned pan-poliovirus assay and real-time PCR platforms for the global poliovirus laboratory network. *PLoS ONE* **2021**, *16*, e0255795. [CrossRef] [PubMed]
10. Burns, C.C.; Kilpatrick, D.R.; Iber, J.C.; Chen, Q.; Kew, O.M. Molecular Properties of Poliovirus Isolates: Nucleotide Sequence Analysis, Typing by PCR and Real-Time RT-PCR. In *Poliovirus: Methods and Protocols*; Martín, J., Ed.; Springer: New York, NY, USA, 2016; pp. 177–212. [CrossRef]
11. Thorley, B.R.; Roberts, J.A. Isolation and Characterization of Poliovirus in Cell Culture Systems. In *Poliovirus: Methods and Protocols*; Martín, J., Ed.; Springer: New York, NY, USA, 2016; pp. 29–53. [CrossRef]
12. Kilpatrick, D.R.; Iber, J.C.; Chen, Q.; Ching, K.; Yang, S.J.; De, L.; Mandelbaum, M.D.; Emery, B.; Campagnoli, R.; Burns, C.C.; et al. Poliovirus serotype-specific VP1 sequencing primers. *J. Virol. Methods* **2011**, *174*, 128–130. [CrossRef] [PubMed]
13. Miles, S.J.; Harrington, C.; Sun, H.; Deas, A.; Oberste, M.S.; Nix, W.A.; Vega, E.; Gerloff, N. Validation of improved automated nucleic acid extraction methods for direct detection of polioviruses for global polio eradication. *J. Virol. Methods* **2024**, *326*, 114914. [CrossRef] [PubMed]

pathogens

MDPI

Review

Immunodeficiency-Related Vaccine-Derived Poliovirus (iVDPV) Infections: A Review of Epidemiology and Progress in Detection and Management

Concepcion F. Estivariz [1,*], Elisabeth R. Krow-Lucal [1,2] and Ondrej Mach [2]

[1] U.S. Centers for Disease Control and Prevention, 1600 Clifton Road, Atlanta, GA 30033, USA; liz.krowlucal@gatesfoundation.org
[2] World Health Organization Headquarters, Av Appia 10, 1211 Geneva, Switzerland; macho@who.int
* Correspondence: cge3@cdc.gov

Abstract: Individuals with certain primary immunodeficiency disorders (PID) may be unable to clear poliovirus infection after exposure to oral poliovirus vaccine (OPV). Over time, vaccine-related strains can revert to immunodeficiency-associated vaccine-derived poliovirus (iVDPVs) that can cause paralysis in the patient and potentially spread in communities with low immunity. We reviewed the efforts for detection and management of PID patients with iVDPV infections and the epidemiology through an analysis of 184 cases reported to the World Health Organization (WHO) during 1962–2024 and a review of polio program and literature reports. Most iVDPV patients (79%) reported in the WHO Registry were residents in middle-income countries and almost half (48%) in the Eastern Mediterranean Region. Type 2 iVDPV was most frequently isolated (53%), but a sharp decline was observed after the switch to bivalent OPV in 2016, with only six cases reported during 2017–2024 compared to 63 during 2009–2016. Patients with common variable immunodeficiency have longer excretion of iVDPV than with other PID types. Implementation of sensitive sentinel surveillance to detect cases of iVDPV infection in high-risk countries and offer antiviral treatment to patients is challenged by competition with other health priorities and regulatory hurdles to the compassionate use of investigational antiviral drugs.

Keywords: immunodeficiency disorders; poliovirus; vaccine-derived poliovirus; vaccine-associated paralytic poliomyelitis

1. Introduction

The use of oral poliovirus vaccine (OPV) worldwide in childhood immunization and vaccination campaigns has been the main strategy of the Global Polio Eradication Initiative (GPEI). This approach has reduced wild poliovirus (WPV) circulation by 99.9%, from >350,000 estimated cases in 125 countries in 1988 to 12 cases in two countries in 2023 [1]. The live, attenuated Sabin strains contained in OPV multiply in oropharyngeal and gastrointestinal mucosae, mimicking natural infection, and induce humoral and mucosal immunity. Upon new exposure to wild or vaccine poliovirus, humoral immunity protects against paralysis whereas mucosal immunity reduces viral replication and excretion through stools or oropharyngeal secretions, thus interrupting person-to-person transmission [2,3]. Additionally, OPV is easy to administer in mass campaigns and vaccine virus can indirectly vaccinate close contacts, which enhances field effectiveness.

However, the genetic instability of Sabin strains leads them to mutate and recombine with other enteroviruses, whereby they may re-acquire the fitness of wild strains [4–6]. Reversion of key mutations associated with neurovirulence can occur shortly after receiving OPV and on rare occasions may result in vaccine-associated poliomyelitis (VAPP) in recipients or close contacts [7,8]. Prolonged replication within one individual or sustained person-to-person transmission within a community with low immunity allows Sabin-related strains to evolve to vaccine-derived poliovirus (VDPVs) which have re-acquired the neurovirulence and transmissibility of wild poliovirus strains [5,6,9,10]. In areas with low population immunity, outbreaks of infections due to circulating VDPVs (cVDPVs) require several immunization campaigns to stop transmission and prevent the establishment of endemic poliovirus transmission [11]. Since 2017, the reported numbers of paralytic polio cases caused by cVDPV have exceeded cases caused by WPV, with a total of 419 WPV cases and 3794 cVDPV cases reported during 2017–2023 (data as of 30 September 2024) [1]. The risks of VAPP and cVDPV outbreaks associated with OPV led the GPEI to conclude that cessation of OPV use is essential to maintain a polio-free world after the eradication of WPV [12].

Individuals with certain primary immunodeficiencies (PID) that severely affect B-cell function may be unable to clear vaccine poliovirus after receiving OPV or having been in contact with a vaccinee, therefore becoming asymptomatic carriers for months or years. With prolonged replication in these individuals, Sabin-related strains evolve to immunodeficiency-associated VDPVs (iVDPVs). Sabin strains or iVDPVs may cause paralytic polio at any time in the immunodeficient individual, resulting in an estimated risk of paralytic polio associated with OPV about 3000-fold higher than that observed for immunocompetent individuals [7,13]. PID patients shedding iVDPVs may also theoretically spread poliovirus in communities with low immunity, posing a potential threat for the re-introduction of poliovirus and outbreaks after the eradication of WPV and cessation of OPV use [14].

To better understand and mitigate the risks posed by iVDPV excretors to global polio eradication, the GPEI has maintained a registry of immunodeficient cases with prolonged shedding of poliovirus or iVDPV since 1961. During the early 2000s, GPEI supported studies to assess the prevalence of prolonged excretion of poliovirus among patients with different types of immunodeficiency disorders in a variety of countries. In the last decade, GPEI has pursued the introduction of sentinel surveillance for the detection of poliovirus among patients with certain PIDs in several higher-middle and lower-middle income countries considered at higher risk for iVDPV emergence. In addition, since the early 2000s, GPEI partners have supported the development of antivirals and monoclonal antibodies that can be used to treat chronic poliovirus infections.

This report summarizes current knowledge on the clinical and epidemiological characteristics of poliovirus infection in immunodeficient individuals. We reviewed the biomedical literature on prevalence studies and case reports published to date and performed an updated epidemiological analysis of patients with iVDPV infection reported to the WHO Registry during 1962–2024. In addition, we describe current GPEI efforts to detect and treat PID patients with iVDPV infection to interrupt shedding and prevent potential community transmission.

2. Materials and Methods

2.1. Study Population

This study analyzes cases reported to the iVDPV Data Registry maintained by the World Health Organization (WHO) from 1962 to June 2024 and cases identified through a literature search. The main sources of cases reported in the WHO iVDPV Registry were focal points for polio surveillance or representatives of the Global Poliovirus Laboratory Network (GPLN) at country and regional levels. Initially, most of the cases were identified through surveillance for Acute Flaccid Paralysis (AFP). Since 2010, a high number of cases with or without paralysis were identified during cross-sectional studies or pilot surveillance projects that screened patients with suspected or diagnosed PID for poliovirus infection.

To identify possible cases missing in the WHO database, we conducted a search of articles published in peer-reviewed journals. We used previous systematic reviews for reference mining on patients with iVDPV infection up to 2016 [5,15,16]. For the years 2014–2024, we conducted a literature search in PubMed using key search terms: VDPV, iVDPV, immunodeficiency, immunocompromised, polio, and "vaccine-associated paralytic poliomyelitis".

Our definition for an iVDPV case for analysis was a laboratory-confirmed VDPV infection in a person of any age with a primary humoral or combined humoral and cellular immunodeficiency disorder. Six cases in the WHO iVDPV Data Registry as of 24 July 2024 were excluded after confirmation of duplicate entry, and two cases were excluded because there was insufficient information to confirm iVDPV (i.e., no genetic sequencing performed).

Testing for poliovirus in stool, oropharyngeal swabs, or other specimens from iVDPV cases was mostly performed in laboratories that are members of the WHO Global Polio Laboratory Network (GPLN), using standardized protocols [17]. Testing usually involves the isolation of poliovirus through growth in cultured cells, followed by an enzyme-linked immunosorbent assay or a reverse transcriptase polymerase chain reaction to identify the serotype and differentiate between wild and vaccine strains. Lastly, sequencing of the genome sequence encoding the major capsid protein, viral protein 1 (VP1), is conducted to distinguish VDPV from Sabin-related strains. Based upon the nucleotide substitution rate of ~1.1% per year in the VP1-coding region, VDPVs are defined as having a VP1 nucleotide divergence from the Sabin strain >1% for types 1 and 3, and >0.6% for type 2. Genetic sequencing of the VP1 region, and in some cases, full poliovirus genome sequencing, allows the assessment of nucleotide divergence between strains and the tracking of pathways of transmission of WPV and VDPVs [5,18].

2.2. Statistical Analysis

Epidemiological data available in the database included the patient's country of residence, patient's date of paralysis onset, date of first positive iVDPV isolation (and additional samples), patient gender, age at paralysis onset or iVDPV detection, polio serotype, and percentage VP1 divergence from the parenteral Sabin strain. If missing, information on type of PID, presence or absence of paralysis, clinical outcome (dead, alive and stopped excreting, alive and continued excreting at the time of reporting), and date of latest positive iVDPV isolate was supplemented with information from case reports in scientific journals and consultation with surveillance focal points, when possible.

Descriptive analysis on demographic and clinical characteristics of iVDPV cases was conducted using R statistical software (v3.4; R Core Team 2018). The duration of excretion under observation was calculated assuming a nucleotide substitution rate of ~1.1% VP1 divergence from Sabin strain per year [18]. Prolonged infection is defined as poliovirus excretion lasting > 6 months and chronic infection as poliovirus excretion > 5 years. Countries are classified by World Bank income level criteria for designation as low, lower-middle, upper-middle, and high income.

3. Results

3.1. Immune Response to OPV and Emergence of VDPVs

3.1.1. Immune Response in Immunocompetent Individuals

Serum neutralizing antibodies are the major determinants of protection against poliomyelitis, although cellular immunity also plays a role [19,20]. Immunity for each of the three poliovirus types is independent although there is some cross-reactivity, especially in early immune responses.

Following natural infection or OPV administration, polioviruses multiply locally the in tonsils, pharyngeal and lower gastrointestinal mucosae, and in gut-associated lymphoid tissue, and then spread to systemic lymphoid tissues and other sites for secondary multiplication, causing transient viremia. Therefore, poliovirus may be detected in oropharyngeal secretions for 1 to 2 weeks and in stools for about 4–8 weeks [21–23]. In immunocompetent individuals, viral replication induces gut-associated CD4+ T helper cells and locally produced cytokines, which drive the development of B-cells that produce poliovirus-neutralizing secretory immunoglobulin (Ig) A. Secretory IgA is transported across the intestinal epithelium into the gut lumen, and its appearance 1–3 weeks after OPV administration is associated with a progressive reduction in viral shedding [24,25]. Cytotoxic CD4 and CD8 T-cell responses also appear to be involved in the clearance of virus-infected cells [20].

Serum IgM and IgG are detected approximately 7–10 days after vaccination. IgM disappears within 2 months whereas IgG persists for years, with titers boosted upon new exposure to live or inactivated poliovirus [26,27]. Even when serum-neutralizing antibody titers go below the limits of detection, immunological memory in B-cells appears to provide life-long protection against paralysis [28]. Mucosal intestinal immunity, provided mostly by secretory IgA, prevents viral replication upon a new infection or vaccine dose, as shown by challenge studies [21,23,29]. However, mucosal immunity is only partial in that subsequent vaccine doses has resulted in the shedding of vaccine poliovirus strains in a portion of immune individuals, although for shorter time and in lower amount than in susceptible individuals. Mucosal immunity also wanes within a few years in the absence of new exposure to poliovirus [3,21,23,29].

3.1.2. Vaccine-Associated Paralysis (VAPP) and Vaccine-Derived Poliovirus (VDPV)

Paralytic poliomyelitis results when poliovirus reaches and destroys motor-neurons in the anterior horn of the spinal cord or in the brainstem, following viremia or through retrograde axonal transport, before neutralizing antibodies have reached protective levels. With WPV, the ratio of paralysis to infection among unvaccinated individuals ranges from 1:200 to 1:2000, with the highest neurovirulence for type 1 and the lowest for type 2 [2,30].

Replication of vaccine-related poliovirus strains in the gastrointestinal tract for several weeks allows genomic changes that modify the Sabin-related strains' genome at a rate of ~1.1% nucleotide substitution per year in the region coding (VP1) [5,18,22]. Those genomic changes often include the reversion of the key mutations attenuating neurovirulence and virus fitness to replicate in infected hosts. There is also intertypic recombination among Sabin-related strains, which may eliminate fitness-decreasing mutations in the parental strain [4,31]. Reversion of neurovirulence sites likely occurs faster for types 2 and 3 than type 1 because they have fewer attenuating substitutions, with post-vaccination shedding of neurovirulent strains observed in up to 75% of infants vaccinated with Sabin type 2 [5,18,32].

Mutations in key attenuated sites in Sabin-related strains are associated with the development of vaccine-associated paralytic poliomyelitis (VAPP) following vaccination. The clinical presentation of VAPP is equivalent to poliomyelitis caused by WPV. Isolation of a vaccine-like virus and/or a temporal link with OPV exposure is usually required for categorization [7,8]. Among immunocompetent patients, recipient VAPP case patients' symptoms usually start 4 to 30–40 days after receiving OPV and 5 to 75 days after exposure to a vaccinee in a contact VAPP case. In the United States, VAPP risk was estimated at about one case per 900,000 for the first OPV doses distributed and declined sharply with subsequent doses in the series [7,8].

Prolonged person-to person transmission of Sabin-related strains in a community or prolonged replication of Sabin strains within a single individual with an immunodeficiency disorder allows the accumulation of reverting mutations and recombination with other enterovirus that increase their fitness to multiply and spread. These vaccine-derived polioviruses (VDPVs) have, by definition, a divergence from the parental Sabin strain in the VP1-coding region of the genome of >1% for types 1 and 3 or >0.6% for type 2 [33] and are assumed to have the transmissibility and neurovirulence of WPV of the same serotype [5,6,9,10]. VDPVs have been classified into three categories based upon their origin status and public health importance. Circulating (cVDPVs), for which community circulation has been demonstrated, emerge in communities with low mucosal immunity to poliovirus because of low vaccination coverage and an absence of WPV circulation. Immunodeficiency-associated poliovirus (iVDPV) is isolated from individuals with PIDs following prolonged replication of Sabin-related strains within the individual. Lastly, ambiguous VDPV (aVDPV) includes isolated detections in samples from a child with AFP or in an environmental sample without demonstration of community circulation [33].

Detection of cVDPVs in a previously polio-free area requires a public health response similar to that used to control WPV outbreaks of the same type, whereas detection of a patient with iVDPV in the absence of community circulation requires case management and follow up [1].

3.1.3. Primary Immunodeficiencies

PIDs result from more than 400 genetic errors regarding functions intrinsic to the cells and tissues of the immune system [34]. Patients with PID have increased susceptibility to infections; recurrent pyogenic and viral infections typically occur with defects of humoral (B-cell) immunity and opportunistic infections with defects of cell-mediated immunity. Patients with PID also have a high risk of autoimmune diseases, allergies, or malignancy. Because the generation of poliovirus-specific neutralizing antibodies plays a major role in clearing enterovirus infections, individuals with pure B-cell deficiencies and combined B- and T-cell deficiencies have a higher risk for prolonged infection by enteroviruses than PIDs affecting other components of the immune system.

B-cell deficiencies are characterized by very low levels of immunoglobulins and B-cells in blood but normal numbers of lymphoid and circulating T-cells and appropriate response to mitogens. B-cell deficiencies are the most common PIDs, with X-linked agammaglobulinemia (AGG) prevalence estimated at 1 per 700,000 individuals and common variable immunodeficiency (CVID) at around 1 per 50,000 individuals in high-income countries [14,35]. X-linked AGG usually presents at 9–12 months of age with recurrent pyogenic infections such as otitis media, sinusitis or pneumonia, unusual and potentially fatal forms of enterovirus infections, or with chronic diarrhea by parasites such as Giardia lamblia. CVID is a heterogeneous collection of conditions with a primary antibody deficiency of at least two immunoglobulin isotypes, caused by different genetic factors. CVID often presents during the second or third decade of life as recurrent sinopulmonary infections, although some patients have infections by unusual pathogens such as *Pneumocystis carini* or mycobacteriae, or chronic diarrheal disease from enterovirus infections or parasitic infestations. CVID also manifests non-infectious complications including autoimmune diseases, non-infectious gastrointestinal disease, granulomatous inflammation, and increased risk of malignancy. Patients with B-cell deficiencies require lifelong replacement therapy with immunoglobulin, antibiotics for treatment and prevention of infections, and appropriate therapy for noninfectious complications [36,37].

Severe combined immunodeficiency (SCID) has multiple genetic causes but presents with a quite uniform phenotype [34]. By three months of age, infants present with a persistent rash, intractable diarrhea, failure to thrive, and, frequently, pneumonia, with profound lymphopenia and absent thymus. Death may occur very quickly from viral infections or adverse outcomes from live vaccines. Bone marrow transplantation as quickly as possible is the only treatment for severe cases; for less severe forms of combined defects, immunoglobulin replacement therapy and management of infections may be successful [37]. Major histocompatibility complex (MHC) class II molecules expressed on antigen-presenting cells and activated T-cells are important for both cell-mediated and humoral immunity. Genetic defects encoding these sites have been found at higher frequency in North African countries [35]. Children present with severe, protracted diarrhea, pneumonia and severe upper respiratory infections, and failure to thrive. Although less severe than SCID, this PID is fatal by the first or second decade of life, but bone marrow transplantation has resulted in long-term survival [37].

3.1.4. Immune Response to Poliovirus in Immunodeficient Individuals

Early studies in the 1960s showed that only a few individuals with immunodeficiencies had a prolonged poliovirus infection following OPV administration, without evident higher risk of poliomyelitis. Among 30 hypogammaglobulinemic patients who received monovalent OPVs sequentially in 1961, only two individuals presented with prolonged infections: a 3-year-old child who shed type 1 virus after monovalent OPV type 1 administration for about 3.5 years, and a 20-year-old woman who shed type 3 virus for about 23 months. The child's shedding was terminated by a Shigella infection whereas the adult's shedding stopped spontaneously [38,39].

As OPV became more widely used, it was confirmed that a small proportion of immunodeficient individuals could have asymptomatic poliovirus infection for months or years following receipt of OPV or exposure to contact vaccinees. Prolonged infection was defined as poliovirus excretion lasting > 6 months and chronic infection as poliovirus excretion > 5 years [2].

With prolonged infection of vaccine poliovirus in immunodeficient individuals, Sabin-related strains evolve to iVDPVs that can be isolated in stools and, occasionally, in oropharyngeal secretions [40]. The iVDPVs are defined by the extent of VP1 nucleotide sequence divergence from their corresponding OPV strain serotype in a similar way as cVDPVs. There are molecular differences between iVDPVs and cVDPVs attributed to the different selective pressures exerted on the virus during prolonged infection within a single individual instead of through multiple individuals [5,6]. Key distinguishing features of iVDPVs from cVDPVs include the presence of multiple lineages within one individual, as polioviruses colonize different areas of the gut that evolve independently, the presence of non-recombinant or vaccine–vaccine recombinant genomes instead of recombinants with other species C enteroviruses, and the presence of more extensive antigen variability than typically observed with cVDPVs of the same age (more non-synonymous nucleotide substitutions vs. synonymous substitutions that code for the same amino acid) [6,41–43]. Despite these differences, iVDPVs are similarly assumed to have lost the attenuated phenotypes for virulence and transmissibility as cVDPVs.

Fortunately, only a very small number of individuals with certain immunodeficiencies are at risk of prolonged infection with Sabin-related strains or with further evolved iVDPVs. Although patients with isolated IgA deficiency may eliminate polioviruses less efficiently than normal individuals [44], a multicentric study in the early 2000s confirmed the very low risk of prolonged poliovirus excretion and of paralytic polio by vaccine-related strains among individuals with mild IgG or IgA deficiencies [45]. Several studies have failed to find prolonged excretors of poliovirus in children or adults with T-cell immunodeficiencies secondary to HIV infection [46–49]. Lastly, the risk also appears to be very small among patients with secondary immunodeficiencies related to cancer or its treatment [46].

Cross-sectional studies conducted in 19 countries during 2008–2021 found only 59 out of 1717 (3%) individuals with B-cell PIDs excreting poliovirus at the time of the study (Table 1). The prevalence of poliovirus shedding reported in these studies ranged from 0–25%, with the highest prevalence observed in a study conducted in Tunisia shortly after an immunization campaign. Only 15 (1%) of the PID patients identified in these studies were shedding iVDPV [45,50–58].

Table 1. Prevalence of poliovirus shedding among patients with primary immunodeficiency disorders (PID) in cross-sectional studies.

Country	Patients with PIDs Studied	Poliovirus Excretors		iVDPV Excretors		Years of Study	Reference
Bangladesh	13	1	8%	0	0%	2008–2013	[54]
Brazil	95	3	3%	0	0%	2001–2002	[45]
China	167	3	2%	0	0%	2008–2013	[54]
China	63	0	0%	0	0%	2014–2015	[50]
Colombia	25	0	0%	0	0%	2014–2015	[50]
Egypt	15	2	13%	0	0%	2006–2009	[59]
Egypt	104	12	12%	6	6%	2011–2014	[51]
India	23	0	0%	0	0%	2014–2015	[50]

Table 1. *Cont.*

Country	Patients with PIDs Studied	Poliovirus Excretors		iVDPV Excretors		Years of Study	Reference
India	42	3	7%	1	2%	2014–2017	[55]
India	154	4	3%	1	1%	2019	[56]
Iran	43	1	2%	0	0%	2008–2013	[54]
Iran	102	4	4%	3	3%	2014–2015	[50]
Israel	24	0	0%	0	0%	2014–2015	[50]
Italy	38	0	0%	0	0%	2001–2002	[52]
Japan	9	0	0%	0	0%	2014–2015	[50]
Mexico	33	1	3%	0	0%	2001–2002	[45]
Mexico	20	0	0%	0	0%	2014–2015	[50]
Poland	0	0	0%	0	0%	2014–2015	[50]
Philippines	70	1	1%	0	0%	2008–2013	[54]
Sri Lanka	51	5	10%	2	4%	2008–2013	[54,60]
Russia	136	0	0%	0	0%	2008–2013	[54]
Russia	83	2	2%	0	0%	2014–2015	[50]
Tunisia	16	4	25%	0	0%	1996–1997	[57]
Tunisia	82	6	7%	0	0%	2008–2013	[54,58]
Tunisia	40	3	8%	1	3%	2014–2015	[50]
Turkey	172	4	2%	1	1%	2014–2015	[50]
United Kingdom	125	0	0%	0	0%	2001–2002	[45]
United States	94	0	0%	0	0%	2001–2002	[45]
Total	**1717**	**59**	**3%**	**15**	**1%**		

Follow-up of immunodeficient patients with iVDPV infection identified through surveillance for acute flaccid paralysis or cross-sectional studies has provided more information about the PIDs at the highest risk for prolonged poliovirus infections. Among the 137 immunodeficient patients with iVDPV infection in the WHO Registry for whom the type of PID was known, 45 patients (33%) had SCID, 23 (17%) had agammaglobulinemia, 22 (16%) had CVID, and 19 (14%) had MHC class II deficiency (Table 2).

Table 2. Characteristics of 184 case patients with immunodeficiency-associated vaccine-derived poliovirus (iVDPV) reported during 1962–2024 (data as of July 2024).

Variable	Categories	iVDPV Cases, n (%)
Gender	Male	103 (56)
	Female	67 (36)
	Missing	14 (8)
Age at onset or first positive specimen	<1 year	83 (45)
	1 to <5 years	64 (34)
	5 to <10 years	11 (6)
	10 to <20 years	7 (4)
	20 to <30 years	3 (2)
	≥30 years	2 (1)
	Missing	14 (8)
Paralysis	Yes	106 (58)
	No	69 (38)
	Unknown	9 (5)

Table 2. *Cont.*

Variable	Categories	iVDPV Cases, n (%)
Country of residence World Bank income classification	High income	38 (21)
	Upper-middle income	77 (42)
	Lower-middle income	68 (37)
	Low income	1 (1)
WHO region of residence	African Region	14 (8)
	Eastern Mediterranean Region	88 (48)
	European Region	24 (13)
	Region of the Americas	18 (10)
	South-East Asian Region	20 (11)
	Western Pacific Region	20 (11)
B-cell immunodeficiencies	CVID	23 (12)
	AGG	23 (12)
	HGG	13 (7)
	Other B-cell immunodeficiencies	2 (1)
Combined B- and T-cell immunodeficiencies	SCID	45 (24)
	MHC class II deficiency	19 (10)
	Other combined immunodeficiencies	9 (5)
Other immune disorders	Other disorders	4 (2)
	Unknown	46 (25)
Poliovirus serotype [a]	1	42 (22)
	2	97 (53)
	3	50 (27)
Outcome status	Dead	74 (40)
	Alive (stopped excreting)	62 (34)
	Alive (excreting at last specimen)	27 (15)
	Unknown	21 (11)

[a] Five patients had co-infection and are counted twice: three patients were co-infected with types 1 and 2, one patient with types 2 and 3, and one patient with types 1 and 3. AGG—agammaglobulinemia, CVID—common variable immunodeficiency disorder, HGG—hypogammaglobulinemia, MHC II—Major histocompatibility complex type 2, SCID—severe combined immunodeficiency disorder.

A number of immunodeficient individuals die shortly after detection of vaccine-like virus or iVDPV infection from complications related to their PID or to poliomyelitis, whereas other patients clear the poliovirus infection after several months or years, resulting in a very small number with chronic infection (>5 years). A study in the US following 37 immunodeficient individuals who developed paralytic polio during 1975–1997 found that 19% were shedding the virus at 6 months, 14% at 1 year, 5% at 4 years, and 0% by 10 years [61]. Among the 98 iVDPV-infected patients in the WHO Registry with follow-up available, the median duration of iVDPV excretion following detection was 3.7 months (ranging <1 month–26 years) and only 10 cases with excretion above 5 years have been reported between 1962 and 2024 (Supplementary Table S1).

Patients with SCID and CVID appear to have the highest difficulty in clearing iVDPV infection, which suggests a significant role for cell-mediated immunity in mounting an adequate immune response to enterovirus infections [16]. However, as opposed to SCID patients, who often die young from infectious complications or stop excreting after bone marrow transplant [16,36], CVID patients are the group with the highest risk of prolonged asymptomatic infection. The median duration of infection between detection and death or clearing among 22 CVID patients with steady follow-up was 0.63 years (range 0.04–26.42), compared to 0.2 years among patients with SCID, or 0.3 years among patients with agammaglobulinemia (Table 3). Of the 10 patients with identified chronic poliovirus excretion, 8 of them had CVID [39,55,62–68] (Supplementary Table S1).

Table 3. Characteristics of case patients with immunodeficiency-associated vaccine-derived poliovirus (iVDPV) reported during 1962–2024 by type of immunodeficiency disorder, clinical outcome, and virus characteristics (data as of July 2024).

Immunodeficiency Disorder	Patients n (%)	Paralysis n (%)	Dead n (%)	Alive (Excreting at Last Specimen) n (%)	Number of Nucleotides at Time of Detection Median (Range)	Length of Excretion in Years Median (Range)	Type 1 n (%)	Type 2 n (%)	Type 3 n (%)
B-cell immunodeficiencies									
AGG	23 (13.2)	22 (96%)	4 (17%)	1 (4%)	1.5 (0.5–3.5)	0.3 (0.05–4.92)	5 (22%)	14 (61%)	4 (17%)
CVID	22 (12.6)	16 (73%)	8 (36%)	1 (5%)	2.2 (0.7–12.3)	0.625 (0.04–26.42)	6 (27%)	13 (59%)	4 (18%)
HGG	13 (7.5)	10 (77%)	8 (62%)	0 (0%)	1.55 (0.6–2.2)	0.485 (0.01–1.83)	2 (15%)	9 (69%)	2 (15%)
Other antibody disorders	2 (1.1)	2 (100%)	0 (0%)	1 (50%)	1.1 (0.6–1.6)	0.45 (0.45–0.45)	1 (50%)	1 (50%)	0 (0%)
Combined B- and T-cell immunodeficiencies									
SCID	45 (25.9)	16 (36%)	30 (67%)	3 (7%)	1.4 (0.66–4.5)	0.2 (0.02–2.13)	11 (24%)	28 (62%)	9 (20%)
MHC class II deficiency	19 (10.9)	7 (37%)	8 (42%)	3 (16%)	1.6 (0.67–4)	0.405 (0.09–1.74)	3 (16%)	9 (47%)	7 (37%)
Other combined immunodeficiencies	9 (5.2)	3 (33%)	3 (33%)	0 (0%)	1.7 (1–2.2)	0.205 (0.05–0.46)	3 (33%)	3 (33%)	3 (33%)
Other immunodeficiency disorders									
Other disorders	4 (2.3)	2 (50%)	1 (25%)	0 (0%)	1 (0.9–1.6)	0.68 (0.07–1.29)	1 (25%)	3 (75%)	0 (0%)
Unknown	47 (27)	28 (60%)	11 (23%)	21 (45%)	1.35 (0.67–7)	0.505 (0.01–3.37)	10 (21%)	17 (36%)	21 (45%)

AGG—Agammaglobulinemia, HGG—Hypogammaglobulinemia, CVID—common variable immunodeficiency disorder, MHC—Major histocompatibility complex, SCID—severe combined immunodeficiency disorder.

In several cases, iVDPV infection was resolved after severe diarrheal disease [39,64,69]. But, other than re-acquisition of immunocompetence with bone marrow transplant [70,71] or treatment with antivirals [66], some cases stop iVDPV excretion after months or years without clear reasons. Unfortunately, we only have anecdotal information on patients' outcomes following treatment from some of the published case reports because this information is not collected in the WHO Registry.

3.2. Epidemiological and Clinical Presentation of Poliovirus Infection in Immunodeficient Patients

3.2.1. Demographic Characteristics of iVDPV Cases Reported to the WHO Registry

As of July 2024, the WHO Registry included 184 cases of iVDPV infection detected during 1962–2024. The predominant type of poliovirus in all cases was type 2, detected in 97 (53%) cases, followed by types 3 and 1 detected in 50 (27%) and 42 (23%) of cases, respectively (Table 2). Figure 1 shows the number of iVDPV cases and serotype reported over time since 1962. The number of iVDPV type 2 isolations decreased after the 2016 global switch from trivalent OPV (tOPV) to bivalent OPV (bOPV), from 36 isolations reported during 2012–2015, to 14 during 2016–2019, and 2 during 2020–2023. Two cases, both detected in 2022 in Egypt, have been linked to novel OPV type 2 (nOPV2, genetically more stable in replication than Sabin-strain OPV type 2), despite the distribution of >900 million doses in outbreak response campaigns during 2021–2024 [72]. Isolation of iVDPV types

1 and 3 among reported cases increased during 2016–2019, with 33 isolations reported, compared to 12 and 13 detected in the 2008–2011 and 2012–2015 periods, respectively; the number for both declined during 2020–2023.

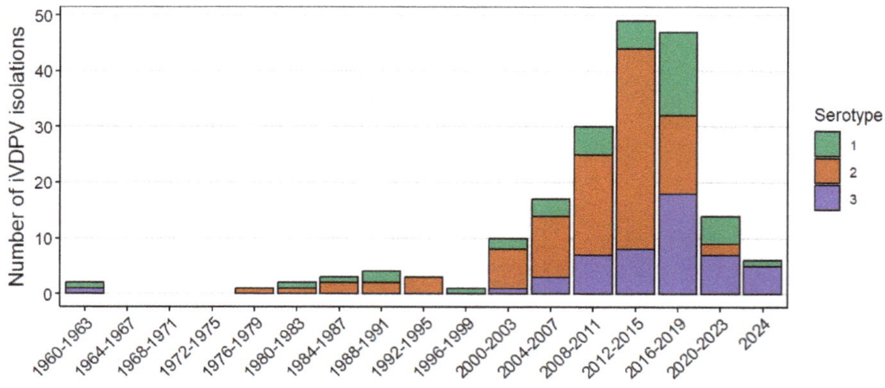

Figure 1. Number of immunodeficiency-associated vaccine-derived poliovirus (iVDPV) isolations reported during 1962–2024 by year of detection and serotype of first positive specimen. The graphic includes 189 isolates in stool specimens from 184 patients with type 1 (n = 42), type 2 (n = 97), and type 3 (n = 50). Five patients with co-infection are counted twice: three patients co-infected with types 1 and 2, one patient with types 2 and 3, and one patient with types 1 and 3.

Since 2008, there has been a shift in reported iVDPV cases from high income countries in the European and the Americas WHO regions to middle income countries in the Eastern Mediterranean Region (Figure 2 and Table 2). As of July 2024, most of the iVDPV cases reported to the WHO Registry (88, 48%) resided in the Eastern Mediterranean WHO Region. Overall, 77 (42%) cases resided in upper-middle income, 68 (37%) in lower-middle income, 38 (21%) in high income countries, and only 1 (1%) in a low-income country (Table 2). Egypt and Iran, with 31 and 30 cases, respectively, are the countries with the highest number of reported cases, followed by China (22) and India (17), as shown on Figure 3.

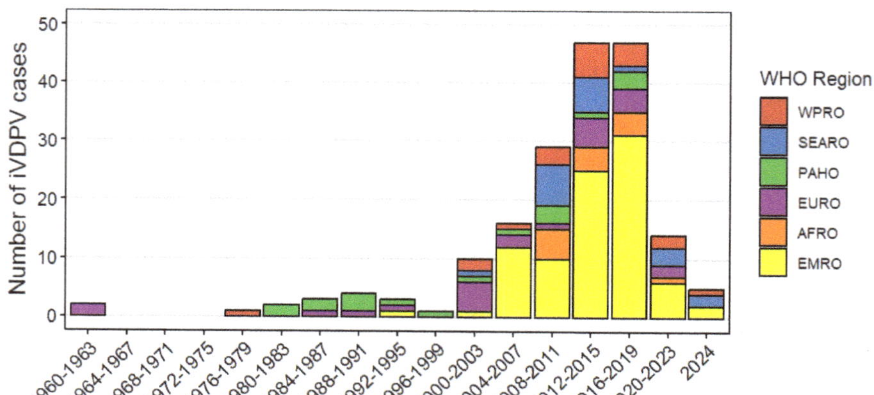

Figure 2. Number of immunodeficiency-associated vaccine-derived poliovirus (iVDPV) cases reported during 1962–2024 by WHO region (N = 184). The x-axis is split in four-year intervals with the total number of cases reported in that year shown as the bar. AFRO—African Region; EMRO—Eastern Mediterranean Region; EURO—European Region; PAHO—Pan-American Health Organization, Region of the Americas; SEARO—South-East Asian Region; WPRO—Western Pacific Region.

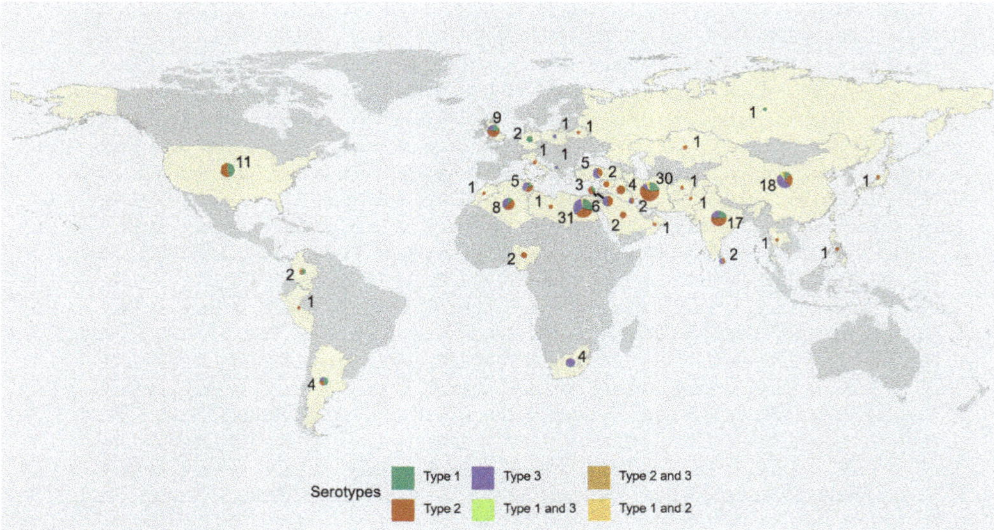

Figure 3. Geographic location of 184 immunodeficiency-associated vaccine-derived poliovirus (iVDPV) cases reported during 1962–2024 by country and serotype. The total number of iVDPV cases by serotype reported over the time period are represented by pie charts proportional to the number of isolations. Five patients had co-infection. Countries that have reported at least one iVDPV case from 1962 to 2024 to date are highlighted in yellow.

Among patients with reported details, males accounted for 103/170 (61%) of iVDPV cases; 83/169 (49%) cases were detected before one year of age (Table 2). At the time of writing this report, 74/184 (40%) patients in the registry had died, 62 (34%) had stopped excreting, and the outcome was unknown for 21 (11%) cases. In addition, 27 patients (15%) were registered as alive and excreting at the latest specimen. However, for 20 of these patients, whose latest specimen was tested for poliovirus between 2011 and 2020, it is likely that they died or stopped shedding, or were lost to follow-up, but the outcome has not yet been reported to the registry.

3.2.2. Risk of Poliomyelitis Among Patients with PID

The risk of poliomyelitis following WPV infection is likely higher among individuals with severe immunodeficiency than in immunocompetent individuals, and potentially they may have more severe disease. However, immunodeficient individuals probably died from poliomyelitis before their immunodeficiency was detected because PIDs were only recognized in the 1950s and the availability of treatment with gamma-globulin was limited to high income countries initially. In reports from three studies conducted in the UK in the early 1960s, eight of 154 (2%) patients with hypogammaglobulinemia developed poliomyelitis, above the expected rate of 0.1–1% among immunocompetent individuals [73].

Studies in the late 20th century showed that immunodeficient individuals had a much higher risk of paralytic poliomyelitis following exposure to OPV, and that paralysis could appear much later after exposure than expected in immunocompetent persons. The categorization as VAPP was considered in immunodeficient individuals even when vaccine exposure occurred well before the upper limits of 30 days (OPV recipients) to 75 days (contacts of recipients), criteria used for categorization as VAPP in immunocompetent individuals [7,13,57,62]. The identification of iVDPVs in the early 2000s showed that some VAPP cases in immunodeficient individuals were associated with iVDPVs infections. Since the early 2000s, some authors have reserved the term VAPP for paralytic poliomyelitis cases in immunodeficient individuals with Sabin-related virus isolated from patients' specimens [68,74] vs. the term iVDPV case when iVDPVs are isolated; other authors have used the term VAPP for both situations [7,13,16,62,75,76].

Among VAPP cases reported during 1980–1991 to the US national poliomyelitis surveillance system, an immunodeficiency disorder was reported in 22 out of 98 cases (22%) and during 1990–2003, in 16 out of 59 cases (27%). The most common underlying immunological defects among the 22 patients reported during 1980–1991 were isolated B-cell deficiencies (73%), whereas combined B- and T-cell deficiencies accounted for 23%, and one patient (4%) was receiving immunosuppressive drugs [7,13]. Based upon estimates of the prevalence of PIDs, the authors projected that infants < 1 year of age with a PID had a risk of VAPP after receiving OPV > 3000 times higher than immunocompetent infants [7,13].

Among the 175 iVDPV case patients in the WHO Registry with a known clinical history, 106 (61%) were paralyzed (Table 2). Paralysis was more frequent in patients with B-cell deficiencies (50/60, 83%) than in patients with combined immunodeficiencies (19/54, 35%) or other categories of immune disorders (9/23, 39%) as reported in previous reviews [16,67,68]. For specific disorders, patients with agammaglobulinemia were most frequently paralyzed (22/23, 96%) followed by patients with hypogammaglobulinemia (10/13, 77%) and CVID (16/22, 73%) (Table 3). Although some authors have hypothesized that variable deficiencies in T-cell function may explain these differences in paralysis outcomes by type of immune disorder [16], it is also possible that longer duration of poliovirus infections of patients with B-cell deficiencies increases the risk of paralysis.

Paralytic poliomyelitis caused by Sabin-related vaccines remains extremely rare among patients with human immunodeficiency virus (HIV) infection, with only two cases reported to date, both likely caused by vaccine-like strains [77,78]. No paralysis related to iVDPV infection has been reported among patients with HIV infection to our knowledge.

3.2.3. Potential Risk of Polio Outbreaks Initiated by Individuals with iVDPV Infection

Th re-introduction of poliovirus transmission into a polio-free country or region by an immunodeficient individual with iVDPV infection is theoretically possible. However, to date, we have very few instances of spread of iVDPV to close contacts and a few other instances when it is difficult to ascertain whether the immunodeficient individual initiated transmission or picked up a cVDPV from the community. In Spain, the same iVDPV isolated in July 2005 from a 14-month-old boy with major histocompatibility class II immunodeficiency (MHC-II) who had developed AFP was isolated in three of the seven family contacts tested. One of the contacts, considered immunocompetent, shed iVDPV for 216 days; no iVDPV was detected in sewage [79]. More recently, in India, genetically linked iVDPVs were isolated from a 9-month-old with SCID and his immunocompetent father in July–August 2022. Specimens collected from 114 additional household contacts and community members were negative. The child died within 3 months of diagnosis and the father presumably stopped shedding poliovirus [80]. In the United States, an iVDPV isolated in an unvaccinated Amish infant with SCID in September 2005 was genetically linked to VDPVs isolated from 8 out of 23 asymptomatic children tested from the same community in Minnesota, US. Phylogenetic analysis suggested that the initiating OPV dose had been given before the child's birth [70]. Lastly, in the Philippines, a type 2 iVDPV detected in August 2019 in a 5-year-old boy with a complex immune disorder had the same genetic distance to parental Sabin-strain (7% divergence) as a cVDPV, causing an outbreak in the Philippines during September 2019–March 2020 [68,81].

The absence of evidence of iVDPV spread from immunodeficient individuals to the wider community has been attributed to: (1) high levels of herd immunity and good hygiene and sanitation in countries where children with PIDs are more likely to survive (high income countries); (2) low survival rate, for lack of treatment, of children with severe PIDs in developing countries where transmission is more likely to occur; and (3) the likelihood that iVDPV excretors may immunize their close contacts before they excrete highly diverged viruses, thus reducing their risk of initiating an outbreak [82]. However, with the decline in population mucosal immunity expected after global interruption of OPV use, the risk of spread of iVDPV will certainly increase with the potential of seeding outbreaks.

Severe PID with combined defects of B- and T-cells, like SCID, are infrequent and patients rarely survive beyond 1 year of age unless they respond to bone marrow transplant which also usually clears any enterovirus, including poliovirus, infection. On the other hand, B-cell immunodeficiencies are the most common PIDs and patients can survive for many years with uninterrupted immunoglobulin therapy and management of infections [36,37]. Considering that most of the chronic poliovirus infections have been detected in patients with CVID (8 out of 10 in our review), this PID group poses a higher risk of becoming a reservoir of neurovirulent poliovirus in the post-eradication era than other iVDPV-infected PID patients.

Estimations and modeling analysis of the risk that long-term iVDPV excretors pose in re-introducing live poliovirus transmission following WPV eradication is complex; very few PID patients present with prolonged poliovirus infection and there is uncertainty of the prevalence and survival rates of PID patients globally at present and in the future. The number of PID patients with iVDPV infection reported to the WHO Registry declined substantially in high-income countries following their shift to exclusive IPV use in the early 2000s but increased in middle income countries that continued to use OPV (Figure 2). In addition to improved detection and availability of therapy in more recent years, the higher number of iVDPV excretors detected in many countries in the Eastern Mediterranean region (e.g., Iran, Egypt, Tunisia) may be partially explained by the higher prevalence of consanguineous marriages compared to other countries that also use bOPV in routine immunization and have similar care opportunities for these patients. The estimated risk of long-term iVDPV excretors is low for PID patients residing in low-income countries, where the life expectancy of such patients is short [50,67,68,83].

Modeling analyses over time changed estimations of the global prevalence of prolonged iVDPV excretors from around 140 in 2006 [84] to about 6 chronic excretors (and 63 paralytic cases) during 2011–2018 [83]. These changes in estimates over time resulted from: (1) updated estimates of prevalence and survival of PIDs; (2) fewer prolonged excretors observed in cross-sectional studies and surveillance pilots conducted during 2000–2015 (~1%, Table 1) compared with earlier studies that followed VAPP case-cohorts during 1975–1997 (up to 10%) [85]; and (3) reductions in the number of iVDPV cases and changes in epidemiology after the shift to IPV-only immunization schedules in high-income and upper-middle income countries in the early 2000s, and after the global withdrawal of type 2 OPV in 2016 [14,83,86].

Following global cessation of OPV use for routine immunization and supplementary campaigns, the prevalence of chronic poliovirus excretors is expected to drop quickly, with very few excretors remaining >10 years after cessation in high- or middle-income countries [14,83,86]. New excretors may also appear if OPV is used in response to VDPV outbreaks post-cessation, as observed in Egypt where two PID patients with iVDPV infection were detected in 2022 following outbreak response campaigns delivering nOPV2 (source: WHO GPLN data). Despite the small number of prolonged excretors expected after OPV cessation, assuming that iVDPVs behave like homotypic WPV, modeling analyses conducted in 2015 and 2017 suggested that chronic iVDPV excretors residing in populations with medium-high infection risk ($R0 > 6$) could be responsible for outbreaks with large numbers of paralytic cases occurring several years after OPV cessation [14,86]. Efforts to identify and treat iVDPV excretors with antiviral drugs before OPV cessation would be cost-effective for the polio eradication initiative because it would reduce the likelihood and number of immunization campaigns required to stop post-cessation outbreaks. The net benefits of iVDPV surveillance and treatment would be considerably reduced, however, if antiviral drugs have low efficacy (i.e., 50% instead of 90%) or if iVDPV strains do not have the same transmissibility as homotypic WPV, which remains an important uncertainty [86].

3.3. Detection and Management of Patients with iVDPV Infection

3.3.1. GPEI Efforts to Identify PID Individuals with iVDPV Infections

During 2008–2020, the GPEI supported surveillance research and pilot interventions that provided estimates of the prevalence of poliovirus excretion among PID patients in low, lower-, and upper-middle income countries. These pilot projects increased awareness among immunologists and physicians treating PIDs that likely contributed to increased case reporting during this period and also provided lessons for the subsequent roll-out of a surveillance platform [50,53–55,59,87–90]. First, a population-based platform that used AFP surveillance human resources to screen all patients admitted to a network hospital for potential PID, using broad clinical criteria for a definition of potential PID, was found to be extremely resource-intensive and not sustainable [91]. In a study conducted in Bangladesh during February 2011 through to January 2013, trained surveillance staff screened 96,000 children admitted to five hospitals for PID using the warning signs from the Jeffrey Model Foundation and found 53 patients who met the clinical definition of potential PID. Of these, 13 (24%) had confirmation of PID based upon a qualitative immunoglobulin assay; only one of 11 patients' stool specimens tested was positive for poliovirus and became negative by 24 months later [87]. A similar project conducted in Egypt demonstrated a sharp decline in patients screened a few months after initiating the project unless frequent monitoring visits and training were implemented. Second, the involvement of physicians specialized in the diagnosis and treatment of PID patients was necessary to ensure coordination with poliovirus surveillance staff for sample collection, transportation, and testing, as well as reporting of results. Third, the availability of therapeutic options for clearing poliovirus infections was an important incentive for patients to accept initial and follow-up sampling and testing. Lastly, ownership by country public health was also essential to facilitate management of community investigations and to facilitate potential access to antiviral drugs.

Based upon the experience from these pilot projects, GPEI opted to support a sentinel-based surveillance platform in a number of low and lower-middle income countries considered at high risk. This platform relies on existing immunization program networks to report potential cases to WHO in countries where immunological diagnostic and treatment centers or experts are available. Parameters used to identify countries at risk for iVDPV emergences and transmission included: (1) predicted annual iVDPV country incidence based upon the high prevalence of consanguineous marriages, mortality among children below 5 years and total population; (2) population susceptibility, based upon coverage with three doses of OPV and one dose of IPV; and (3) risk of high poliovirus transmission, based upon mortality from diarrhea among children under 5 years old. The risk score was combined with information about the availability of care for PID patients and previous experience in detecting iVDPV infections. Countries with high scores included Pakistan, Iran, Egypt, Tunisia, China, Indonesia, India, Brazil, and Mexico.

During 2020–2024, GPEI guidelines and training modules for implementing poliovirus surveillance among patients with PID were developed and adapted by different WHO regional offices [92]. In addition, a data management system linking patient information with laboratory results was integrated within the WHO Polio information System (POLIS). Advocacy meetings and workshops were conducted with immunologists and surveillance focal points. As of June 2024, India and Pakistan have successfully transitioned from research-based surveillance projects to systematic surveillance with 21 and 98 sites, respectively. Egypt, Tunisia, and Iran are in transition and China continues a research-related surveillance project in three provinces, active since 2021. Program-based PID poliovirus surveillance was also initiated in Nigeria and Senegal in 2022 and in Cuba and Colombia in 2023.

However, implementation of poliovirus surveillance of PID patients has been hampered by several challenges in the last five years. Surveillance activities were markedly curtailed during the COVID-19 pandemic. Program and country perception of the risk of iVDPV carriers and urgency in establishing surveillance have declined as the GPEI and country programs have had to respond to outbreaks of type 2 cVDPV in >35 countries, endemic WPV1 circulation continues in Afghanistan and Pakistan, and country authorities are preoccupied with other urgent country health priorities. The GPEI has insufficient funding to sustain iVDPV surveillance in low-income countries with no immunology diagnostic capacity and there are no adequate mechanisms to transfer funds to middle-income countries transitioning from research projects. Lack of implementation of data sharing protocols and an absence of adequate data platform systems at the regional levels results in ad hoc reporting of iVDPV cases without systematic follow-up of patients to monitor the duration of iVDPV excretion and outcome of infection. Lastly, delays in the clinical development of an effective antiviral combination therapy and regulatory obstacles in some countries to the use of available antivirals are barriers to participation by parents of children with PID or by immunologists treating these patients.

All these challenges have reduced the sensitivity of poliovirus surveillance among PID individuals, which may be partly responsible for the observed reduction in the total iVDPV cases reported to the WHO Registry during 2019–2024. As an example, before submitting this manuscript, we found a case-report of a Pakistani patient, resident in Spain, with CVID and asymptomatic co-infection by iVDPV types 1 and 3 (divergence from parent Sabin strain 2.7% for type 1 and 1.5% for type 3). The case patient was identified in May 2019 but not reported to the WHO registry and our literature search missed it because it was reported as an "imported" VDPV case instead of an immunodeficiency-related VDPV case. The patient was still excreting iVDPV as of February 2020, after treatment with the antiviral pocapavir failed to interrupt infection [93].

3.3.2. Management and Control Measures Recommended for PID Patients with iVDPV Infection

The GPEI guidelines for poliovirus surveillance in PID patients recommend testing for poliovirus infection those patients with low immunoglobulin levels for the age for whom transitory or secondary immunodeficiency (i.e., severe malnutrition, infection by HIV) have been excluded, and for whom a specialized physician confirms a diagnosis of a PID associated with risk of prolonged poliovirus excretion. Virologic testing is not recommended for patients with isolated immunoglobulin deficiencies (i.e., Ig A deficiency) [92].

Stool specimens should be sent to a global polio network laboratory for testing and, if necessary, genetic sequencing of poliovirus using the transportation logistics and GPLN resources available for AFP surveillance. Patients with negative specimens are recommended to have annual testing for potential new infection after exposure to vaccinees in essential immunization or campaigns [40,57,94]. For patients with specimens positive for poliovirus (vaccine-like strain or VDPV), a polio surveillance officer will conduct an investigation to assess the patient's potential source of exposure and contact networks, polio vaccination status and potential infection among close contacts, and risk of transmission in the community (i.e., vaccination coverage, population density, sanitation). Collection of stool samples from household contacts and from a sample of young children in the community are recommended to rule out circulation.

Management of the PID patient with poliovirus infection includes counseling and education for the patient and family on hand and toilet hygiene to prevent transmission to contacts, vaccination of close contacts with IPV if required, and vaccination of health staff and adherence to standard precautions for infection control in health care facilities. Monthly stool specimen collections are recommended to monitor clearance of vaccine-like poliovirus or evolution to iVDPV.

Treatment with regular immunoglobulin therapy or bone marrow transplant, in addition to management of infections, depends on the type of PID and the country level of care. Treatment with antivirals is to be considered in PID individuals excreting WPV or iVDPV in any stool specimen and in patients excreting vaccine-like virus for longer than 2 months. As of April 2023, a total of 12 patients had received Pocapavir (a capsid inhibitor), with successful clearance of the iVDPV infection observed in six patients (50%), and the development of resistant poliovirus strains in the remaining patients. A combination of Pocapavir with Imocitrelvir, a protease inhibitor, is still under clinical development. In addition to the emergence of viral resistance with a single agent, a major challenge for the provision of antiviral drugs for more patients with iVDPV infection has been the absence of regulatory mechanisms that allow their use as an investigational drug or for compassionate use in a number of countries, like Egypt or India.

4. Conclusions and Future Directions

Prolonged poliovirus infection following exposure to OPV in patients with certain primary immunodeficiencies is associated with high risk of paralysis for the individual and an uncertain risk of re-introduction of poliovirus in a polio-free world. Surveillance for poliovirus infection among PID patients and prompt treatment with effective antiviral drugs, when available, is crucial to reduce the risk posed by patients with iVDPV infection for their own health and for the global eradication endgame. In this updated analysis of the WHO Registry of patients with iVDPV infection, we observed a sharp reduction in the number of type 2 iVDPV cases reported during 2020–2024, as expected after the global switch from tOPV to bOPV that removed OPV type 2 from use. However, because reported cases with iVDPV types 1 and 3 also increased in this period, the actual decline in total iVDPV cases was small. This analysis also confirmed the trend of a higher proportion of cases reported from middle income countries than from high income countries, because OPV remains in use in the former and where there is capacity for PID diagnosis and treatment. The higher number of cases reported from specific countries such as Egypt or Iran are explained by the higher prevalence of certain PIDs associated with consanguineous marriages, and their high population/number of births.

The GPEI supports establishing sensitive surveillance for the detection of iVDPV infection among patients with PIDs in sentinel sites in countries considered at a higher risk for the emergence and potential transmission of iVDPVs. However, following successful pilots in certain countries, efforts to roll out a program-based surveillance for poliovirus infections in PIDs have been challenged by competing health priorities in high-risk countries and within the GPEI and by the lack of availability of highly effective antiviral drugs. The development of resistance to a single drug and bureaucratic challenges to using antiviral agents for investigational use or under compassionate use limits timely access for a number of patients in some countries; the small number of patients available for testing new antivirals or combinations further slows their clinical development.

Despite the challenges, the GPEI plans to continue advocating and supporting the implementation of surveillance for poliovirus infections among patients with PID and ultimate access to antiviral treatment. In collaboration with PATH, a new study is comparing, in Pakistan, the accuracy of a rapid screening tests for the detection of patients with low IgG levels, which may facilitate the implementation of surveillance in low-income countries without high diagnostic capacity. A combination therapy of Pocapavir, a capsid inhibitor, with Imocitrelvir, a protease inhibitor, less likely to induce resistance, has completed Phase 1 clinical trials and is expected to go into further clinical trials in India in 2025 (further information in a separate article in this supplement).

Supplementary Materials: The following supporting information can be downloaded at: https://www.mdpi.com/article/10.3390/pathogens13121128/s1, Table S1: Characteristics of iVDPV cases in the WHO Registry as of June 2023; Figure S1: VP1 divergence of isolated iVPDV from parental Sabin strains, by serotype and category of immunodeficiency [95–127].

Author Contributions: Conceptualization, C.F.E., E.R.K.-L. and O.M.; methodology, C.F.E. and E.R.K.-L.; software, E.R.K.-L.; validation, C.F.E. and E.R.K.-L.; formal analysis, E.R.K.-L.; investigation, C.F.E. and E.R.K.-L.; data curation, E.R.K.-L.; writing—original draft preparation, C.F.E.; writing—review and editing, C.F.E., E.R.K.-L. and O.M. All authors have read and agreed to the published version of the manuscript.

Funding: This research received no external funding.

Institutional Review Board Statement: Not applicable.

Informed Consent Statement: Not applicable.

Data Availability Statement: No new data were created for this review; data used for this review are available in the published peer preview literature and Supplementary Materials.

Conflicts of Interest: The authors declare no conflicts of interest.

References

1. Global Polio Eradication Initiative. List of Wild Poliovirus by Country and Year. Available online: http://polioeradication.org/polio-today/polio-now/wild-poliovirus-list (accessed on 20 November 2022).
2. Estivariz, C.F.; Burns, C.C.; Macklin, G.R. Poliovirus Vaccine—Live. In *Vaccines*, 8th ed.; Orenstein, W.A., Offit, P.A., Edwards, K.M., Plotkin, S.A., Eds.; Elsevier: Philadelphia, PA, USA, 2023; pp. 914–968.
3. Sutter, R.W.; Patriarca, P.A. Inactivated and live, attenuated poliovirus vaccines: Mucosal immunity. In *Measles and Poliomyelitis*; Kurstak, E., Ed.; Springer: Friesach, Austria, 1993; pp. 279–293.
4. Agol, V.I. Vaccine-derived polioviruses. *Biologicals* **2006**, *34*, 103–108. [CrossRef] [PubMed]
5. Burns, C.C.; Diop, O.M.; Sutter, R.W.; Kew, O.M. Vaccine-derived polioviruses. *J. Infect. Dis.* **2014**, *210* (Suppl. S1), S283–S293. [CrossRef]
6. Kew, O.M.; Wright, P.F.; Agol, V.I.; Delpeyroux, F.; Shimizu, H.; Nathanson, N.; Pallansch, M.A. Circulating vaccine-derived polioviruses: Current state of knowledge. *Bull. World Health Organ.* **2004**, *82*, 16–23.
7. Alexander, L.N.; Seward, J.F.; Santibanez, T.A.; Pallansch, M.A.; Kew, O.M.; Prevots, D.R.; Strebel, P.M.; Cono, J.; Wharton, M.; Orenstein, W.A.; et al. Vaccine policy changes and epidemiology of poliomyelitis in the United States. *JAMA* **2004**, *292*, 1696–1701. [CrossRef]
8. Platt, L.R.; Estivariz, C.F.; Sutter, R.W. Vaccine-associated paralytic poliomyelitis: A review of the epidemiology and estimation of the global burden. *J. Infect. Dis.* **2014**, *210* (Suppl. S1), S380–S389. [CrossRef]
9. Estivariz, C.F.; Watkins, M.A.; Handoko, D.; Rusipah, R.; Deshpande, J.; Rana, B.J.; Irawan, E.; Widhiastuti, D.; Pallansch, M.A.; Thapa, A.; et al. A large vaccine-derived poliovirus outbreak on Madura Island–Indonesia, 2005. *J. Infect. Dis.* **2008**, *197*, 347–354. [CrossRef]
10. Jenkins, H.E.; Aylward, R.B.; Gasasira, A.; Donnelly, C.A.; Abanida, E.A.; Koleosho-Adelekan, T.; Grassly, N.C. Effectiveness of immunization against paralytic poliomyelitis in Nigeria. *N. Engl. J. Med.* **2008**, *359*, 1666–1674. [CrossRef]
11. Global Polio Eradication Initiative. Responding to a Poliovirus Event or Outbreak Part 2: Protocol for Poliovirus Type 2 (V 2.4). *Geneva: World Health Organization.* Available online: https://terrance.who.int/mediacentre/data/sage/SAGE_Docs_Ppt_April2018/4_session_polio/April2018_session4_poliovirus_event_procedure_SOP.pdf (accessed on 5 June 2018).
12. Global Polio Eradication Initiative. Polio Eradication & Endgame Strategic Plan 2013–2018. *WHO/POLIO/13.02. Geneva, Switzerland.* Available online: https://www.archive.polioeradication.org/who-we-are/strategic-plan-2013-2018/ (accessed on 12 December 2024).
13. Sutter, R.W.; Prevots, D.R. Vaccine-Associated Paralytic Poliomyelitis Among Immunodeficient Persons. *Infect. Med.* **1994**, *11*, 426–438.
14. Duintjer Tebbens, R.J.; Pallansch, M.A.; Thompson, K.M. Modeling the prevalence of immunodeficiency-associated long-term vaccine-derived poliovirus excretors and the potential benefits of antiviral drugs. *BMC Infect. Dis.* **2015**, *15*, 379. [CrossRef]
15. Macklin, G.; Liao, Y.; Takane, M.; Dooling, K.; Gilmour, S.; Mach, O.; Kew, O.M.; Sutter, R.W.; The iVDPV Working Group. Prolonged Excretion of Poliovirus among Individuals with Primary Immunodeficiency Disorder: An Analysis of the World Health Organization Registry. *Front. Immunol.* **2017**, *8*, 1103. [CrossRef] [PubMed]
16. Shaghaghi, M.; Soleyman-Jahi, S.; Abolhassani, H.; Yazdani, R.; Azizi, G.; Rezaei, N.; Barbouche, M.R.; McKinlay, M.A.; Aghamohammadi, A. New insights into physiopathology of immunodeficiency-associated vaccine-derived poliovirus infection; systematic review of over 5 decades of data. *Vaccine* **2018**, *36*, 1711–1719. [CrossRef]
17. World Health Organization. Department of Immunization, Vaccines and Biologicals. In *Polio laboratory Manual*, 4th ed.; World Health Organization: Geneva, Switzerland, 2004; Available online: https://www.medbox.org/document/polio-laboratory-manual (accessed on 5 November 2024).
18. Jorba, J.; Campagnoli, R.; De, L.; Kew, O. Calibration of multiple poliovirus molecular clocks covering an extended evolutionary range. *J. Virol.* **2008**, *82*, 4429–4440. [CrossRef] [PubMed]
19. Hammon, W.M.; Coriell, L.L.; Ludwig, E.H.; Mc, A.R.; Greene, A.E.; Sather, G.E.; Wehrle, P.F. Evaluation of Red Cross gamma globulin as a prophylactic agent for poliomyelitis. 5. Reanalysis of results based on laboratory-confirmed cases. *J. Am. Med. Assoc.* **1954**, *156*, 21–27. [CrossRef] [PubMed]
20. Wahid, R.; Cannon, M.J.; Chow, M. Virus-specific CD4+ and CD8+ cytotoxic T-cell responses and long-term T-cell memory in individuals vaccinated against polio. *J. Virol.* **2005**, *79*, 5988–5995. [CrossRef] [PubMed]
21. Ghendon, Y.; Sanakoyeva, I.I. Comparison of the resistance of the intestinal tract ot poliomyelitis virus (Sabin's strains) in persons after naturally and experimentally acquired immunity. *Acta Virol.* **1961**, *5*, 265–273.

22. Alexander, J.P., Jr.; Gary, H.E., Jr.; Pallansch, M.A. Duration of poliovirus excretion and its implications for acute flaccid paralysis surveillance: A review of the literature. *J. Infect. Dis.* **1997**, *175* (Suppl. S1), S176–S182. [CrossRef]
23. Onorato, I.M.; Modlin, J.F.; McBean, A.M.; Thoms, M.L.; Losonsky, G.A.; Bernier, R.H. Mucosal immunity induced by enhanced-potency inactivated and oral polio vaccines. *J. Infect. Dis.* **1991**, *163*, 1–6. [CrossRef]
24. Ogra, P.L. Mucosal immune response to poliovirus vaccines in childhood. *Rev. Infect. Dis.* **1984**, *6* (Suppl. S2), S361–S368. [CrossRef] [PubMed]
25. Valtanen, S.; Roivainen, M.; Piirainen, L.; Stenvik, M.; Hovi, T. Poliovirus-Specific Intestinal Antibody Responses Coincide with Decline of Poliovirus Excretion. *J. Infect. Dis.* **2000**, *182*, 1–5. [CrossRef] [PubMed]
26. Ogra, P.L.; Fishaut, M.; Gallagher, M.R. Viral vaccination via the mucosal routes. *Rev. Infect. Dis.* **1980**, *2*, 352–369. [CrossRef]
27. Ghendon, Y.; Robertson, S.E. Interrupting the transmission of wild polioviruses with vaccines: Immunological considerations. *Bull. World Health Organ.* **1994**, *72*, 973–983.
28. Abbink, F.; Buisman, A.M.; Doornbos, G.; Woldman, J.; Kimman, T.G.; Conyn-van Spaendonck, M.A. Poliovirus-specific memory immunity in seronegative elderly people does not protect against virus excretion. *J. Infect. Dis.* **2005**, *191*, 990–999. [CrossRef] [PubMed]
29. Faden, H.; Duffy, L.; Sun, M.; Shuff, C. Long-term immunity to poliovirus in children immunized with live attenuated and enhanced-potency inactivated trivalent poliovirus vaccines. *J. Infect. Dis.* **1993**, *168*, 452–454. [CrossRef]
30. Nathanson, N.; Kew, O.M. From emergence to eradication: The epidemiology of poliomyelitis deconstructed. *Am. J. Epidemiol.* **2010**, *172*, 1213–1229. [CrossRef] [PubMed]
31. Macadam, A.J.; Pollard, S.R.; Ferguson, G.; Skuce, R.; Wood, D.; Almond, J.W.; Minor, P.D. Genetic basis of attenuation of the Sabin type 2 vaccine strain of poliovirus in primates. *Virology* **1993**, *192*, 18–26. [CrossRef] [PubMed]
32. Georgescu, M.M.; Balanant, J.; Macadam, A.; Otelea, D.; Combiescu, M.; Combiescu, A.A.; Crainic, R.; Delpeyroux, F. Evolution of the Sabin type 1 poliovirus in humans: Characterization of strains isolated from patients with vaccine-associated paralytic poliomyelitis. *J. Virol.* **1997**, *71*, 7758–7768. [CrossRef]
33. Global Polio Eradication Initiative. Classification and Reporting of Vaccine-Derived Polioviruses (VDPVs). Available online: http://polioeradication.org/wp-content/uploads/2016/09/Reporting-and-Classification-of-VDPVs_Aug2016_EN.pdf (accessed on 4 April 2021).
34. Tangye, S.G.; Al-Herz, W.; Bousfiha, A.; Cunningham-Rundles, C.; Franco, J.L.; Holland, S.M.; Klein, C.; Morio, T.; Oksenhendler, E.; Picard, C.; et al. Human Inborn Errors of Immunity: 2022 Update on the Classification from the International Union of Immunological Societies Expert Committee. *J. Clin. Immunol.* **2022**, *42*, 1473–1507. [CrossRef]
35. Abolhassani, H.; Azizi, G.; Sharifi, L.; Yazdani, R.; Mohsenzadegan, M.; Delavari, S.; Sohani, M.; Shirmast, P.; Chavoshzadeh, Z.; Mahdaviani, S.A.; et al. Global systematic review of primary immunodeficiency registries. *Expert Rev. Clin. Immunol.* **2020**, *16*, 717–732. [CrossRef]
36. Yong, P.F.K.; Grimbacher, B.; Thaventhiran, J.E.D. "A Rose is a Rose is a Rose," but CVID is Not CVID. *Adv. Immunol.* **2011**, *111*, 47–107. [PubMed]
37. Rosen, F.S.; Cooper, M.D.; Wedgwood, R.J. The primary immunodeficiencies. *N. Eng. J. Med.* **1995**, *333*, 431–440. [CrossRef] [PubMed]
38. MacCallum, F.O. Hypogammaglobulinaemia in the United Kingdom. VII. The role of humoral antibodies in protection against and recovery from bacterial and virus infections in hypogammaglobulinaemia. *Spec. Rep. Ser. Med. Res. Counc.* **1971**, *310*, 72–85.
39. Martín, J. Vaccine-derived poliovirus from long term excretors and the end game of polio eradication. *Biologicals* **2006**, *34*, 117–122. [CrossRef] [PubMed]
40. Weil, M.; Shulman, L.M.; Heiman, S.; Stauber, T.; Alfandari, J.; Weiss, L.; Silberstein, I.; Indenbaum, V.; Mendelson, E.; Sofer, D. Prolonged excretion of type-2 poliovirus from a primary immune deficient patient during the transition to a type-2 poliovirus-free world, Israel, 2016. *Eurosurveillance* **2016**, *21*, 30408. [CrossRef] [PubMed]
41. Odoom, J.K.; Yunus, Z.; Dunn, G.; Minor, P.D.; Martin, J. Changes in population dynamics during long-term evolution of sabin type 1 poliovirus in an immunodeficient patient. *J. Virol.* **2008**, *82*, 9179–9190. [CrossRef] [PubMed]
42. Yang, C.F.; Chen, H.Y.; Jorba, J.; Sun, H.C.; Yang, S.J.; Lee, H.C.; Huang, Y.C.; Lin, T.Y.; Chen, P.J.; Shimizu, H.; et al. Intratypic recombination among lineages of type 1 vaccine-derived poliovirus emerging during chronic infection of an immunodeficient patient. *J. Virol.* **2005**, *79*, 12623–12634. [CrossRef] [PubMed]
43. Kew, O.M.; Sutter, R.W.; Nottay, B.K.; McDonough, M.J.; Prevots, D.R.; Quick, L.; Pallansch, M.A. Prolonged replication of a type 1 vaccine-derived poliovirus in an immunodeficient patient. *J. Clin. Microbiol.* **1998**, *36*, 2893–2899. [CrossRef]
44. Savilahti, E.; Klemola, T.; Carlsson, B.; Mellander, L.; Stenvik, M.; Hovi, T. Inadequacy of mucosal IgM antibodies in selective IgA deficiency: Excretion of attenuated polio viruses is prolonged. *J. Clin. Immunol.* **1988**, *8*, 89–94. [CrossRef] [PubMed]
45. Halsey, N.A.; Pinto, J.; Espinosa-Rosales, F.; Faure-Fontenla, M.A.; da Silva, E.; Khan, A.J.; Webster, A.D.; Minor, P.; Dunn, G.; Asturias, E.; et al. Search for poliovirus carriers among people with primary immune deficiency diseases in the United States, Mexico, Brazil, and the United Kingdom. *Bull. World Health Organ.* **2004**, *82*, 3–8. [PubMed]
46. Asturias, E.J.; Grazioso, C.F.; Luna-Fineman, S.; Torres, O.; Halsey, N.A. Poliovirus excretion in Guatemalan adults and children with HIV infection and children with cancer. *Biologicals* **2006**, *34*, 109–112. [CrossRef] [PubMed]
47. Hennessey, K.A.; Lago, H.; Diomande, F.; Akoua-Koffi, C.; Caceres, V.M.; Pallansch, M.; Kew, O.; Nolan, M.; Zuber, P. Poliovirus vaccine shedding among persons with HIV in Abidjan, Cote d'Ivoire. *J. Infect. Dis.* **2005**, *192*, 2124–2128. [CrossRef] [PubMed]

48. Pavlov, D.N.; Van Zyl, W.B.; Kruger, M.; Blignaut, L.; Grabow, W.O.; Ehlers, M.M. Poliovirus vaccine strains detected in stool specimens of immunodeficient children in South Africa. *Diagn. Microbiol. Infect. Dis.* **2006**, *54*, 23–30. [CrossRef] [PubMed]
49. Ryder, R.W.; Oxtoby, M.J.; Mvula, M.; Batter, V.; Baende, E.; Nsa, W.; Davachi, F.; Hassig, S.; Onorato, I.; Deforest, A.; et al. Safety and immunogenicity of bacille Calmette-Guerin, diphtheria-tetanus-pertussis, and oral polio vaccines in newborn children in Zaire infected with human immunodeficiency virus type 1. *J. Pediatr.* **1993**, *122*, 697–702. [CrossRef] [PubMed]
50. Aghamohammadi, A.; Abolhassani, H.; Kutukculer, N.; Wassilak, S.G.; Pallansch, M.A.; Kluglein, S.; Quinn, J.; Sutter, R.W.; Wang, X.; Sanal, O.; et al. Patients with Primary Immunodeficiencies Are a Reservoir of Poliovirus and a Risk to Polio Eradication. *Front. Immunol.* **2017**, *8*, 685. [CrossRef] [PubMed]
51. El-Sayed, Z.A.; Mach, O.; Hossny, E.; Galal, N.M.; El-Sawy, I.; ElMarsafy, A.; Reda, S.M.; Moussa, I.; Sibak, M.A.; Bassiouni, L.; et al. Poliovirus excretion among persons with Primary Immune Deficiency disorders: Summary of data from enhanced poliovirus surveillance in Egypt, 2011–2014. *J. Vaccines Vaccin.* **2016**, *7*, 1000331. [CrossRef]
52. Fiore, L.; Novello, F.; Simeoni, P.; Amato, C.; Vellucci, L.; De Stefano, D.; Grandolfo, M.E.; Luzzi, I. Surveillance of acute flaccid paralysis in Italy: 1996–1997. AFP Study Group. Acute flaccid paralysis. *Eur. J. Epidemiol.* **1999**, *15*, 757–763. [CrossRef]
53. Galal, N.M.; Meshaal, S.; ElHawary, R.; Nasr, E.; Bassiouni, L.; Ashghar, H.; Farag, N.H.; Mach, O.; Burns, C.; Iber, J.; et al. Poliovirus excretion following vaccination with live poliovirus vaccine in patients with primary immunodeficiency disorders: Clinicians' perspectives in the endgame plan for polio eradication. *BMC Res. Notes* **2018**, *11*, 717. [CrossRef] [PubMed]
54. Li, L.; Ivanova, O.; Driss, N.; Tiongco-Recto, M.; da Silva, R.; Shahmahmoodi, S.; Sazzad, H.M.; Mach, O.; Kahn, A.L.; Sutter, R.W. Poliovirus excretion among persons with primary immune deficiency disorders: Summary of a seven-country study series. *J. Infect. Dis.* **2014**, *210* (Suppl. S1), S368–S372. [CrossRef]
55. Mohanty, M.C.; Madkaikar, M.R.; Desai, M.; Taur, P.; Nalavade, U.P.; Sharma, D.K.; Gupta, M.; Dalvi, A.; Shabrish, S.; Kulkarni, M.; et al. Poliovirus Excretion in Children with Primary Immunodeficiency Disorders, India. *Emerg. Infect. Dis.* **2017**, *23*, 1664–1670. [CrossRef] [PubMed]
56. Mohanty, M.C.; Desai, M.; Mohammad, A.; Aggarwal, A.; Govindaraj, G.; Bhattad, S.; Lashkari, H.P.; Rajasekhar, L.; Verma, H.; Kumar, A.; et al. Assessment of Enterovirus Excretion and Identification of VDPVs in Patients with Primary Immunodeficiency in India: Outcome of ICMR-WHO Collaborative Study Phase-I. *Vaccines* **2023**, *11*, 1211. [CrossRef]
57. Triki, H.; Barbouche, M.B.; Bahri, O.; Bejaoui, M.; Dellagi, K. Community-acquired poliovirus infection in children with primary immunodeficiencies in Tunisia. *J. Clin. Microbiol.* **2003**, *41*, 1203–1211. [CrossRef] [PubMed]
58. Driss, N.; Ben-Mustapha, I.; Mellouli, F.; Ben Yahia, A.; Touzi, H.; Bejaoui, M.; Ben Ghorbel, M.; Triki, H.; Barbouche, M.R. High susceptibility for enterovirus infection and virus excretion features in Tunisian patients with primary immunodeficiencies. *Clin. Vaccine Immunol.* **2012**, *19*, 1684–1689. [CrossRef] [PubMed]
59. Galal, N.M.; Bassiouny, L.; Nasr, E.; Abdelmeguid, N. Isolation of poliovirus shedding following vaccination in children with antibody deficiency disorders. *J. Infect. Dev. Ctries.* **2012**, *6*, 881–885. [CrossRef] [PubMed]
60. de Silva, R.; Gunasena, S.; Ratnayake, D.; Wickremesinghe, G.D.; Kumarasiri, C.D.; Pushpakumara, B.A.; Deshpande, J.; Kahn, A.L.; Sutter, R.W. Prevalence of prolonged and chronic poliovirus excretion among persons with primary immune deficiency disorders in Sri Lanka. *Vaccine* **2012**, *30*, 7561–7565. [CrossRef]
61. Khetsuriani, N.; Prevots, D.R.; Quick, L.; Elder, M.E.; Pallansch, M.; Kew, O.; Sutter, R.W. Persistence of vaccine-derived polioviruses among immunodeficient persons with vaccine-associated paralytic poliomyelitis. *J. Infect. Dis.* **2003**, *188*, 1845–1852. [CrossRef]
62. Centers for Disease Control and Prevention. Prolonged poliovirus excretion in an immunodeficient person with vaccine-associated paralytic poliomyelitis. *MMWR Morb. Mortal. Wkly. Rep.* **1997**, *46*, 641–643.
63. Centers for Disease Control and Prevention. Update on vaccine-derived polioviruses. *MMWR Morb. Mortal. Wkly. Rep.* **2006**, *55*, 1093–1097.
64. Bellmunt, A.; May, G.; Zell, R.; Pring-Akerblom, P.; Verhagen, W.; Heim, A. Evolution of poliovirus type I during 5.5 years of prolonged enteral replication in an immunodeficient patient. *Virology* **1999**, *265*, 178–184. [CrossRef]
65. MacLennan, C.A.; Huissoon, A.P.; Kumararatne, D.S. Vaccine-derived poliomyelitis 12 years after infection. *N. Engl. J. Med.* **2011**, *365*, 1355. [CrossRef] [PubMed]
66. Bermingham, W.H.; Canning, B.; Wilton, T.; Kidd, M.; Klapsa, D.; Majumdar, M.; Sooriyakumar, K.; Martin, J.; Huissoon, A.P. Case report: Clearance of longstanding, immune-deficiency-associated, vaccine-derived polio virus infection following remdesivir therapy for chronic SARS-CoV-2 infection. *Front. Immunol.* **2023**, *14*, 1135834. [CrossRef] [PubMed]
67. Guo, J.; Bolivar-Wagers, S.; Srinivas, N.; Holubar, M.; Maldonado, Y. Immunodeficiency-related vaccine-derived poliovirus (iVDPV) cases: A systematic review and implications for polio eradication. *Vaccine* **2015**, *33*, 1235–1242. [CrossRef] [PubMed]
68. Macklin, G.; Diop, O.M.; Humayun, A.; Shahmahmoodi, S.; El-Sayed, Z.A.; Triki, H.; Rey, G.; Avagyan, T.; Grabovac, V.; Jorba, J.; et al. Update on Immunodeficiency-Associated Vaccine-Derived Polioviruses—Worldwide, July 2018–December 2019. *MMWR Morb. Mortal. Wkly. Rep.* **2020**, *69*, 913–917. [CrossRef] [PubMed]
69. Mohanty, M.C.; Madkaikar, M.R.; Desai, M.; Aluri, J.; Varose, S.Y.; Taur, P.; Sharma, D.K.; Nalavade, U.P.; Rane, S.V.; Gupta, M.; et al. Natural Clearance of Prolonged VDPV Infection in a Child With Primary Immunodeficiency Disorder. *Front. Immunol.* **2019**, *10*, 1567. [CrossRef]

70. Alexander, J.P.; Ehresmann, K.; Seward, J.; Wax, G.; Harriman, K.; Fuller, S.; Cebelinski, E.A.; Chen, Q.; Jorba, J.; Kew, O.M.; et al. Transmission of imported vaccine-derived poliovirus in an undervaccinated community in Minnesota. *J. Infect. Dis.* **2009**, *199*, 391–397. [CrossRef] [PubMed]
71. Singanayagam, A.; Klapsa, D.; Burton-Fanning, S.; Hand, J.; Wilton, T.; Stephens, L.; Mate, R.; Shillitoe, B.; Celma, C.; Slatter, M.; et al. Asymptomatic immunodeficiency-associated vaccine-derived poliovirus infections in two UK children. *Nat. Commun.* **2023**, *14*, 3413. [CrossRef] [PubMed]
72. Bandyopadhyay, A.S.; Zipursky, S. A novel tool to eradicate an ancient scourge: The novel oral polio vaccine type 2 story. *Lancet Infect. Dis.* **2023**, *23*, e67–e71. [CrossRef]
73. Wyatt, H.V. Poliomyelitis in hypogammaglobulinemics. *J. Infect. Dis.* **1973**, *128*, 802–806. [CrossRef]
74. Jorba, J.; Diop, O.M.; Iber, J.; Sutter, R.W.; Wassilak, S.G.; Burns, C.C. Update on Vaccine-Derived Polioviruses—Worldwide, January 2015–May 2016. *MMWR Morb. Mortal. Wkly. Rep.* **2016**, *65*, 763–769. [CrossRef]
75. Shaghaghi, M.; Parvaneh, N.; Ostad-Rahimi, P.; Fathi, S.M.; Shahmahmoodi, S.; Abolhassani, H.; Aghamohammadi, A. Combined immunodeficiency presenting with vaccine-associated paralytic poliomyelitis: A case report and narrative review of literature. *Immunol. Investig.* **2014**, *43*, 292–298. [CrossRef]
76. Shahmahmoodi, S.; Mamishi, S.; Aghamohammadi, A.; Aghazadeh, N.; Tabatabaie, H.; Gooya, M.M.; Zahraei, S.M.; Mousavi, T.; Yousefi, M.; Farrokhi, K.; et al. Vaccine-associated paralytic poliomyelitis in immunodeficient children, Iran, 1995–2008. *Emerg. Infect. Dis.* **2010**, *16*, 1133–1136. [CrossRef]
77. Ion-Nedelcu, N.; Dobrescu, A.; Strebel, P.M.; Sutter, R.W. Vaccine-associated paralytic poliomyelitis and HIV infection. *Lancet* **1994**, *343*, 51–52. [CrossRef]
78. Chitsike, I.; van Furth, R. Paralytic poliomyelitis associated with live oral poliomyelitis vaccine in child with HIV infection in Zimbabwe: Case report. *BMJ* **1999**, *318*, 841–843. [CrossRef]
79. Avellon, A.; Cabrerizo, M.; de Miguel, T.; Perez-Brena, P.; Tenorio, A.; Perez, J.L.; de Aragon, M.V.; Trallero, G. Paralysis case and contact spread of recombinant vaccine-derived poliovirus, Spain. *Emerg. Infect. Dis.* **2008**, *14*, 1807–1809. [CrossRef] [PubMed]
80. Mohanty, M.C.; Govindaraj, G.; Ahmad, M.; Varose, S.Y.; Tatkare, M.; Shete, A.; Yadav, S.; Joshi, Y.; Yadav, P.; Sharma, D.; et al. Immunodeficiency-Related Vaccine-Derived Poliovirus (iVDPV) Excretion in an Infant with Severe Combined Immune Deficiency with Spillover to a Parent. *Vaccines* **2024**, *12*, 759. [CrossRef] [PubMed]
81. Snider, C.J.; Boualam, L.; Tallis, G.; Takashima, Y.; Abeyasinghe, R.; Lo, Y.R.; Grabovac, V.; Avagyan, T.; Aslam, S.K.; Eltayeb, A.O.; et al. Concurrent outbreaks of circulating vaccine-derived poliovirus types 1 and 2 affecting the Republic of the Philippines and Malaysia, 2019–2021. *Vaccine* **2023**, *41* (Suppl. S1), A58–A69. [CrossRef]
82. Dowdle, W.R.; De Gourville, E.; Kew, O.M.; Pallansch, M.A.; Wood, D.J. Polio eradication: The OPV paradox. *Rev. Med. Virol.* **2003**, *13*, 277–291. [CrossRef] [PubMed]
83. Kalkowska, D.A.; Pallansch, M.A.; Thompson, K.M. Updated modelling of the prevalence of immunodeficiency-associated long-term vaccine-derived poliovirus (iVDPV) excreters. *Epidemiol. Infect.* **2019**, *147*, e295. [CrossRef] [PubMed]
84. Tebbens, R.J.; Sangrujee, N.; Thompson, K.M. The costs of future polio risk management policies. *Risk Anal.* **2006**, *26*, 1507–1531. [CrossRef]
85. Khetsuriani, N.; Helfand, R.; Pallansch, M.; Kew, O.; Fowlkes, A.; Oberste, M.S.; Tukei, P.; Muli, J.; Makokha, E.; Gary, H. Limited duration of vaccine poliovirus and other enterovirus excretion among human immunodeficiency virus infected children in Kenya. *BMC Infect. Dis.* **2009**, *9*, 136. [CrossRef]
86. Duintjer Tebbens, R.J.; Thompson, K.M. Comprehensive screening for immunodeficiency-associated vaccine-derived poliovirus: An essential oral poliovirus vaccine cessation risk management strategy. *Epidemiol. Infect.* **2017**, *145*, 217–226. [CrossRef]
87. Sazzad, H.M.; Rainey, J.J.; Kahn, A.L.; Mach, O.; Liyanage, J.B.; Alam, A.N.; Kawser, C.A.; Hossain, A.; Sutter, R.; Luby, S.P. Screening for long-term poliovirus excretion among children with primary immunodeficiency disorders: Preparation for the polio posteradication era in Bangladesh. *J. Infect. Dis.* **2014**, *210* (Suppl. S1), S373–S379. [CrossRef]
88. Shaghaghi, M.; Shahmahmoodi, S.; Abolhassani, H.; Soleyman-Jahi, S.; Parvaneh, L.; Mahmoudi, S.; Chavoshzadeh, Z.; Yazdani, R.; Zahraei, S.M.; Ebrahimi, M.; et al. Vaccine-Derived Polioviruses and Children with Primary Immunodeficiency, Iran, 1995–2014. *Emerg. Infect. Dis.* **2016**, *22*, 1712–1719. [CrossRef]
89. Shaghaghi, M.; Shahmahmoodi, S.; Nili, A.; Abolhassani, H.; Madani, S.P.; Nejati, A.; Yousefi, M.; Kandelousi, Y.M.; Irannejad, M.; Shaghaghi, S.; et al. Vaccine-Derived Poliovirus Infection among Patients with Primary Immunodeficiency and Effect of Patient Screening on Disease Outcomes, Iran. *Emerg. Infect. Dis.* **2019**, *25*, 2005–2012. [CrossRef] [PubMed]
90. Yao, N.; Liu, Y.; Xu, J.W.; Wang, Q.; Yin, Z.D.; Wen, N.; Yang, H.; Rodewald, L.E.; Zhang, Z.Y. Detection of a Highly Divergent Type 3 Vaccine-Derived Poliovirus in a Child with a Severe Primary Immunodeficiency Disorder—Chongqing, China, 2022. *MMWR Morb. Mortal. Wkly. Rep.* **2022**, *71*, 1148–1150. [CrossRef]
91. World Health Organization. Meeting of the Strategic Advisory Group of Experts on immunization, October 2016—Conclusions and recommendation. *Wkly. Epidemiol. Rec.* **2016**, *91*, 561–584.
92. Global Polio Eradication Initiative. *Guidelines for Implementing Polio Surveillance Among Patients with Primary Immunodeficiency Disorders (PIDs)*; Global Polio Eradication Initiative: Geneva, Switzerland, 2022.
93. Álamo-Junquera, D.; Politi, J.; Simón, P.; Dieli-Crimi, R.; Borrell, R.P.; Colobran, R.; Martínez-Gallo, M.; Campins, M.; Antón, A.; Esperalba, J.; et al. Coordinated Response to Imported Vaccine-Derived Poliovirus Infection, Barcelona, Spain, 2019–2020. *Emerg. Infect. Dis.* **2021**, *27*, 1513. [CrossRef] [PubMed]

94. DeVries, A.S.; Harper, J.; Murray, A.; Lexau, C.; Bahta, L.; Christensen, J.; Cebelinski, E.; Fuller, S.; Kline, S.; Wallace, G.S.; et al. Vaccine-derived poliomyelitis 12 years after infection in Minnesota. *N. Engl. J. Med.* **2011**, *364*, 2316–2323. [CrossRef] [PubMed]
95. Kew, O.M.; Sutter, R.W.; de Gourville, E.M.; Dowdle, W.R.; Pallansch, M.A. Vaccine-derived polioviruses and the endgame strategy for global polio eradication. *Ann. Rev. Microbiol.* **2005**, *59*, 587–635. [CrossRef]
96. Minor, P. Vaccine-derived poliovirus (VDPV): Impact on poliomyelitis eradication. *Vaccine* **2009**, *27*, 2649–2652. [CrossRef]
97. Labadie, K.; Pelletier, I.; Saulnier, A.; Martin, J.; Colbere-Garapin, F. Poliovirus mutants excreted by a chronically infected hypogammaglobulinemic patient establish persistent infections in human intestinal cells. *Virology* **2004**, *318*, 66–78. [CrossRef] [PubMed]
98. Yoneyama, T.; Hagiwara, A.; Hara, M.; Shimojo, H. Alteration in oligonucleotide fingerprint patterns of the viral genome in poliovirus type 2 isolated from paralytic patients. *Infect. Immun.* **1982**, *37*, 46–53. [CrossRef] [PubMed]
99. Hara, M.; Saito, Y.; Komatsu, T.; Kodama, H.; Abo, W.; Chiba, S.; Nakao, T. Antigenic analysis of polioviruses isolated from a child with agammaglobulinemia and paralytic poliomyelitis after Sabin vaccine administration. *Microbiol. Immunol.* **1981**, *25*, 905–913. [CrossRef]
100. Abo, W.; Chiba, S.; Yamanaka, T.; Nakao, T.; Hara, M.; Tagaya, I. Paralytic poliomyelitis in a child with agammaglobulinemia. *Eur. J. Pediatr.* **1979**, *132*, 11–16. [CrossRef]
101. Misbah, S.A.; Lawrence, P.A.; Kurtz, J.B.; Chapel, H.M. Prolonged faecal excretion of poliovirus in a nurse with common variable hypogammaglobulinaemia. *Postgrad. Med. J.* **1991**, *67*, 301–303. [CrossRef] [PubMed]
102. Minor, P. Characteristics of poliovirus strains from long-term excretors with primary immunodeficiencies. *Dev. Biol.* **2001**, *105*, 75–80.
103. MacLennan, C.; Dunn, G.; Huissoon, A.P.; Kumararatne, D.S.; Martin, J.; O'Leary, P.; Thompson, R.A.; Osman, H.; Wood, P.; Minor, P.; et al. Failure to clear persistent vaccine-derived neurovirulent poliovirus infection in an immunodeficient man. *Lancet* **2004**, *363*, 1509–1513. [CrossRef]
104. Dunn, G.; Klapsa, D.; Wilton, T.; Stone, L.; Minor, P.D.; Martin, J. Twenty-Eight Years of Poliovirus Replication in an Immunodeficient Individual: Impact on the Global Polio Eradication Initiative. *PLoS Pathog.* **2015**, *11*, e1005114. [CrossRef]
105. Shahmahmoodi, S.; Parvaneh, N.; Burns, C.; Asghar, H.; Mamishi, S.; Tabatabaie, H.; Chen, Q.; Teimourian, S.; Gooya, M.M.; Esteghamati, A.R.; et al. Isolation of a type 3 vaccine-derived poliovirus (VDPV) from an Iranian child with X-linked agammaglobulinemia. *Virus Res.* **2008**, *137*, 168–172. [CrossRef] [PubMed]
106. Hidalgo, S.; Garcia Erro, M.; Cisterna, D.; Freire, M.C. Paralytic poliomyelitis caused by a vaccine-derived polio virus in an antibody-deficient Argentinean child. *Pediatr. Infect. Dis. J.* **2003**, *22*, 570–572. [CrossRef]
107. Centers for Disease Control and Prevention. Laboratory surveillance for wild and vaccine-derived polioviruses—worldwide, January 2007–June 2008. *MMWR Morb. Mortal. Wkly. Rep.* **2008**, *57*, 967–970.
108. Buttinelli, G.; Donati, V.; Fiore, S.; Marturano, J.; Plebani, A.; Balestri, P.; Soresina, A.R.; Vivarelli, R.; Delpeyroux, F.; Martin, J.; et al. Nucleotide variation in Sabin type 2 poliovirus from an immunodeficient patient with poliomyelitis. *J. Gen. Virol.* **2003**, *84*, 1215–1221. [CrossRef] [PubMed]
109. Tharmaphornpilas, P. Vaccine-derived poliovirus, Thailand, 2003. *Emerg. Infect. Dis.* **2005**, *11*, 777–778. [CrossRef]
110. Parvaneh, N.; Shahmahmoudi, S.; Tabatabai, H.; Zahraei, M.; Mousavi, T.; Esteghamati, A.R.; Gooya, M.M.; Mamishi, S.; Nategh, R.; Kew, O.M.; et al. Vaccine-associated paralytic poliomyelitis in a patient with MHC class II deficiency. *J. Clin. Virol.* **2007**, *39*, 145–148. [CrossRef] [PubMed]
111. Centers for Disease Control and Prevention. Poliovirus infections in four unvaccinated children—Minnesota, August–October 2005. *MMWR Morb. Mortal. Wkly. Rep.* **2005**, *54*, 1053–1055.
112. Centers for Disease Control and Prevention. Update on vaccine-derived polioviruses—worldwide, January 2006-August 2007. *MMWR Morb. Mortal. Wkly. Rep.* **2007**, *56*, 996–1001.
113. Mamishi, S.; Shahmahmoudi, S.; Tabatabaie, H.; Teimourian, S.; Pourakbari, B.; Gheisari, Y.; Yeganeh, M.; Salavati, A.; Esteghamati, A.-R.; Gooya, M.M.; et al. Novel BTK mutation presenting with vaccine-associated paralytic poliomyelitis. *Eur. J. Pediatr.* **2008**, *167*, 1335–1338. [CrossRef]
114. Driss, N.; Mellouli, F.; Ben Yahia, A.; Touzi, H.; Barbouche, M.R.; Triki, H.; Bejaoui, M. Sequential asymptomatic enterovirus infections in a patient with major histocompatibility complex class II primary immunodeficiency. *J. Clin. Microbiol.* **2014**, *52*, 3486–3489. [CrossRef]
115. Centers for Disease Control and Prevention. Update on Vaccine-Derived Polioviruses—Worldwide, January 2008–June 2009. *MMWR Morb. Mortal. Wkly. Rep.* **2009**, *58*, 1002–1006.
116. Burgos, M.E.; Elkik, S.; Barbosa, P.; Oleastro, M.; Freire, C.; Parra, A.; Caparelli, M.; Sarkis, C. A vaccine derived poliovirus case in an immunocompromised argentinian child. *Int. J. Infect. Dis.* **2010**, *14*, e450–e451. [CrossRef]
117. Centers for Disease Control and Prevention. Update on Vaccine-Derived Polioviruses—Worldwide, July 2009–March 2011. *MMWR Morb. Mortal. Wkly. Rep.* **2011**, *60*, 846–850.
118. Centers for Disease Control and Prevention. Update on vaccine-derived polioviruses—worldwide, April 2011–June 2012. *MMWR Morb. Mortal. Wkly. Rep.* **2012**, *61*, 741–746.
119. Diop, O.M.; Burns, C.C.; Wassilak, S.G.; Kew, O.M. Update on vaccine-derived polioviruses—Worldwide, july 2012–december 2013. *MMWR Morb. Mortal. Wkly. Rep.* **2014**, *63*, 242–248. [PubMed]

120. Wang, H.-B.; Luo, H.-M.; Li, L.; Fan, C.-X.; Hao, L.-X.; Ma, C.; Su, Q.-R.; Yang, H.; Reilly, K.H.; Wang, H.-Q.; et al. Vaccine-derived poliovirus surveillance in China during 2001–2013: The potential challenge for maintaining polio free status. *BMC Infect. Dis.* **2017**, *17*, 742. [CrossRef]
121. Gumede, N.; Muthambi, V.; Schoub, B.D. Immunodeficiency-associated vaccine-derived poliovirus type 3 in infant, South Africa, 2011. *Emerg. Infect. Dis.* **2012**, *18*, 992–994. [CrossRef]
122. Diop, O.M.; Burns, C.C.; Sutter, R.W.; Wassilak, S.G.; Kew, O.M. Update on Vaccine-Derived Polioviruses—Worldwide, January 2014–March 2015. *MMWR Morb. Mortal. Wkly. Rep.* **2015**, *64*, 640–646. [PubMed]
123. Schubert, A.; Bottcher, S.; Eis-Hubinger, A.M. Two Cases of Vaccine-Derived Poliovirus Infection in an Oncology Ward. *N. Engl. J. Med.* **2016**, *374*, 1296–1298. [CrossRef] [PubMed]
124. Trimble, R.; Atkins, J.; Quigg, T.C.; Burns, C.C.; Wallace, G.S.; Thomas, M.; Mangla, A.T.; Infante, A.J. Vaccine-Associated Paralytic Poliomyelitis and BCG-osis in an Immigrant Child with Severe Combined Immunodeficiency Syndrome—Texas, 2013. *MMWR Morb. Mortal. Wkly. Rep.* **2014**, *63*, 724–741.
125. Jorba, J.; Diop, O.M.; Iber, J.; Henderson, E.; Sutter, R.W.; Wassilak, S.G.F.; Burns, C.C. Update on Vaccine-Derived Polioviruses—Worldwide, January 2016-June 2017. *MMWR Morb. Mortal. Wkly. Rep.* **2017**, *66*, 1185–1191. [CrossRef]
126. Jorba, J.; Diop, O.M.; Iber, J.; Henderson, E.; Zhao, K.; Sutter, R.W.; Wassilak, S.G.F.; Burns, C.C. Update on Vaccine-Derived Polioviruses—Worldwide, January 2017–June 2018. *MMWR Morb. Mortal. Wkly. Rep.* **2018**, *67*, 1189–1194. [CrossRef]
127. Howard, W.; Moonsamy, S.; Seakamela, L.; Jallow, S.; Modiko, F.; du Plessis, H.; Sibiya, R.; Kamupira, M.; Maseti, E.; Suchard, M. Sensitivity of the acute flaccid paralysis surveillance system for poliovirus in South Africa, 2016–2019. *J. Med. Microbiol.* **2021**, *70*, 001441. [CrossRef]

MDPI AG
Grosspeteranlage 5
4052 Basel
Switzerland
Tel.: +41 61 683 77 34

Pathogens Editorial Office
E-mail: pathogens@mdpi.com
www.mdpi.com/journal/pathogens

www.ingramcontent.com/pod-product-compliance
Lightning Source LLC
Chambersburg PA
CBHW061548210926
51850CB00009B/2035
9783725855278